P9-CQT-519

# Communication and Language Acquisition

# Communication and Language Acquisition

## Discoveries from Atypical Development

edited by

**Lauren B. Adamson, Ph.D.**

and

**Mary Ann Romski, Ph.D.**

Georgia State University
Atlanta

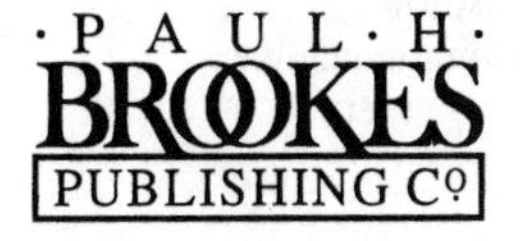


Baltimore • London • Toronto • Sydney

**Paul H. Brookes Publishing Co.**
Post Office Box 10624
Baltimore, Maryland 21285-0624



Typeset by Wilsted & Taylor, Oakland, California.
Manufactured in the United States of America by
Thomson-Shore, Dexter, Michigan.

**Library of Congress Cataloging-in-Publication Data**

Communication and language acquisition : discoveries from atypical development / [edited] by Lauren B. Adamson and Mary Ann Romski.
p. cm.
Includes bibliographical references and index.
ISBN 1-55766-279-7
1. Language disorders in children. 2. Language acquisition. 3. Developmentally disabled children—Language. 4. Communicative disorders in children—Patients—Language. I. Adamson, Lauren, 1948– . II. Romski, Mary Ann, 1952–
RJ496.L35C652 1997
618.92′855—DC21 96-37329
CIP

British Library Cataloguing in Publication data are available from the British Library.

# Contents

# About the Authors

**Lauren B. Adamson, Ph.D.**, Professor, Department of Psychology, and Associate Dean, College of Arts and Sciences, Georgia State University, Atlanta, GA 30303. Dr. Adamson's research interests include the development of shared attention during the first 3 years of life and patterns of atypical communication development.

**Mary Ann Romski, Ph.D.**, Professor, Departments of Communication, Psychology and Educational Psychology & Special Education, Georgia State University, Atlanta, GA 30303. Dr. Romski's research focuses on language development and intervention for children and youth with mental retardation who do not speak.

---

**Roger Bakeman, Ph.D.**, Professor, Department of Psychology, Georgia State University, Atlanta, GA 30303. Dr. Bakeman is a developmental psychologist with interests in quantitative methods that best unlock the stories latent in quantitative data. He is especially interested in methods of coding and analyzing videotaped materials.

**Jacquelyn Bertrand, Ph.D.**, Psychologist, Division of Birth Defects and Developmental Disabilities, Centers for Disease Control, Atlanta, GA 30341. Dr. Bertrand conducts research on the developmental and behavioral profiles of individuals with genetic disorders.

**Antoinette Gomes, Ph.D.**, Intern, Philadelphia Child Guidance Clinic, 34th Street and Civic Center, Philadelphia, PA 19104. Dr. Gomes' research and clinical interests focus on the early identification and prevention of psychopathology in children from minority backgrounds.

**Mikael Heimann, Ph.D.**, Associate Professor, Department of Psychology, Goteborg University, Haraldsgatan 1, Goteborg, S-41314, Sweden. Dr. Heimann is a licensed psychologist and psychotherapist. His research interests include infancy, autism, and the language development of, and computer-assisted instruction for, children with disabilities.

**Mary Louise Hemmeter, Ph.D.**, Research Assistant Professor, Department of Special Education, University of Kentucky, 229 Taylor Educational Building, Lexington, KY 40506. Dr. Hemmeter's research interests include transition and early language intervention. She is particularly interested in interventions that are implemented by parents and/or other family members and the generalized effects of these interventions in the school and the home.

**Peggy P. Hester, Ph.D.**, Research Assistant Professor, Department of Special Education, Vanderbilt University, Box 328 Peabody, Nashville, TN 37203. Dr. Hester has extensive clinical and research experience in parent implementation and generalization of naturalistic language training strategies, as well as training of professionals to teach parents to utilize these strategies.

**Ann P. Kaiser, Ph.D.**, Professor, Department of Special Education, Vanderbilt University, Box 328 Peabody, Nashville, TN 37203. Dr. Kaiser has published extensively in the areas of early childhood special education and early language acquisition and intervention, most specifically, the implementation and generalized effects of naturalistic language training procedures. She is currently serving as Chair of the Department of Special Education at Vanderbilt University.

**Amy R. Lederberg, Ph.D.**, Associate Professor, Department of Educational Psychology and Special Education, Georgia State University, Atlanta, GA 30303. Dr. Lederberg's research has focused on social and language development of deaf children. She has been particularly interested in how language delay affects social and symbolic development.

**William J. McIlvane, Ph.D.**, Director of the Mental Retardation Research Center at the Eunice Kennedy Shriver Center for Mental Retardation, Inc., 200 Trapelo Road, Waltham, MA 02254. Dr. McIlvane holds academic appointments at the Massachusetts General Hospital, Harvard Medical School, and Northeastern University. His research interests concern the experimental and theoretical analysis of both human and nonhuman behavior, with a primary emphasis on processes involved in discrimination learning and formation of stimulus classes.

**Carolyn B. Mervis, Ph.D.**, Professor of Psychology, Emory University, Atlanta, GA 30322. Dr. Mervis's research has focused on early language and cognitive development by children who are developing typically and by children with mental retardation.

**Peter Mundy, Ph.D.**, Professor, Departments of Psychology and Pediatrics, Psychology Annex, University of Miami, 5665 Ponce De Leon Blvd., Coral Gables, FL 33146. Dr. Mundy is the Director of the University of Miami Psychological Services and the University's Center for Autism and Related Disorders. His research focuses on understanding the applied and basic science implications of developments in social-communication skills in young children.

**Keith E. Nelson, Ph.D.**, Professor, Department of Psychology, Pennsylvania State University, University Park, PA 16802. Dr. Nelson's interests include applied and theoretical issues related to the improvements of speech, literacy, and sign language skills in children with disabilities.

**Byron F. Robinson, M.A.**, Program in Cognition and Development, Department of Psychology, Emory University, Atlanta, GA 30322. Mr. Robinson's interests focus on language and cognition relations in a developmental context, as well as the methods used for uncovering such relations.

**Rose A. Sevcik, Ph.D.**, Assistant Research Professor, Department of Psychology, Georgia State University, Atlanta, GA 30303. Dr. Sevcik's research has focused on the language and communication development of children and youth with mental retardation, developmental reading disorders, and symbol acquisition by great apes.

**Patricia Elizabeth Spencer, Ph.D.**, Associate Professor, Department of Social Work, Gallaudet University, HMB 334S, 800 Florida Avenue NE, Washington, D.C. 20002. Dr. Spencer's research addresses contributions of early interactive experiences on social, communicative, and symbolic development of deaf children.

**Helen Tager-Flusberg, Ph.D.**, Professor, Department of Psychology, University of Massachusetts, Boston, MA 02125-3393. Dr. Tager-Flusberg conducts research on language and cognition in typically developing children and in children and adolescents with neurodevelopmental disorders.

**Tomas Tjus, M.Sc.**, Instructor and doctoral student, Department of Psychology, Goteborg University, Haraldsgatan 1, Goteborg, S-41314, Sweden. Mr. Tjus is a licensed psychologist and psychotherapist. His research interests include developmental psychopathology and the language development of, and computer-assisted instruction for, children with disabilities.

**Ruth V. Watkins, Ph.D.**, Assistant Professor, Department of Speech and Hearing Science, University of Illinois, 901 S. Sixth Street, Champaign, IL 61820. Dr. Watkins' research examines the linguistic challenges facing children with language impairment, as well as effective approaches to intervention for young children with language-learning difficulties.

**Grover J. Whitehurst, Ph.D.**, Professor of Psychology and Pediatrics, State University of New York, Stony Brook, NY 11794-2500. Dr. Whitehurst conducts applied research on the development of language and reading, with particular emphasis on children from low-income families and with a continuing interest in children with early language delays. He also pursues interests in the use of computer technologies in higher education.

**Krista M. Wilkinson, Ph.D.**, Assistant Scientist, Eunice Kennedy Shriver Center for Mental Retardation, Inc., and Instructor at Northeastern University, 200 Trapelo Road, Waltham, MA 02254. Dr. Wilkinson conducts an interdisciplinary research program with the dual purpose of exploring basic processes in lexical acquisition and intervention techniques for individuals with communication impairments.

# Preface

The idea for *Communication and Language Acquisition: Discoveries from Atypical Development* grew out of two symposia that we organized: "Language Learning Research and Mental Retardation: Contributions to Developmental Research," which was presented at the 1993 Gatlinburg Conference on Research and Theory in Mental Retardation and Developmental Disabilities in Gatlinburg, Tennessee, and "Early Language Acquisition: Basic Research with Children with Developmental Disabilities," which was presented at the 1993 biennial meeting of the Society for Research in Child Development in New Orleans, Louisiana. We organized these symposia because we wanted to discuss the impact of findings from atypical language and communication development on theories of development in general.

The positive response to these symposia revealed that the time was well past due for drawing together researchers who have the conceptual courage to design studies of language and communication disabilities with basic, as well as applied, concerns in mind. In addition to the majority of the original participants, other contributors were invited, in each case hoping to locate yet another example of the extraordinary benefits that can accrue when atypical phenomena are considered relevant to debates about basic issues.

The editing of this volume was made possible by funding from a Georgia State University Research Enhancement Grant and from National Institute of Child Health and Human Development Grant No. 06016 to Georgia State University's Language Research Center. We are grateful for the administrative support we received from Tawanna Tookes as well as the Dean's Office and the Departments of Communication and Psychology, College of Arts and Sciences. We thank our colleague Rose A. Sevcik for her ongoing support and encouragement during the completion of this project. We also acknowledge Carol Hollander, our original acquisitions editor, for urging us to embark on this project and Melissa A. Behm for her continuing wise counsel.

To Daniel and Thomas Adamson

and

Benjamin and Brian Romski

# Introduction

*Communication and Language Acquisition: Discoveries from Atypical Development* is a collective effort to open a new avenue of basic research, one that draws information about communication and language disabilities into contemporary debates about fundamental issues related to development and learning. Thus, the purpose is not so much to review a field as to revise traditional notions about where it contains challenging data. Although each chapter can stand on its own as a significant contribution to a specific area, when read together they amplify an exciting new theme: Research on atypical communication and language is an invaluable source of knowledge about how children become accomplished communicators.

This theme is not often sounded in the field of language and communication development, which is routinely split into the basic realm of normative theory and the applied realm of language and communication disorders. Traditionally, the flow of influence between these areas has been unidirectional. Although researchers in the applied realm have often mined the basic realm for crucial insights that might guide intervention efforts or provide explanations for difficulties, theorists have, with rare exception, not searched the applied realm for empirical information or conceptual inspiration. The authors in this volume move against this expected flow. Each draws fascinating findings from his or her research programs to illustrate how research with children who do not acquire language rapidly and smoothly can help to answer questions essential to the entire field of language and communication development.

This book is divided into three complementary sections. The first section focuses attention on the broad theoretical and methodological frames that surround research programs in order to help locate some of the issues and strategies that arise when researchers attempt to bridge the divide between the basic and the applied realms. The final two sections draw on contemporary research programs that focus on insights that may be gained through the study, in turn, of particular forms of atypical development and of the context of these paths.

The first section provides a reconsideration of theories and methods and a challenge to contemporary scholars of child language and communication development. Each of the chapters addresses questions that typically go unasked, much less unanswered, by researchers focused on the content of communication. By examining classical theories of development, Adamson (Chapter 1) uses a historical perspective to explore how a consideration of atypical communication and language development has contributed to the thinking of three classical developmental theorists, Piaget, Vygotsky, and Werner. Her findings indicate that developmentalists have a long history—but a short memory—of theorizing what atypical communication and language development might reveal about normative developmental processes.

Wilkinson and McIlvane in Chapter 2 provide a behavioral framework, rooted in atypical development, with which to consider psycholinguistic theories of early vocabulary development and delay. By highlighting points of vulnerability and modifiability, this framework emphasizes significant lexical milestones, or cusps, that children must master to continue on the path to adult language competence. In Chapter 3, Bakeman and Robinson rose to the challenge of our question: What is a researcher to do methodologically when questions are asked about low-incidence populations? They suggest two complementary approaches for analyzing data sets with few subjects such as those often found in studies of children with atypical language and communication development. These two approaches, the graphic presentation of data and permutation tests, permit careful examination of "small-*N*" data sets that also have utility for scholars of typical development.

In each of the six chapters in Section II, the authors gain clarity on perennial developmental issues by observing unusual patterns. These chapters share important characteristics: the judicious selection of participants, the careful description of the researchers' actions at several developmental points, and the explicit articulation of a conceptual frame that helps to highlight the theoretical significance of the researchers' observations. In addition, they each provide a compelling view of extraordinary ways that language and communication may develop.

In Chapter 4, Mervis and Bertrand detail the sequencing of several cognitive and language milestones along the developmental path followed by children whose achievements in the domains of language and cognition appear dissociated when compared with typically developing children. Their studies of children with Williams syndrome, who display relative strength in language, and children with Down syndrome, who display relative strength in cognition, provide a rigorous test for claims of universality in developmental sequences. Their findings suggest that some links that regularly occur during typical development, such as those between canonical babbling and rhythmic banging and those between spontaneous exhaustive sorting and fast mapping of object labels, occur even under conditions of dissociation whereas others, such as the link between pointing and the onset of the referential production of words, do not.

In Chapter 5, Mundy and Gomes also compare two distinctive patterns of atypical acquisition. By focusing specifically on the paths taken by young children with autism and young children with Down syndrome, they are able to document a variety of ways in which the many nonverbal communication skills that involve and integrate various cognitive, affective, and self-regulatory processes develop and prepare the way for subsequent language development.

Tager-Flusberg (Chapter 6) likewise compares children with autism with other children, including typically developing preschoolers and children with Down syndrome. She sets up her contrasts to discern how "the joints between two cognitive domains—language and theory of mind—can be carved." Of particular note is that she views the relation from both directions, asking not only about the influence of phenomena related to cognition on language development but also about how language acquisition might influence the development of theory of mind. The view that results provides compelling evidence for developmental changes in the way linguistic and cognitive processes may interact.

In Chapter 7, Watkins reviews the burgeoning research on how the unusual linguistic profile of children with specific language impairment (SLI) differs from that of typical children in hopes of revealing the operations of the linguistic system. She makes clear how valuable these studies are to our understanding of such central issues as the modularity of language as well as underlying genetic contributions to language acquisition.

The last two chapters in Section II shift perspective slightly by focusing attention not only on the paths followed by children with contrasting etiologies but also on informative differences that appear within a specific group. Sevcik and Romski (Chapter 8) seek to identify differences in how youth with severe language delays that are concomitant to mental retardation acquire early language skills through augmented means. Their research reveals the importance of comprehension to several aspects of language acquisition and suggests how differences in comprehension abilities may lead children down different routes to the same endpoint, the production of new vocabulary. In Chapter 9, Spencer and Lederberg distinguish deaf children who are reared by signing deaf parents from those who are reared by speaking hearing parents. This grouping adds fascinating new information to the perennial debates related to "universality" and "resiliency" in early language and communication development. In particular, their findings highlight the importance of the availability of rich and consistent language input to early communication and language development.

In the third section, the theme of the importance of input is highlighted as the focus shifts from the child to the environment. When language development proceeds both rapidly and smoothly, it is reasonable to credit the young child with a robust acquisition mechanism. When it does not, the impact of a specific disability on language and communication development can be assessed, as is done in Section II. Two other approaches are also feasible. One approach involves examining extreme variation of environment to gain a fuller view of the role of context in language development. The second approach entails observing the effects of various environmental interventions that might enhance a child's mastery of language and communication.

Whitehurst, in Chapter 10, takes the first approach. He characterizes the role of an impoverished social/cultural environment on early language development and reports differences in the quality and rate of language and literacy development in these young children. His careful analyses of the impact of this type of context provides strong evidence of how important the consideration of diverse interactional influences is to a full accounting of language development.

Using the second approach, Chapters 11 (Kaiser, Hemmeter, and Hester) and 12 (Nelson, Heimann, and Tjus) employ carefully crafted language interventions that support the language development of children with a range of developmental disabilities. The authors discuss how the outcomes of these interventions provide invaluable information about the role that different forms of language input may play during early development. In Chapter 11, Kaiser and her colleagues examine the effects of a specific type of social language input, enhanced milieu teaching, on the development of children with delays. They argue that their approach permits a more holistic view of how communication influences other aspects of development and how the course of development is affected by changes to any one of the component domains. Nelson, Heimann, and Tjus, in Chapter 12, use findings from their computer-based reading intervention with a broad range of children with atypical language development to refine their Rare Event Learning (REL) theory of language development.

We encourage the readers to scan "out of order" as well as in sequence. Each new juxtaposition will, we hope, give rise to new notions about the importance of understanding the vast array of different ways that communication and language develop. Traditionally, researchers have applied their understanding of typical language development to atypical populations in hopes of facilitating the language development of children with developmental disabilities. This goal is surely a most important aim that all the contributors of this volume fully endorse. In addition, these authors direct their attention to fundamental developmental issues in order to demonstrate the benefits of considering how children with communication and language disorders can provide us with extraordinary findings that can help sharpen the cutting edge of theory.

# I

# RECASTING THEORIES AND METHODS

# 1

# Order and Disorder

## Classical Developmental Theories and Atypical Communication Development

Lauren B. Adamson

Developmental psychologists are gathered around their field's traditional margins, seeking to describe and explain phenomena related to language and communication disorders (e.g., Tager-Flusberg, 1994); psychopathology (Keating & Rosen, 1991); and mental retardation (Hodapp & Burack, 1990). They are focusing on extreme variations of development in hopes of strengthening the understanding of both normal and abnormal processes. But as they expand the scope of their investigations, they risk losing contact with the field's conceptual foundation that was laid out following grand plans of developmental order proposed decades ago by theorists such as Jean Piaget, Heinz Werner, and Lev Vygotsky. Although they may find that this foundation of images, questions, and methods provides a solid starting point for efforts to understand normative developmental progressions, they are likely to find that it offers only weak support for new investigations of developmental disorders.

I experienced this uneasy situation when I began to study extreme variations of early language use (Adamson, 1992, 1996). As I observed a toddler with aphonia due to a tracheostomy acquiring language (Adamson & Dunbar, 1991) and older children who were augmenting their limited expressive speech with graphic symbols (Adamson, Romski, Deffebach, & Sevcik, 1992), I was dismayed by how little explicit guidance classical developmental theorists had to offer in the area of disorders, especially communication-related disorders. I

This work was supported in part by a grant from the Chancellor's Research Initiative Fund of Georgia State University. The author gratefully thanks Duncan McArthur for his assistance during the writing of this chapter.

considered their neglect a serious matter that risked not only the oversight of details about unusual forms of behavior but also the slighting of crucial information about developmental change. At the time, I turned to Roman Jakobson's (1960) nondevelopmental perspective on variations in communication to supplement the normative developmental views provided by Piaget, Werner, and Vygotsky. Nevertheless, I remained puzzled by this curious gap in the developmental legacy.

Given the breadth and brilliance of developmental theorizing in Europe during the interwar period of the 1920s and 1930s, it struck me as improbable that issues related to disorders did not arise. Furthermore, the historical record suggests that early developmentalists often took interest in applied problems (Sears, 1975) and were surrounded by colleagues who sought to learn about the human condition from the study of atypical experiences. For example, they all admired the work of Kurt Goldstein, who demonstrated repeatedly that "the observation and analyses of pathological phenomena often yield greater insight into the processes of the organism than that of the normal" (1934/1939, p. 9).

These observations led me to ask whether traditional theorists of developmental order were really silent about disorders. Rather, might the problem be one of reception? Could it be that most English-speaking developmentalists, educated after developmental issues were absorbed into psychology's mainstream and concern about applied issues had temporarily waned (Parke, Ornstein, Rieser, & Zahn-Waxler, 1992; Sears, 1975), were not sufficiently aware of traditional theorists' suggestions? If so, what guidance would classical developmental theorists offer about integrating information on disorders into theories of communication development and language acquisition?

Spurred by such questions, I decided to review developmental psychology's theoretical foundation. To this end, I scanned many early texts searching for missing gems, peculiar slants, and unmined veins related to atypical communication and language development. In this chapter, I summarize what I encountered during my foray into developmental psychology's past. In the first section, I briefly introduce Piaget, Werner, and Vygotsky as three developmentalists who, during the early part of the 20th century, simultaneously provided designs for a new discipline of developmental psychology. In the second section, I summarize what each of these theorists wrote about development and about disorders, particularly those involving communication and language. I describe how each approached the study of atypical phenomena that may occur during a child's transition to language but none investigated these phenomena thoroughly enough to determine how they might clarify or challenge reigning notions of development. In the final section, I argue that despite the lack of a buried treasure, developmental psychology's past does contain a store of suggestions about how atypical phenomena may elaborate and ultimately alter claims about language and communication development.

## THE CLASSICAL DEVELOPMENTAL PERSPECTIVE

Developmental psychology's roots are spread throughout late 19th-century European scientific thought. Thus, when developmental notions began to flourish in the early 20th century, they sprang forth simultaneously in several locations. From our perspective in 1997, three sites appear to have been particularly fertile: bourgeois Geneva, pre-Nazi Hamburg, and revolutionary Moscow. At each of these places, a grand theorist—Piaget, Werner, and Vygotsky, respectively—formulated a comprehensive design for developmental psychology.

In much of this chapter, each theorist's design is presented separately to demonstrate the range of agendas that were proposed for, and still inform, developmental psychology. But first it is important to review why these three designs are often considered together. In some surveys of developmental theories, Piaget and Werner are grouped together under the common rubric of organicism (e.g., Langer, 1969) while Vygotsky is placed close by, as a feisty relative who shared fundamental commitments to development yet flirted with mechanistic-sounding notions. In other surveys (e.g., Glick, 1983; Morss, 1990), all three share the same heading.

This grouping has a compelling conceptual basis. Piaget, Werner, and Vygotsky each sought to describe and explain directional change. Each focused primarily on changes during childhood, although each also extended the scope of theory to encompass changes on other scales, including brief time periods (microgenesis), the entire life cycle, and even cultural change and species evolution. Each strove to understand the orderliness, sequentiality, and apparent lawfulness of change regardless of its content. In doing so, each tended to focus on qualitative shifts that occur during periods of rapid change rather than on developmental milestones, age norms, or quantifiable growth. Furthermore, all three agreed that an extremely important transformational moment, the emergence of symbols at the end of infancy, occurred during early childhood, and each tried to understand how such symbol formation influenced thought.

This grouping also has broad historical validity. Piaget, Werner, and Vygotsky were all born in the 1890s. They entered an intellectual world permeated with notions of evolution and energized by hopes of progress (Kessen, 1990; Morss, 1990). Each was broadly educated in the continental intellectual tradition of Kant, Freud, and Marx, and each initially had access to the works of scholars throughout Europe. Within this tradition, they all were similarly situated. Each was attracted to Gestalt psychology with its emphasis on perception and problem solving, and each took interest in but stood independent of psychoanalysis.

Finally, Piaget, Werner, and Vygotsky all worked far from the mainstream of American psychology with its relatively atheoretical and pro-behaviorist approach to the science of psychology. As they began to publish in the 1920s and early 1930s, they received immediate acclaim from their European colleagues. But, like Gestalt psychologists such as Kohler and Wertheimer (Sokal, 1984), their work was difficult to place within American disciplinary boundaries. Only fragments of the European developmentalists' works were imported into American academic discussions, and when they were, it was usually to address issues and audiences involved with children and education, concerns that were not considered by Americans to be central to psychology. When Werner fled Hitler's Germany in 1933, his classic work on developmental psychology, *Comparative Psychology of Mental Development* (1926/1948), had not yet been translated into English, and it took him more than a decade to secure a permanent academic position (at Clark University; see Witkin, 1965). Piaget's vast corpus of mature writings remained untranslated and virtually unknown until the 1960s when cognitive psychologists such as Flavell (1963) introduced them en masse. Many of Vygotsky's writings, including his remarkable works on abnormal psychology and learning disabilities (Rieber & Carton, 1993), are only becoming available in the 1990s after being clouded for decades by the turbulent storms of Soviet psychology (Joravsky, 1987; Kozulin, 1984; Luria, 1979).

## THREE DEVELOPMENTALIST AGENDAS

Against this shared conceptual and historical backdrop, Piaget, Werner, and Vygotsky worked independently. They did know of and respect some of one another's writings, but their paths rarely crossed, much less penetrated into each others' spheres. Vygotsky and Piaget's famous debate about the fate of egocentric speech illustrates their distance. In *Thought and Language* (1962, 1986), Vygotsky used Piaget's first book, *The Language and Thought of the Child* (1923/1959), as a point of departure. Piaget was apparently apprised by Luria of Vygotsky's criticisms. But he did not read them for decades, and when he did, he began his belated response with a poignant statement:

> It is not without sadness that an author discovers, twenty-five years after its publication, the work of a colleague who has died in the meantime, when that work contains so many points of immediate interest to him which should have been discussed personally and in detail. (Piaget, 1962a, p. 1)

Around this time, Werner entered the fray briefly (see Werner & Kaplan, 1963, pp. 321–325), ascribing much of the supposed debate to a mere misconstrual by Vygotsky of Piaget's concept of egocentrism.

The separations within European developmental psychology were not due solely to geographic distance. When the basic premises of various developmental theories are compared with each other rather than contrasted to behaviorism, the fundamental differences are striking. Each theorist proposed a distinctive agenda that ultimately led him to distinct notions about what an understanding of atypical development might contribute to theory building.

Before embarking on this exposition, a caveat is in order. What follows is the report of a modest project: a presentist reading of selected works centered on the specific concern for the theoretical importance of disorders involving communication and language development. To provide a fuller rendering of each theorist's project in the context of American developmental psychology would require constructing an intellectual biography true to the time and path of each theorist's development. Furthermore, it would be necessary to place specific works within a changing context because authors update works (e.g., Werner released many editions of *Comparative Psychology of Mental Development*); translators transform them (cf. the 1962 and 1986 versions of Vygotsky's *Thought and Language*); and readers undoubtedly personalize them. Fortunately, there are several excellent biographies available that provide such historically sensitive accounts; I refer to them often in the following sections.

### Piaget's Search for the Universal Epistemic Subject

American psychologists are now well aware that Piaget proposed and kept close to his own agenda as a genetic epistemologist who took passionate interest in understanding the nature of knowledge and, more specifically, the ways in which knowledge develops (Chapman, 1988; Flavell, 1963). He adopted this epistemological position first and foremost; he asked only secondarily what this position might imply about developmental variations. He expressed this position clearly and often, even when probed directly by psychologists concerned with other matters. For example, during a dialogue with Robert Rieber on the psychology of language and thought, Piaget (1983) explained the following:

> It should be remembered that we have essentially dealt from a structural point of view with an "epistemic" subject where the individual differences are not at the center of such analysis. . . . Stages deal with normative characteristics of development; they deal with the description of behaviors that children have in common at a given moment of their development and as such transcend individual differences. (pp. 111–112)

Given this agenda, it is not surprising that Piaget wrote relatively little about language disorders (Elliot & Donaldson, 1982; Sinclair, 1982). He tended to treat both developmental disorders and language as areas peripheral to cognition, and he usually delegated their investigation to his collaborators in Geneva where they were mined primarily for the evidence they might provide about the "epistemic subject." In his own writings, he tended to draw sharp divisions between cognition and language and between developmental delay and deviance. (For a cogent critique of Piaget's analytic tendencies, see Kamhi and Masterson, 1989.) Moreover, as Rosenberg (1984) lamented in his essay on disorders of first-language development, Piaget never developed a substantial model of language or proposed mechanisms that might map cognitive achievements onto language structures. Even in *Play, Dreams, and Imitation in Childhood* (1945/1962b), where he presents a sustained analysis of how symbols emerge as an "epistemic subject" actively adapts to the environment, Piaget does not address issues related to individual differences in either path or process.

Nonetheless, in his general writings, Piaget repeatedly noted two ways that information about children with disabilities might be relevant to his theory-building efforts. First, he suggested that children with mental retardation might reveal whether the progressive development of logical thought proceeds in a universal and invariant sequence. Barbel Inhelder's (1943/1968) *The Diagnosis of Reasoning in the Mentally Retarded* is, as Piaget noted in his prefaces to both of its editions, an outstanding exemplar of how the study of children with developmental disabilities might be theoretically interesting. (For an extensive review of related work, see Modgil and Modgil, 1976.) Inhelder explored whether difficulties in developing more advanced operative structures are best understood in terms of delay or deviancy. To the extent that development was delayed rather than deviant, Piaget's theory would receive support.

Inhelder's central question was, "Do the reflections of retardates during physical experiments constitute abnormal phenomena as well as simple arrestations at certain levels of development?" (1943/1968, p. 217). Her method was to record activities during Piagetian tasks that assessed concepts such as conservation and then "to seek signs which indicate normal intelligence through the study of relative failures and insufficiencies in cases where individuals have been diagnosed by other methods as being abnormal and slightly deficient (p. 299). Inhelder's results, although introduced as "contrary to what was expected," were clearly theory confirming: "No process of reasoning has been observed thus far . . . that has escaped the evolutionary structures of operatory groupments" (p. 217). The theoretical import of this conclusion is then forcefully stated: "The fact that there is found in these subjects, who suffer from intellectual and behavioral problems, the existence of a common operatory construction which obeys the same laws of integration illustrates the profound unity between the logical and the psychological" (p. 299). Even when differences are noted, they are interpreted as more evidence for one path of development. For example, the observation that the level of reasoning of some children with mental retardation tends to be relatively homogeneous is ascribed either to slower speed or premature fixation at a final level and interpreted as additional indication that "the operatory stages appear to be a natural psychological fact" (p. 301).

Piaget also endorsed examining individuals with atypical abilities because it might help establish the precedence of operative over figurative development. Piaget (1923/1959) persistently claimed from his earliest book, *The Language and Thought of the Child*, to his last summary statements (Piaget, 1964/1967, 1970) and research volumes (e.g., Piaget & Inhelder, 1971) that new operative knowledge is constructed as the epistemic subject acts and that it is not received through language. Furthermore, changes in operative knowledge precede and influence the subject's figurative knowledge. Although the relation between figurative and operative development was studied most often in typically developing children, Piaget argued that "the study of individuals suffering from pathological conditions of language and thought is essential—specifically when studying results which indicate that language does not constitute the framework of logic, but rather is molded by logic" (Rieber & Voyat, 1983, p. 17). In this regard, he cited studies of logical thinking in deaf children, particularly those of Furth (1966), where "thinking" may develop "without language." Generally, Piaget's strategy of relating operative and figurative accomplishments has prompted many researchers to pose questions about the relation between cognitive and linguistic accomplishments by children with developmental disorders (e.g., Mervis, 1990; see also Chapter 5) and to design intervention strategies consistent with his theory (e.g., Morehead & Morehead, 1974).

In summary, traditional Piagetian treatments of disorders were essentially theory-confirming exercises. These exercises did not happen often, particularly in the area of language and communication development. When they did, Piaget and his colleagues emphasized the orderliness of developmental progress and the primacy of operative development over figurative development. Language per se was often viewed as a secondary formation, dependent on thought that was developmentally derived from a subject's actions.

### Werner's Proposal for a Comparative-Developmental Vocabulary

American developmental psychologists best know Werner as a champion of the concept of development to whose explication he devoted both a significant book (1926/1948) and a seminal chapter (1957). At the center of these works was the suggestion that developmentalists "search out organized forms, those processes and structures, which lie behind and govern overt behavioral outcomes, and then try to discover how these forms, processes, or structures grow and change" (Flavell, 1966, p. 26). Contemporary developmentalists rarely acknowledge Werner's influence as they study language development and developmental disorders. However, as Glick recently remarked, Werner's "theoretical ideas are linked to emerging ideas in a somewhat subterranean way[;] a more careful conceptualization of his contemporary relevance may open up some issues that have remained buried under decades of disciplinary practice" (1992, p. 565).

To compare organized forms across developmental levels, Werner formulated an innovative theoretical language (Glick, 1983). This language contains a vocabulary rich with contrastive categories such as *syncretic-discrete* and *diffuse-articulated* that describe connections, dynamics, and forces within psychological organizations (Werner, 1926/1948). Such terms, Werner argued, would help researchers take a holistic view of phenomena as diverse as children, cultures, species, and psychopathology and make comparisons across levels of organization without reference to an external scale such as age

(Langer, 1970; Morss, 1990). Werner infused his words into his own theoretical proposals, the best known of which is his orthogenetic principle that "wherever development occurs it proceeds from a state of relative globality and lack of differentiation to a state of increasing differentiation, articulation, and hierarchic integration" (1957, p. 126).

Werner's vocabulary also permeated his empirical studies, which included extensive investigations of both language acquisition and developmental disorders. Yet despite a consistent vocabulary, he rarely spoke of language and disorders simultaneously. Even in his collective work (Barton & Franklin, 1978), the content of his chapters in the section (Part 3) on mental retardation and brain injury barely overlaps with that of his essays on language and symbolization (Part 4). Furthermore, although Werner's work on normative development was well received by American developmental psychologists, his investigations of developmental disabilities were all but overlooked; they were not even mentioned in summaries of his views in *Carmichael's Manual of Child Psychology* (Langer, 1970) and in developmental theory textbooks (e.g., Baldwin, 1967).

This disjuncture between language development and mental disorder can be explained partly by Werner's mid-career dislocation. His lifelong interests in cognitive development, perception, music, and language were evident in his earliest writing. (See Witkin, 1965, for a chronological list of Werner's publications, which includes his first article, "A genetic table of conceptual forms" [1912], and a monograph, *The Origins of the Metaphor* [1919], that reports a series of studies on the aesthetic-expressive aspects of speech.) This line of inquiry flourished during Werner's 15-year tenure in Hamburg, which he began in 1917 as a research associate at William Stern's Psychological Institute and continued as a member of the Faculty of Philosophy once the University of Hamburg was established in 1921. In 1933, this work was abruptly interrupted when the Nazis terminated Werner's appointment. For Werner, the next decade was a horrific period of "uncertainty, radical readjustment, and personal sorrow" (Witkin, 1965, p. 307).

By 1937, at the Wayne County Training School in Michigan, Werner had begun to establish a "second career" focused on the study of perceptual and conceptual processes in children with mental retardation (Witkin, 1965). Many of his studies from this era (e.g., Strauss & Werner, 1942; Werner, 1945) sought to demonstrate that developmental principles could differentiate between "retardation," which he thought could be explained by developmental psychology, and "defect" that results from brain "injury"or damage. This work was very influential, particularly through Werner's collaboration with fellow emigrant and neuropsychologist Alfred A. Strauss, whose book *Psychopathology and Education of the Brain-Injured Child* (Strauss & Lehtinen, 1947) helped establish the area of learning disabilities as a comprehensive field of study. But it was not an area that seemed to sustain Werner's interest. Once Werner secured academic appointments (first in 1943 as an instructor at Brooklyn College and then in 1947 as professor at Clark University where he was soon appointed as the G. Stanley Hall Professor of Genetic Psychology and the chair of the new, separate Department of Psychology; see Franklin, 1990), he returned to the study of the normative development of language and thought (e.g., Werner & Kaplan, 1952; Werner & Kaplan, 1963).

The seams between Werner's work on language development and his work on mental retardation may reflect conceptual, as well as personal, difficulties. In much of his work, Werner's central theoretical interest was the delineation of the unfolding of universal ideal forms. In the area of language development, this interest flourished in the detailed discussion of the complexity and scope of a child's early accomplishments that Werner and Kaplan (1963) presented in *Symbol Formation*. Their approach was clearly pathbreaking, moving studies of early language beyond simple inventories of vocabulary size and sentence length to the study of organized sets of rules that generate utterances (Flavell, 1966). Werner situated the process of language development within a broad context of psychological and social processes. Moreover, he challenged traditional assumptions about the relation between phenomena. For example, he suggested that a division between processes such as cognition and affect or cognition and perception might reflect an advanced developmental status, not an inevitable split (Glick, 1983), and that the separation between an organism and its context (or its vital field of *Umwelt*) might change qualitatively with development (Langer, 1969).

Despite the breadth of Werner's analysis of development, it was only near the end of his career that he began to show interest in the theoretical challenges presented by variations in developmental processes. He introduced words into his comparative-developmental vocabulary, such as *multilinearity* and *horizontal differentiation*, that invoked images of different developmental paths and different patterns of specialization, respectively (see Flavell, 1966; Witkin, 1965). Furthermore, he began to urge developmentalists to pay attention to problems of individuality or "differential" psychology. For example, he closed his classic essay on the concept of development with the observation that "the conviction has been growing in recent years that developmental conceptualization, in order to reaffirm its truly organismic character, has to expand its orbit of interest to include as a central problem the study of individuality" (Werner, 1957, p. 146).

When Werner discussed how an appreciation of atypical development might enrich understandings of language development, he tended to focus on "special states" such as dreaming and the "special orientations" taken by, for example, adults with schizophrenia (Werner & Kaplan, 1963) or aphasia (Werner, 1956), rather than on phenomena related to early language development. When he did consider early language disorders, it was primarily to illustrate how they conform to his developmental laws. For example, Werner and Kaplan summarized Helen Keller's (1903) "beautiful description" of her insight into symbolization as an example of "the very *shift of function* from signal to symbol which, in the normally growing child, can rarely be directly observed but must be inferred from his behavior" (1963, p. 111, emphasis in original). They remarked further that the study of successful language therapy for "deaf-blind children" might provide "information of great significance for the problem of early development of symbolization" because their steps toward grasping the representative function of names occur "in exactly the way that organismic theory of symbol formation would predict" (p. 112).

Werner also recognized the usefulness of articulating the relation between developmental processes and intervention. He made a particularly compelling case at a conference held at Clark University in 1959 on "The Relationship Between Rehabilitation and Psychology" (Werner, 1978). He began this presentation with a summary of how his general experimental psychology differed from many others, including presumably that of his American audience. He introduced his view as organismic (rather than elementaristic) and developmental (rather than agenetic) and explained that it was field oriented (rather than concerned with organisms in isolation) and focused on dynamic, vectorial functioning (and not on static functioning). He then argued that his approach to psychology might profitably inform the conceptualization of rehabilitation, which he defined as "essentially a dynamic and genetic process of the formation of interdependent functioning which takes place through interpersonal activity"(pp. 328–329).

In *Symbol Formation*, Werner and Kaplan (1963) reiterated the developmental significance of interpersonal activity. In their discussion of normative development, they proposed that the proper unit of analysis for the study of early symbolization was an interpersonal one, the "primordial sharing situation" (p. 42). In addition, they referred repeatedly to a case report by Luria and Yudovich (1959) of 5-year-old identical twin boys with speech retardation whose successful therapy Werner and Kaplan attributed to processes that occur within the "normal social intercourse" that is found in a "natural social habitat" (p. 121). By separating twins who previously had been enmeshed in a "closely knit companionship, ostensibly so gratifying as to forestall any pressure towards communication with the surrounding world" (p. 118) and placing them with other children, Luria and Yudovich found that in only 3 months' time, each twin was "compelled to develop and articulate his speech in order to achieve open commerce with others" (p. 121). Werner and Kaplan (1963) reported that the language development of each twin raced along a normative course from "speech forms characteristic of very early levels to speech forms of a genetically more advanced level" (p. 118). For example, names that were initially "contextualized," "quite diffuse and equivocal in their reference," and lacking in "articulateness and specificity of meaning" rapidly became more "decontextualized" (pp. 119–120). Syntax that was at first "predominantly amorphous sentential forms" was transformed into "grammatically and functionally differentiated sentence structures" (p. 319).

In summary, Werner strove to provide developmentalists with a way to conceptualize the forms of change. His theoretical writings provide a vocabulary that emphasizes differences across developmental levels. He argued that development occurred in an orderly manner regardless of time, place, or organism. Werner often used his developmental principles to elaborate phenomena related to the transition to symbolization, which included many aspects of language development. He rarely focused specifically on disorders of language development. When he did, his conclusion was that successful development always started within an interpersonal context and then traced a course toward increased differentiation and hierarchical integration.

### Vygotsky's Discovery of the Historical Child

To contemporary developmental psychologists, Vygotsky appears both as a romantic historic figure (for short biographies, see Kozulin, 1986, and Wertsch, 1985, both of whom call him the "Mozart of Psychology") and a fresh theoretical inspiration for both basic and applied efforts (see, respectively, Kessen, 1979, and Schneider & Watkins, 1996). This dual identity stems from Vygotsky's personal and professional tragedies. Soon after the Russian Revolution, Vygotsky started to make major contributions to the reshaping of Soviet psychology. By 1930, his influence was extensive, particularly in the areas of paedology and defectology, and his reputation was international. But in 1934 he died of tuberculosis. Then, 2 years later, the 1936 Decree on Paedology outlawed his primary field of study. His work was repressed in the Soviet Union until the 1950s, and many of his writings remained unpublished in Russian until the 1980s. Only in the 1990s has a full range of these works been translated into English (see, e.g., Vygotsky & Luria, 1930/1993, and volumes of his work edited by Rieber & Carton, 1993; van der Veer & Valsiner, 1994). However, American developmentalists had received earlier tastes in the form of intriguing suggestions from a narrow circle of European-trained psychologists that included Werner and Goldstein (Kozulin, 1986) and in selective translations (e.g., Vygotsky, 1934/1962, 1978).

From the start, Vygotsky sought to challenge developmentalists' universalist conception of their project. Vygotsky's critique of the traditional psychology of his era was stinging. For example, in one of his earliest books, *The Historical Meaning of the Crisis in Psychology* (1926; cited in Kozulin, 1986), he argued that all the then-current schools of psychology—introspectionism, behaviorism, and psychoanalysis—were doomed to be separate, closed spheres of inquiry and that only a new Marxist methodology could lead to a unified scientific psychology. Vygotsky's alternative psychology was inspired by his insight that "the task of psychology . . . is not the discovery of the eternal child. The task of psychology is the discovery of the historical child" (1934/1987, p. 91).

In an attempt to understand the "historical child," Vygotsky sketched and elaborated a theoretical perspective whose fundamental aim was to depict how individual consciousness emerges from relations with others and how "culture becomes a part of each person's nature" (Cole & Scribner, 1978, p. 6). Although this perspective changed considerably over his short career (see van der Veer & Valsiner, 1991), it always included both developmental and cultural-historical aspects. Furthermore, Vygotsky drew these aspects together by emphasizing that human beings' contact with their physical surroundings, unlike that of other animals, is mediated by the use of sociocultural artifacts such as tools and language.

Vygotsky produced several compelling images of how culture becomes internalized as children master the use of tools and signs (Glick, 1983; Wertsch, 1985). One interesting image consists of intersecting developmental lines. Vygotsky often located key moments of developmental transformation at the point when two lines of development—the line of natural or biological development and the line of cultural-historical development—converge. For example, he argued that "the very essence of cultural development" may be contained in occasions that allow a "collision of mature cultural forms of behavior with the primitive forms that characterize the child's behavior" so that culture is superimposed on and radically transforms the biological functioning (1981, p. 151). Speech is presumably situated at one of these points. Developmentally it transforms thought and is transformed itself as it becomes internalized.

A second and related image, that of a zone of proximal development, depicts the process of interpersonal guidance or instruction that Vygotsky theorized was a crucial developmental mechanism. Generally, Vygotsky argued that children are first lent and then acquire their culture's signs and tools as they interact with more culturally sophisticated partners such as parents, teachers, and older peers. With his concept of the zone of proximal development (1978), he sharpened this claim, focusing attention on events that occur when a culturemate supports "good learning," that is, learning that nurtures development. Within the zone, the educator meets the child at the edge of current development and "sets in motion a variety of developmental processes that would [otherwise] be impossible" (Vygotsky, 1978, p. 90). Early in life, language is a crucial aspect of these encounters for, in Vygotsky's words, "it is first and foremost a means of social interaction, a means of pronouncement and understanding" (1934; quoted in Wertsch, 1985, p. 94).

For our purposes, it is interesting that Vygotsky drew from these images a strong rationale for including issues related to developmental disorders within his new psychology. He envisioned a unified field of study, paedology, which would encompass both the scientific study of development and its application. Defectology was an important part of this unified field, and Vygotsky was devoted to building an appropriate institutional structure. In 1925, he began to organize the Laboratory of Psychology for Abnormal Children in Moscow. This institute became, in 1929, the Experimental Defectological Institute of Narakompros (People's Commisariat for Education) and, after Vygotsky's death, the Scientific Research Institute of Defectology of the Academy of Pedagogical Sciences (van der Veer & Valsiner, 1991; Wertsch, 1985). Vygotsky also wrote extensively about "defective children," particularly children with sensory impairments, at the same time that he was investigating issues relating to the language development and psychology of all children. Although he often argued that the same fundamental laws governed the cognitive and psychological development of all children, he also recognized that the study of children with disabilities might provide invaluable insight into broad problems of learning and development (Knox & Stevens, 1993).

Like much of his work, Vygotsky's writings about atypical development tended to be broad treatments of general issues; thus, we do not have examples of case histories or detailed discussions of experimental results (van der Veer & Valsiner, 1991). Nevertheless, we are offered many provocative suggestions about how the study of atypical development might provide critical insight into developmental and cultural processes. For example, he argued that, as with typical development, the development of a child with a disability should be considered a sociocultural process and should be understood "primarily in terms of how it changes a complex system of development" (Wertsch, 1985, p. 18). This insight led him to focus not only on the child's "defect" but also on how his or her culture provided support for development. In such discussions, Vygotsky was particularly interested in situations where a biological function, such as vision or hearing, fails and thus creates an "experiment of nature" that might help demonstrate the flexibility of the cultural forms of behavior. Moreover, he argued that these experiments might provide insight into the relation between natural and cultural lines of development. For example, he suggested that as researchers tried to articulate the "qualitative uniqueness" of a development that is impeded by a defect, they may see how, with the support of special sociocultural tools such as braille, a second line of cultural development can enlist other biological functions to circumvent the weak point and build a psychological superstructure over it so that a bypass could be created around the "defect" (Knox & Stevens, 1993, p. 13; see also van der Veer & Valsiner, 1991).

The impact of this analysis of atypical development can be seen throughout Vygotsky's writings. For example, van der Veer and Valsiner (1991) argued convincingly that Vygotsky's early work in defectology influenced his overarching conception of development, leading him to formulate the idea of mediation and to distinguish explicitly between signs and meanings. Moreover, this analysis was central to Vygotsky's notion that interventions might be located at the juncture between culture and biology. He and his colleagues strove to adjust cultural tools so that they might better fit the child with a developmental disorder and to train children with disorders to use cultural means more effectively. In this regard, his focus was on the entire child, rather than merely on the defect itself. Thus, Vygotsky (1931/1993a) wrote about assessment that "for us it is important to know not only what kind of defect has been diagnosed in a given child and how the assessed child has been affected, but also what kind of child possesses the given defect" (p. 125). This view also takes into account "not only the child's negative characteristics, not only his minuses, but also a positive contour of his personality" (1993b, p. 169).

Vygotsky often focused his discussion of intervention on the development of speech. In his general theory, he argued that speech is extraordinarily important for it is "not only a tool of communication, but also a tool of thinking; consciousness develops mainly with the help of speech and originates in social experience" (1924; cited in van der Veer & Valsiner, 1991, p. 64). This dual function of speech led Vygotsky to suggest that the type of symbol system should not matter, as long as meaning is retained. The key is that the system allows a child to internalize language and develop those higher mental functions for which language serves as the basis (Knox & Stevens, 1993). This realization led him to advocate for intervention methods that emphasized meaning and against those that emphasized the technical aspects of tool use (such as "pronunciation"). For example, he sought to design specific tools such as "a special system of cultural signs and symbols which are adapted to the specific psychophysiological characteristics of an abnormal child" (Vygotsky, 1993b, p. 168). Moreover, he praised methods that integrated the teaching of speech into social experiences such as games that might elicit speech (van der Veer & Valsiner, 1991). It is interesting to note that this analysis was later to inspire Luria and Yudovich's (1959) treatment of nonspeaking twins that, in turn, was discussed by Werner and Kaplan (1963; also see previous section on Werner) in support of their analysis of the social context of symbol formation.

In summary, Vygotsky attempted to focus psychology on the historical child whose mind is embedded in society. This agenda led him to construct images, such as intersecting developmental lines and the zone of proximal development, that highlight the social relation between developing children and their educators, including parents and teachers. Moreover, it drew attention to the role of speech as a tool both of social interaction and of thought. As he formulated a cultural-historical psychology, Vygotsky often considered the development of children with disabilities, drawing out implications for both his general principles of development and his views of effective education and intervention.

## CONCLUSIONS: FROM THEORETICAL FOUNDATIONS TO CONTEMPORARY RESEARCH

The study of language and communication disorders has rarely informed the theoretical core of contemporary developmental psychology. In the beginning of this chapter, I suggested that one explanation for this slight might lie in the normative slant of traditional developmental theories that focus primarily on the orderly emergence of phenomena such as symbols and concepts. However, I also raised a second possibility: Perhaps early developmental theorists did consider the implications of atypical development but, due to the vagrancies of history, we, their English-speaking heirs, have not been well positioned to hear their suggestions. Intrigued by this latter prospect, I reviewed the publications of Piaget, Werner, and Vygotsky in hopes of locating discussions in which these seminal theorists investigated atypical development. My main findings, reported in detail in the preceding sections of this chapter, are summarized in Table 1.

In this concluding section, I consider what this historical exercise might contribute to contemporary theories of language and communication development. This assessment is motivated by my basic conviction that researchers should periodically revisit their theoretical foundation. As I argue in the following sections, such review can help ground our current work by reminding us of the limitations and promises of early visions of our field's projects, by locating previously overlooked material that can inspire new views, and by stimulating fresh attempts to formulate heuristic theoretical notions.

## Reminding Ourselves of Our Roots

The classical theoretical texts of developmental psychology proposed ambitious projects that sought to address a broad range of issues related to patterns of directed change. However, only some issues, such as the emergence of symbols and concept acquisition in typically developing children, were widely discussed. Such selectivity is, of course, necessary. (For a fascinating discussion of the relation between theoretical scope and precision, see Pepper, 1942.) Nonetheless, it means that other issues are addressed more narrowly than those of focal concern. This appears to be the case when classical developmentalists considered the spheres of language acquisition and developmental disorders, as well as their intersection. For example, when they focused on language acquisi-

Table 1. Three classic agendas for developmental psychology

| Agenda | Theorist | Lifespan | Primary location | Study of atypical populations |
|---|---|---|---|---|
| Search for the epistemic subject | Jean Piaget | 1896–1980 | Geneva | At edge of interest |
| Articulate a developmental vocabulary | Heinz Werner | 1890–1964 | Hamburg<br>Wayne County, Michigan<br>Clark University | Periodical concern |
| Discover the cultural-historical child | Lev Vygotsky | 1896–1934 | Moscow | Integral to defectology and paedology |

tion, they almost always emphasized the development of meaning. And when atypical patterns of acquisition were mentioned, it was rarely as a source of important information about development in general and language acquisition in specific.

To a large degree, Piaget is responsible for the boundaries on the range of concerns perceived as central by American developmental psychologists. Although he inspired a research renaissance by raising new topics and articulating provocative themes, his contributions shifted attention toward universals and away from variations. Furthermore, the performance of children who were experiencing severe developmental difficulties was often described primarily in normative terms and discussed within the terms of the reigning theoretical frame. This perspective fueled the possibility that, as Inhelder (1943/1968) once mused, "the normal child can be discovered in the pathological child" (p. 299). Moreover, it blocked from view a range of important theoretical problems and challenging empirical phenomena. Thus, as Fincham (1982) pointedly suggested in his critical analysis of the implications of Piaget's views for the understanding of learning disabilities, disabilities related to language might appear as a mere "epiphenomenon of operative immaturity" (p. 381).

It is important to recognize traditional theoretical tendencies that limit movement into new areas of research. Acknowledging them may help to explain the unidirectional flow from theory to application that has characterized much of the research literature on language and communication disabilities. Furthermore, it may inspire us to counter this flow by reexamining prior studies that were conceived of as primarily "applied" in hopes of locating theory-broadening information.

### Locating New Findings in Old Texts

A second reason for reviewing the corpus of classic texts is to uncover ideas that may have been overlooked previously. Returning to a "narrow" historical base might seem paradoxical, but, as the results of our review confirm, this is a most auspicious time to revisit the writings of classical developmental theorists in hopes of gathering fresh information. In particular, there are two interesting twists in historical narrative that may help us locate new material.

First, developmentalists in the 1990s are well positioned to use new data to elaborate and challenge assumptions in these texts. As we sharpen our focus on more applied concerns (a shift displayed in new journals such as *Applied Developmental Psychology* and *Applied Developmental Science*), I think it is particularly important that we enter into two-way dialogues about developmental processes, including dialogues with familiar texts. For example, each rereading of Piaget's writings of the origin of intelligence (1936/1963) and the formation of symbols (1945/1962b) provides not only a review of the sequences of sensorimotor structures but also a reminder of how closely he observed infants' active attempts to adapt to daily challenges. In short, it might reinstate Piaget's functionalism at a time when his structuralism dominates our collective memory of his work. This reminder might, in turn, stimulate interest in the importance of expanding the range of observations to include children with communication and language disorders not only to document their movement through developmental sequences but also to contribute important insights into the complex process of adaptation that Piaget sought to understand (see Cohen, 1983).

Second, developmental psychologists can now gain access to material that has been hidden in the folds of our field's history. Several texts, such as Werner's writings on mental retardation, have escaped notice. Others, such as Vygotsky's rich volumes on "defectology," are just being exposed in the 1990s. These works reveal developmental theories that are amenable to atypical phenomena. When circumstances led Werner to the study of children with mental retardation, he readily used his broad comparative frame and abstract developmental vocabulary as a heuristic source of questions about various developmental forms. When Vygotsky puzzled over the complex relation between natural and cultural processes, he championed the central conceptual value of examining how children with disabilities develop in various educational contexts.

## Stimulating Theoretical Efforts

This chapter is motivated by the desire to contribute to a fuller understanding of how research on atypical patterns of communication and language development might challenge and clarify notions about development. Unfortunately, we did not find fully worked examples in the writings of Piaget, Werner, and Vygotsky that might serve as a model for new investigations. However, two positive discoveries were made that might guide our efforts. First, our historical base does contain compelling rationales for such work. Second, it also contains several points that may be sharpened through the study of atypical developmental courses. For example, Piaget's account of how symbolic representation is first manifest in the "epistemic subject's" activity might be enhanced by observations of young children whose spoken language is delayed. Werner's "developmental vocabulary" might be enriched by expanding the range of exemplars for terms such as multilinearity that refer to diverse patterns of development. Vygotsky's sketch of the intersection of culture and biology, as well as his claims about the importance of cultural tools in fostering the development of children with communication disorders, might be clarified through observations of the use of new technologies such as computer-based speech output communication devices.

However, such "theory-mending" exercises are only of limited value if the result is merely a more complete version of a stale theory. Rather, we must admit the possibility that the addition of new information about atypical communication and language development may challenge the premises and stretch the boundaries of a classical theory. Although it is beyond the scope of this chapter to undertake such "theory-revitalizing" work, I hope that it helps to lay the groundwork for such efforts by bringing to the fore the traditional theories of developmental order. This review revealed that the field's backdrop is a tapestry of varied agendas, interesting concepts, and difficult debates that would be greatly enriched by systematic consideration of developmental disorders.

## REFERENCES

Adamson, L.B. (1992). Variations of early language use. In L.T. Winegar & J. Valsiner (Eds.), *Children's development within social contexts: Vol. 1. Metatheory and theory* (pp. 123–141). Hillsdale, NJ: Lawrence Erlbaum Associates.

Adamson, L.B. (1996). *Communication development during infancy.* Boulder, CO: Westview.

Adamson, L.B., & Dunbar, B. (1991). Communication development of young children with tracheostomies. *Augmentative and Alternative Communication, 7,* 275–283.

Adamson, L.B., Romski, M.A., Deffebach, K., & Sevcik, R.A. (1992). Symbol vocabulary and the focus of conversations: Augmenting language development for youth with mental retardation. *Journal of Speech and Hearing Research, 35,* 1333–1343.

Baldwin, A.L. (1967). *Theories of child development.* New York: John Wiley & Sons.

Barton, S.S., & Franklin, M.B. (Eds.) (1978). *Developmental processes: Heinz Werner's selected writings: Vol. 2. Cognition, language, and symbolization.* New York: International Universities Press.

Chapman, M. (1988). *Constructive evolution.* Cambridge, England: Cambridge University Press.

Cohen, D. (1983). *Piaget: Critique and reassessment.* London: Croom Helm.

Cole, M., & Scribner, S. (1978). Introduction. In M. Cole, V. John-Steiner, S. Scribner, & E. Souberman (Eds.), *Mind in society* (pp. 1–14). Cambridge, MA: Harvard University Press.

Elliot, A., & Donaldson, M. (1982). Piaget on language. In S. Modgil & C. Modgil (Eds.), *Jean Piaget: Consensus and controversy* (pp. 157–166). New York: Praeger.

Fincham, F. (1982). Piaget's theory and the learning disabled: A critical analysis. In S. Modgil & C. Modgil (Eds.), *Jean Piaget: Consensus and controversy* (pp. 369–390). New York: Praeger.

Flavell, J. (1963). *The developmental psychology of Jean Piaget.* Princeton, NJ: Van-Nostrand.

Flavell, J.H. (1966). Heinz Werner on the nature of development. In S. Wapner & B. Kaplan (Eds.), *Heinz Werner, 1890–1964, papers in memoriam* (pp. 25–31). Worcester, MA: Clark University Press.

Franklin, M.B. (1990). Reshaping psychology at Clark: The Werner era. *Journal of the History of the Behavioral Sciences, 26,* 176–189.

Furth, H.G. (1966). *Thinking without language: Psychological implications of deafness.* New York: Free Press.

Glick, J.A. (1983). Piaget, Vygotsky, and Werner. In S. Wapner & B. Kaplan (Eds.), *Toward a holistic developmental psychology* (pp. 35–52). Hillsdale, NJ: Lawrence Erlbaum Associates.

Glick, J.A. (1992). Heinz Werner's relevance for contemporary developmental psychology. *Developmental Psychology, 28,* 558–565.

Goldstein, K. (1939). *The organism: A holistic approach to biology derived from pathological data in man.* New York: American Books. (Original work published 1934)

Hodapp, R.M., & Burack, J.A. (1990). What mental retardation teaches us about typical development: The examples of sequences, rates, and cross-domain relations. *Development and Psychopathology, 2*, 213–226.

Inhelder, B. (1968). *The diagnosis of reasoning in the mentally retarded.* New York: John Day. (Original work published 1943; 2nd edition, 1963)

Jakobson, R. (1960). Linguistics and poetics. In T.A. Sebeok (Ed.), *Style in language* (pp. 350–377). New York: John Wiley & Sons.

Joravsky, D. (1987). L.S. Vygotskii: The muffled deity of Soviet psychology. In M.G. Ash & W.R. Woodward (Eds.), *Psychology in twentieth-century thought and society* (pp. 189–212). Cambridge, England: Cambridge University Press.

Kamhi, A.G., & Masterson, J.J. (1989). Language and cognition in mentally handicapped people: Last rites for the difference-delay controversy. In M. Beveridge, G. Conti-Ramsden, & I. Leudar (Eds.), *Language and communication in mentally handicapped people* (pp. 83–111). London: Chapman & Hall.

Keating, D.P., & Rosen, H. (1991). *Constructivist perspectives on developmental psychopathology and atypical development.* Hillsdale, NJ: Lawrence Erlbaum Associates.

Keller, H. (1903). *The story of my life.* New York: Doubleday, Page.

Kessen, W. (1979). The American child and other cultural inventions. *American Psychologist, 34*, 815–820.

Kessen, W. (1990). *The rise and fall of development.* Worcester, MA: Clark University Press.

Knox, J.E., & Stevens, C.B. (1993). Vygotsky and Soviet Russian defectology: An introduction. In R.W. Rieber & A.S. Carton (Eds.), *The collected works of L.S. Vygotsky: Vol. 2. The fundamentals of defectology* (pp. 1–25). New York: Plenum.

Kozulin, A., (1984). *Psychology in utopia: Toward a social history of Soviet psychology.* Cambridge: MIT Press.

Kozulin, A. (Ed.). (1986). Vygotsky in context. In L. Vygotsky, *Thought and language* (pp. xi–lvi). Cambridge: MIT Press.

Langer, J. (1969). *Theories of development.* New York: Holt, Rinehart & Winston.

Langer, J. (1970). Werner's comparative organismic theory. In P.H. Mussen (Ed.), *Carmichael's manual of child psychology* (3rd ed.) (Vol. 1, pp. 733–771). New York: John Wiley & Sons.

Luria, A.R. (1979). *The making of mind: A personal account of Soviet psychology.* Cambridge, MA: Harvard University Press.

Luria, A.R., & Yudovich, F.Ia. (1959). *Speech and the development of mental processes in the child.* London: Staples Press.

Mervis, C.B. (1990). Early conceptual development of children with Down syndrome. In D. Cicchetti & M. Beeghly (Eds.), *Children with Down syndrome: A developmental perspective* (pp. 252–301). Cambridge, England: Cambridge University Press.

Modgil, S., & Modgil, C. (1976). *Piagetian research: Compilation and commentary: Vol. 5. Part II: Reasoning among handicapped children.* Windsor, England: NFER Publishing.

Morehead, D.M., & Morehead, A. (1974). From signal to sign: A Piagetian view of thought and language during the first two years. In R.L. Schiefelbusch & L.L. Lloyd (Eds.), *Language perspectives: Acquisition, retardation, and intervention* (pp. 153–190). Baltimore: University Park Press.

Morss, J.R. (1990). *The biologising of childhood: Developmental psychology and the Darwinian myth.* Hillsdale, NJ: Lawrence Erlbaum Associates.

Parke, R.D., Ornstein, P.A., Rieser, J.J., & Zahn-Waxler, C. (1992). The past as prologue: An overview of a century of developmental psychology. In R.D. Parke, P.A. Ornstein, J.J. Rieser, & C. Zahn-Waxler (Eds.), *A century of developmental psychology* (pp. 1–70). Washington, DC: American Psychological Association.

Pepper, S.C. (1942). *World hypotheses: Study in evidence*. Berkeley: University of California.

Piaget, J. (1959). *The language and thought of the child*. New York: Humanities Press. (Original work published 1923)

Piaget, J. (1962a). *Comments on Vygotsky's critical remarks concerning The Language and Thought of the Child, and Judgment and Reasoning in the Child*. Cambridge: MIT Press.

Piaget, J. (1962b). *Play, dreams, and imitation in childhood*. New York: Norton. (Original work published 1945 [*La formation de symbole*])

Piaget, J. (1963). *The origins of intelligence in children*. New York: Norton. (Original work published 1936)

Piaget, J. (1967). *Six psychological studies*. New York: Random House. (Original work published 1964)

Piaget, J. (1970). Piaget's theory. In P.H. Mussen (Ed.), *Carmichael's manual of child psychology* (3rd ed.) (Vol. 1, pp. 703–732). New York: John Wiley & Sons.

Piaget, J. (1983). Dialogue III: Jean Piaget's views on the psychology of language and thought. In R.W. Rieber (Ed.), *Dialogues on the psychology of language and thought: Conversations with Noam Chomsky, Charles Osgood, Jean Piaget, Ulric Neisser, & Marcel Kinsbourne* (pp. 103–120). New York: Plenum.

Piaget, J., & Inhelder, B. (1971). *Mental imagery in the child: A study of the development of imaginal representation*. New York: Basic Books.

Rieber, R.W., & Carton, A.S. (Eds.). (1993). *The collected works of L.S. Vygotsky: Vol. 2. The fundamentals of defectology*. New York: Plenum.

Rieber, R.W., & Voyat, G. (1983). Introduction: An overview of the controversial issues in the psychology of language and thought. In R.W. Rieber (Ed.), *Dialogues on the psychology of language and thought: Conversations with Noam Chomsky, Charles Osgood, Jean Piaget, Ulric Neisser, & Marcel Kinsbourne* (pp. 7–26). New York: Plenum.

Rosenberg, S. (1984). Disorders of first-language development: Trends in research and theory. In E.S. Gollin (Ed.), *Malformation of development: Biological and psychological sources and consequences* (pp. 195–237). New York: Academic Press.

Schneider, P., & Watkins, R.V. (1996). Applying Vygotskian developmental theory to language intervention. *Language, Speech, and Hearing Services in Schools, 27*, 157–170.

Sears, R.R. (1975). Your ancients revisited: A history of child development. In E.M. Hetherington (Ed.), *Review of child development research* (Vol. 5, pp. 1–73). Chicago: University of Chicago Press.

Sinclair, H. (1982). Piaget on language: A perspective. In S. Modgil & C. Modgil (Eds.), *Jean Piaget: Consensus and controversy* (pp. 167–177). New York: Praeger.

Sokal, M.M. (1984). The Gestalt psychologists in behaviorist America. *The American Historical Review, 12*, 1240–1263.

Strauss, A.A., & Werner, H. (1942). Disorders of conceptual thinking in brain-injured children. *Journal of Nervous Mental Disease, 96*, 153–171.

Strauss, A.A., & Lehtinen, L.E. (1947). *Psychopathology and education of the brain-injured child*. New York: Grune & Stratton.

Tager-Flusberg, H. (Ed.). (1994). *Constraints on language acquisition: Studies of atypical children*. Hillsdale, NJ: Lawrence Erlbaum Associates.

van der Veer, R., & Valsiner, J. (1991). *Understanding Vygotsky: A quest for synthesis.* Oxford, England: Blackwell.

van der Veer, R., & Valsiner, J. (Eds.). (1994). *The Vygotsky reader.* Oxford, England: Blackwell.

Vygotsky, L.S. (1962). *Thought and language.* Cambridge: MIT Press. (Original work published 1934)

Vygotsky, L.S. (1978). *Mind in society: The development of higher psychological processes.* Cambridge, MA: Harvard University Press. (Collected writings, some original work published 1935, 1960, and 1966 and some previously unpublished original work)

Vygotsky, L.S. (1981). The genesis of higher mental functions. In J.V. Wertsch (Ed.), *The concept of activity in Soviet psychology* (pp. 144–188). Armonk, NY: Sharpe.

Vygotsky, L.S. (1986). *Thought and language,* revised and edited by Alex Kozulin. Cambridge: MIT Press.

Vygotsky, L.S. (1987). Thinking and speech. In R.W. Reiber & A.S. Carton (Eds.), *The Collected Works of L.S. Vygotsky: Vol. 1. Problems of general psychology* (pp. 39–285). New York: Plenum. (Original work published 1934)

Vygotsky, L.S. (1993a). Compensatory processes in the development of the retarded child. In R.W. Rieber & A.S. Carton (Eds.), *The collected works of L.S. Vygotsky: Vol. 2. The fundamentals of defectology* (pp. 122–138). New York: Plenum. (Original work presented 1931)

Vygotsky, L.S. (1993b). Defectology and the study of the development and education of abnormal children. In R.W. Rieber & A.S. Carton (Eds.), *The collected works of L.S. Vygotsky: Vol. 2. The fundamentals of defectology* (pp. 164–170). New York: Plenum.

Vygotsky, L.S. , & Luria, A.R. (1993). *Studies on the history of behavior: Ape, primitive, and child* (V.I. Golod & J.E. Knox, Trans.) Hillsdale, NJ: Lawrence Erlbaum Associates. (Original work published 1930)

Werner, H. (1945). Perceptual behavior of brain-injured children: An experimental study by means of the Rorschach technique. *Genetic Psychology Monographs, 31,* 51–111.

Werner, H. (1948). *Comparative psychology of mental development.* New York: International Universities Press. (Original work published 1926)

Werner, H. (1956). Microgenesis and aphasia. *The Journal of Abnormal and Social Psychology, 52,* 347–353.

Werner, H. (1957). The concept of development from a comparative and organismic point of view. In D. Harris (Ed.), *The concept of development* (pp. 125–148). Minneapolis: University of Minnesota Press.

Werner, H. (1978). Significance of general experimental psychology for the understanding of abnormal behavior and its correction or prevention. In S.S. Barton & M.B. Franklin (Eds.), *Developmental processes: Heinz Werner's selected writings: Vol. 2. Cognition, language, and symbolization* (pp. 327–345). New York: International Universities Press.

Werner, H., & Kaplan, B. (1963). *Symbol formation.* New York: John Wiley & Sons.

Werner, H., & Kaplan, E. (1952). The acquisition of word meanings: A developmental study. *Monographs of the Society for Research in Child Development, 15* (Serial no. 51).

Wertsch, J.V. (1985). *Vygotsky and the social formation of mind.* Cambridge, MA: Harvard University Press.

Witkin, H.A. (1965). Heinz Werner: 1890–1964. *Child Development, 30,* 307–328.

# 2

# Contributions of Stimulus Control Perspectives to Psycholinguistic Theories of Vocabulary Development and Delay

Krista M. Wilkinson and William J. McIlvane

Language-related research encompasses a variety of topics, including social-transactional processes, cognitive and symbolic processes, and the logical operations of syntax. Since the 1960s, psycholinguists, linguists, philosophers, and other interested parties have recorded, analyzed, and debated a comprehensive database of developmental language phenomena (e.g., Kessel, 1988; Slobin, 1985). Over this time, we have come to appreciate the implications of individual variation within language learners of a single community and across different language communities (Adamson, 1992; Bates & MacWhinney, 1987; Nelson, 1981; Slobin, 1985). Variations among typical language learners provide one window into the course of development. Understanding the extremes of variation, delayed or deviant development, also seems necessary for a comprehensive account of language acquisition and use. Furthermore, the processes involved in typical development may be elucidated by study of how development "breaks down" (e.g., Mervis & Bertrand, 1993b).

To capture the diversity of developmental variations, language researchers have historically integrated information from different approaches to the study of behavior. In this chapter, we consider how theoretical and empirical advances in behavior-analytic studies of mental retardation can contribute to our understanding of early word learning. The traditional focus of behavior

Funding for the research and preparation of this chapter was supported by NICHD Grant No. HD25995 and by a contract from the Commonwealth of Massachusetts (100220023SC).

The authors thank their colleagues at the Shriver Center for their insights during the conceptualization of this chapter.

analysis is the study of factors that influence acquisition and modification of behavior, often through the study of individuals whose development has not followed the typical path (i.e., individuals diagnosed with autism, mental retardation, or other disorders). This interest reflects the long-standing strength of the discipline in developing effective teaching and communication methods for these individuals. We illustrate some of the ways theoretical advances in behavior analysis (e.g., Sidman, 1993) from the 1990s can offer new perspectives on issues being debated by language researchers. However, before proceeding, we offer two caveats about our terminology. First, we refer to behavior analysis and psycholinguistics as two disciplines within the more general field of psychology. Although these disciplines share at least one goal (to explain language-related behavior), there are clear differences in theory and methodology. We contend that these differences are useful, providing multiple perspectives on the same phenomena. Second, we have selected terms that will communicate to psycholinguists the basic analytical approach of behavior analysis. Unfortunately, the two disciplines sometimes express the same idea with different words; other times they use the same words to express different ideas. We recognize that some of our terminological choices (and interpretations of findings) may differ from customary practice in behavior analysis. We believe, however, that this chapter accurately reflects contemporary thinking in the discipline in the 1990s.

## BACKGROUND OF BEHAVIOR ANALYSIS

One main goal of behavior analysis is to understand how an individual's behavior is influenced by contingencies in the environment. The father of modern behavior analysis, B.F. Skinner (1969), distinguished two types of contingencies: 1) ontogenic contingencies of reinforcement and 2) phylogenic contingencies of survival. Ontogenic contingencies affect behavior within the lifetime of the individual. The proposition states that when given behavior in a given environment is followed by positive (or negative) consequences, the probability that the behavior will occur under similar circumstances becomes more (or less) likely. By contrast, phylogenic contingencies are those represented in the Darwinian process of evolution, contingencies that operate over many lifetimes to select physical and behavioral characteristics that increase the probability of survival and reproduction. In a contemporary behavior-analytic account, behavior is viewed as the joint product of ontogenic and phylogenic contingencies. Because phylogenic contingencies cannot be experimentally controlled under most circumstances, behavior analysts tend to focus on ontogenic contingencies for experimental study. The action of phylogenic contingencies is inferred when behavioral phenomena cannot be experimentally related (nor plausibly attributed) to ontogenic contingencies.

In behavior analysis in the 1990s, one extremely active subdiscipline focuses on stimulus control. The term *stimulus control* refers to the probability that an individual will behave in a certain way given a certain set of (environmental) conditions (McIlvane, 1992). Consider the following elementary example. When a young child hears her father say, "It's cookie time," she behaves in one of the many ways appropriate to the words spoken (e.g., running to the cookie jar; holding out her hand; saying "No, I want cake"). She would likely behave differently, however, if her father said, "It's bath time." The child's differential response to "cookie" versus "bath" is an example of stimulus control. As behavior analysts say, the various behaviors were under the control of the words spoken.

Stimulus control may be evident even when the controlling stimuli are not present in the immediate external environment. Slightly altering our example, consider the child's likely behavior when she wants another cookie but her father has gone out of the room. Looking about the room and not seeing him, she calls out "Daddy!" which causes her father to reenter the room. Saying "Daddy" as opposed to "Mommy" (who also gives out cookies) shows control by a recently present stimulus. Not all word production under stimulus control need be "referential," however. One may have, for example, explicitly taught, nongenerative responses (paired associates; see discussion of reference on p. 29).

Stimulus control research has many parallels with cognitively oriented analyses of attention, memory, categorization, executive functioning, and so forth (Sidman, 1979). Furthermore, interpretive and philosophical research in behavior analysis has taken on an increasingly broader range of problems that connect with more traditional analyses of word learning (e.g., processes of observational learning [MacDonald, Dixon, & LeBlanc, 1986; Whitehurst, 1978]). Notably, the mechanistic S–R (stimulus–response) psychologies that were fashionable in the middle of the 20th century bear almost no relationship to behavior analysis in the 1990s. Rather than conceptualizing learning in terms of discrete S–R relations, behavior analysts speak instead of learning relations among environmental events (Sidman, 1986) and even of learning relations among relations (Lipkens, Hayes, & Hayes, 1993).

As in psycholinguistic accounts, stimulus control analyses suggest that children acquire new behaviors by noting regularities in the environment and the consequences of their own actions. Perhaps the main difference in the perspectives is the status of processes that may mediate the effects of differential reinforcement. Traditional behavior-analytic accounts have postulated that direct experience and differential reinforcement dictate word use. Although psycholinguists have criticized such accounts (see discussion of reference, p. 29), we describe developments in the field of behavior analysis that might prove less vulnerable to this type of argument.

## OVERVIEW OF LEXICAL PRINCIPLES

To accomplish our interdisciplinary analysis, we will adopt the lexical principles framework proposed within psycholinguistics by Golinkoff, Mervis, and Hirsh-Pasek (1994). Briefly, this is a developmental framework of six principles, or strategies, that may guide children's word learning. The principles are organized into two tiers, to reflect conceptual relations between the principles within each tier and a hierarchical relationship between the principles of the first and second tiers. In this chapter, we define each of the principles and discuss the implications of related work in behavior analysis for each principle.

This framework suits our purposes for several reasons. First, it provides an excellent structure for organizing the comprehensive psycholinguistic evidence. Second, it permitted Golinkoff and colleagues to identify some of the most relevant, and often unresolved, issues within psycholinguistics. Third, the framework is flexible enough to accommodate different approaches to these unresolved issues, including those germane to an integration of behavior-analytic perspectives. For instance, an ongoing debate concerns whether the proposed principles are somehow innate to the language-learning child ("primitive"; Macnamara, 1982; Markman, 1989), are more likely constructed by the child through social interactions within a language-rich community (Bruner, 1983; Golinkoff et al., 1994), or are actually not necessary (e.g., Nelson, 1988). We see the framework as a helpful descriptive framework even if one believes that the principles are unnecessary or metaphors for describing behavior (as a behavior analyst might). Finally, the framework permits us to identify specific ways in which empirical evidence from behavior analysis and mental retardation research can contribute to ongoing discussions about word learning.

Although this chapter identifies points of convergence within each of the six proposed principles, readers will note that some of these convergences are treated in greater detail than others. The discussion of the N3C (novel name–nameless category) principle includes an in-depth analysis of both the theoretical and the empirical convergences across the disciplines. In contrast, the discussion of conventionality limits itself to identifying several points that might warrant future discussion. This asymmetric treatment reflects the relative novelty of the interdisciplinary effort and the inherent challenges of bridging two theoretically distinct programs. For instance, the extensive treatment of N3C reflects the existence of an active interdisciplinary effort that has resulted in a detailed theoretical overview of this particular topic (Wilkinson, Dube, & McIlvane, 1996). Our intention in this chapter is to extend such interdisciplinary discussion to the other five areas of analysis by offering ideas and avenues for discussion and research. By identifying where convergences might occur, we hope to reduce obstacles introduced by terminological differences, thereby stimulating discussion within and across both disciplines.

## TIER 1: EARLIER-DEVELOPING PRINCIPLES

### Reference

The first principle in the lexical principles framework, *reference,* states that "words map to objects, actions, and attributes" (Golinkoff et al., 1994, p. 130). As Golinkoff and colleagues noted, this principle "is the first and most fundamental insight children must attain . . . while children must learn exactly which words people use to refer to which objects or events, they first must know *that* people use words to refer" (p. 130). Ultimately, children move from the general concept of reference (i.e., that symbol-based referential relations can and do exist) to the subsequent sorting of which specific symbol relates to which specific referent.

Because the principle of reference specifically concerns word learning (compared with nonsymbolic forms of referencing objects or events, such as pointing), it involves symbolic or linguistic relations that are arbitrary, that is, they do not depend on shared physical characteristics. With respect to the establishment of such symbolic relations, psycholinguists have persuasively demonstrated that most children begin to learn word meanings through participation in social event routines. (Whether this phenomenon involves or requires an "innate" characteristic is still debated; see Golinkoff et al., 1994; Macnamara, 1982; Nelson, 1988.) Such routines permit learners to predict upcoming events and their associated word forms; conventionalize prelinguistic communications into words; and show decontextualized word use outside of the initial context of acquisition, with different partners, across multiple exemplars, and for referents that are distant in either time or space (Bruner, 1983; Nelson, 1986). The grounding of word learning within the systems of its natural occurrence has been critical to understanding the role of preverbal behaviors, such as turn taking (Bruner, 1983); imitation (Clark, 1977; Corrigan, 1980; Snow, 1981); and joint attention (Dunham, Dunham, & Curwin, 1993; Tomasello, 1988).

Despite our increased understanding of the systemic bases of reference, Golinkoff and colleagues (1994) succinctly restated two fundamental, yet unanswered, problems: 1) distinguishing true linguistic relations (also termed referential or symbolic) from arbitrary paired associate relations, and 2) "figuring out how the form gets 'hooked up' with the meaning" (p. 131). Several components of research in behavior analysis may provide some avenues for approaching these two issues.

***Distinguishing Reference from Paired Associate Learning: Stimulus Control and Equivalence*** Although the distinction between the limited paired associate and the flexible referential symbol has received extensive treatment in philosophical (Gauker, 1990), psycholinguistic (Bates, 1979; Macnamara, 1982), and comparative language literatures (Savage-Rumbaugh,

1986; Terrace, 1985), a clear framework for organizing and defining operational differences has remained elusive (Golinkoff et al., 1994). From the perspective of many psycholinguists, the test for referential symbol use is decontextualized word use (e.g., Bates, 1979). Decontextualization is evident in the following example: A young child visits the zoo with her babysitter and hears the names of several exotic animals. When her grandmother later asks her what she saw there, she says, "A zebra" and proceeds to describe "a horse with stripes." The use of "zebra" is decontextualized insofar as its referent is absent and the context is dissimilar to that in which the original learning occurred. When decontextualized word use is routine, reference is inferred.

A problem with this conceptualization, however, is encountered if decontextualized word use is observed sometimes but not always. Perhaps this problem has gone unresolved because typically developing children rarely show context-bound word use beyond the beginning stages of word learning (Bates, 1979; Dromi, 1987; Mervis & Bertrand, 1993a). The distinction assumes considerable importance, however, for children who do not learn language readily. For example, difficulties experienced in teaching fully developed functional language skills to nonverbal humans and nonhumans emphasize the need to distinguish referential symbols from less flexible paired associates (see Terrace, 1985, for a discussion of this issue).

Despite many impressive successes (e.g., Lovaas, 1977), early behaviorally oriented language instruction work attracted considerable criticism; detractors argued that children were merely taught arbitrary responses to stimuli that lacked referential character (Terrace, 1985). With the benefit of hindsight, such limitations of language instruction efforts seem partly attributable to unsophisticated strategies. Certain widely used language instruction methods, for example, were straightforward adaptations of the reinforcement procedures that had taught nonverbal behavior to rats, pigeons, and monkeys. However, more recent research (in the 1990s) in the area of stimulus control has led to a broader empirical and conceptual framework that is less prone to criticism of this sort. Specifically, behavior analysts have come to differentiate between mere *if. . . then* relations and the flexible relations that provide a basis for emergent or generative behavior (Mackay & Sidman, 1984; Sidman & Tailby, 1982). This framework and its emerging database may prove useful to operationalization of the processes underlying the principle of reference.

Within the area of stimulus control, Sidman's (1993) ***equivalence paradigm*** has most clearly articulated the distinction between paired associate and referential relations. Sidman differentiated between a mere *conditional* relation and an *equivalence* relation. A conditional relation is a restricted if . . . then relation that exists solely between one specific stimulus and another. In an equivalence relation, however, a stimulus (e.g., a word or other symbol) stands in the place of, or is equivalent to, its referent and other related stimuli. (See Sidman & Tailby, 1982, for a technical definition of stimulus equivalence and Sidman, 1993, for a general introduction to equivalence research and its applications.) The key difference between the two rests on the generativity of the relations. To illustrate the critical difference, consider three "sets" of stimuli: spoken words, everyday objects, and arbitrary depictions of everyday objects (icons or written words). In behavior analysis, common notation is to assign letters to represent each set of stimuli: thus, spoken words might be considered set A; objects might be set B; and icons, set C. Suppose the child learns that the word "cookie," when uttered by her mother, is usually followed by her mother offering the appropriate sweet snack. This learning would reflect what might be called a conditional AB relation between the word "cookie" (set A) and the relevant item (set B). Independently, the child learns that the snack items can be retrieved from a jar labeled with the written word *cookie* (as opposed to the one labeled *flour*). This second relation would be called a conditional CB relation, between the written word (set C) and the cookie found inside (set B). Alone, each of these relations is a simple nongenerative conditional relation. Equivalence relations would be demonstrated if, without instruction, the child showed the emergent ability to produce the spoken name to obtain the item (BA relations), to find the cookie jar when asked to put a cookie away (BC relations), and, most important, to match the spoken word "cookie" with the written depiction *cookie*, even in the absence of the treats themselves (CA and AC relations). If these BA, BC, CA, and AC relations emerge without explicit instruction, the stimuli A, B, and C (the word, object, and written depiction) are said to constitute an *equivalence class*. The emergent relations show that A, B, and C are not mere paired associates, but rather bear generative symbolic relations to each other ("one stimulus has acquired the same meaning as another" [McIlvane, Dube, Green, & Serna, 1993, p. 266]).

The validity of this conceptual distinction has received empirical support through evidence of the distinction between humans' symbol comprehension and pigeons' remarkably sophisticated key-pecking performances (see Epstein, Lanza, & Skinner, 1980). The remarkable and well-documented capability of pigeons and other nonhumans to learn multiple, perhaps thousands of, conditional discriminations has been likened by some researchers to human verbal behavior (e.g., Epstein et al., 1980). Although other researchers have taken issue with this comparison (Savage-Rumbaugh, 1984; Terrace, 1985), it remains a challenge for them to operationalize precisely what constitutes the fundamental differences. However, the conceptual distinction between conditional and equivalence relations appears to provide one avenue for such an effort: Equivalence research has suggested that only humans, and possibly some symbol-using nonhumans (e.g., sea lions [Schusterman & Kastak, 1993]), show the emergent generative relations of equivalence (Sidman et al., 1982). Perhaps this distinction, derived from the program that originally raised questions of the continuity of behavior, may provide a framework for an operational definition that explicitly and empirically incorporates the generative features of referential symbols.

***Establishing Relations Between Word Forms and Their Referents*** The second unresolved issue raised by Golinkoff and colleagues (1994) concerning reference is how the form gets "hooked up" with the meaning. Typically developing children appear to identify salient features of their environment labeled by words with little trouble, and their occasional errors do not interfere with language acquisition. Bruner (1974/1975, 1983) and others (e.g., Nelson, 1986; Trevarthen, 1980) have discussed how symbol learning may be presaged and aided by social routines. Certain children with disabilities, however, do not learn words even after exposure to such routines. Why do these children, many of whom demonstrate prelinguistic forms of reference (McLean, McLean, Brady, & Etter, 1991), fail to benefit from apparently appropriate social environments?

One exploration of this relational process in word learning is the analysis of breakdowns. For example, Rincover and Koegel's (1975) study of generalization by children with autism illustrates how stimulus control analysis can elucidate issues in development. In this study, 10 children were taught simple motor responses to verbal cues in one setting. When transfer to a different setting was tested, six children responded appropriately to the cues, but four did not show generalization. For these four children, stimulus control analyses revealed that control by the cues depended on incidental aspects of the original teaching setting. When these incidental stimuli were also included in the new setting, generalization was observed.

Rincover and Koegel's (1975) study concerned generalization of explicitly taught conditional (nonreferential) relations. The outcomes, though, highlight a critical issue: Acquisition and generalization could and did occur for all children. The stimuli that came to control responding, however, were not always the ones intended by the teachers (see Schreibman & Koegel, 1982; Schreibman & Lovaas, 1973; and our discussion of object scope on p. 34). Similar findings have also been reported with young children (Eimas, 1969). These data demonstrate that the learning of conditional relations can and does deviate from expectations, even in very highly structured situations. Given that conditional relations may provide the foundation for emergent equivalence (referential) relations, the deviations in their acquisition suggest that new words will not always be hooked up with the correct referents. In fact, the occurrence of such atypical stimulus control highlights the importance of Quine's (1960) often-cited dilemma concerning children's ability to discriminate between the multiple referential possibilities inherent in any word-learning event. (See our discussion of object scope on p. 34 for elaboration of Quine's dilemma.)

These observations of highly restricted stimulus control in both typically and atypically developing children lead one to ask about the determinants (i.e., the stimulus control) of children's decontextualized word use. The literature on behavior analysis addresses this in two ways. The first is in its analysis of primary stimulus generalization, that is, the observation that behavior learned under one set of circumstances may also be exhibited in situations that are similar but not identical to the original conditions of learning (Stokes & Baer, 1977). However, mere transfer of training does not capture fully the essence of decontextualization. Therefore, a second broader concept of transfer of stimulus functions seems necessary. The child must use the symbol in a manner that is consistent with a referential function. The topic of primary stimulus generalization is germane to the principle of extendability, and the topic of transfer of stimulus functions relates to the second-tier principles of categorical scope and conventionality (addressed later in this chapter).

### Extendability

The process of decontextualization has often been the hallmark for inferring referential symbol use. Although children may initially learn by rote to extend a word, ultimately the generativity of referential symbol use requires that a more general strategy (principle) be operative. The most basic of those principles proposed by Golinkoff and colleagues (1994) is *extendability*, which states that children learn that "a word can be used to label referents other than exemplars which someone else has previously labeled" (p. 134). Potential bases for extension include, but are not limited to, shape, sound, thematic relation, or a shared attribute or feature (Golinkoff et al., 1994; these are termed "situational bases" for extension by Mervis & Bertrand, 1993a). This principle is "an important insight into the ways words work: they do not label unique referents" (Golinkoff et al., 1994, p. 134). Although at this level there is no restriction on the possible bases for extension, extension appears to depend primarily on some perceived similarity between exemplars, compared to potentially more abstract category-based relations (see the section on categorical scope in Tier 2). The evidence that children do indeed extend new words to previously unlabeled referents, most often based on shape, is extensive (reviewed by Golinkoff et al., 1994).

***Stimulus Classes and Extendability*** The observation that children almost immediately extend new labels to new exemplars is paralleled by the observation in behavior analysis that "discrimination training typically establishes control by stimulus classes rather than merely by specific stimuli" (McIlvane et al., 1993, p. 245; see also Fields, Reeve, Adams, & Verhave, 1991). Stimulus classes are groups of stimuli that, due to some similarity (physical or functional) among the members of the class, serve as functionally equivalent. In psycholinguistic terms, the category "food" may function as a coherent stimulus class partly on the basis that all foods are (or could be) edible. In their psycholinguistic studies of children's acquisition of categories, Mervis and Bertrand (1993a) discussed how children's classifications may shift as they learn more about the bases for adult categories. For example, Mervis and Bertrand noted that a child may label a round piggy bank a "ball," focusing on shape and ignoring the slot hole for coins, until he learns that it is not throwable. This example (among others) illustrates two aspects of what behavior analysts call stimulus classes: 1) Stimulus class membership can be contextually influenced (i.e., influenced both by feature as well as functional characteristics), and 2) stimulus class membership may be subject to revision.

***Stimulus Generalization and Extendability*** Stimulus classes based on feature similarities may be most relevant to our analysis of the principle of extension. Within behavior analysis (and experimental psychology in general), there is an extensive literature on how stimulus similarity may determine performance, especially with nonhuman subjects (e.g., Guttman & Kalish, 1956). Studies that seem most relevant to language development are those that have examined the performance of typically developing young children. These studies have found that children often (but not always) generalize on the basis of shape similarity (Stoddard & McIlvane, 1989), which is consistent with the developmental research.

Perhaps the clearest example of methodologies for examining how physical feature similarity interacts with other processes to determine performance was contributed by Fields and colleagues (1991). They studied a population of convenience (college students) to evaluate whether perceptual variants of exemplars already established within specific equivalence classes would also be spontaneously incorporated into the equivalence class. The perceptual variants were derived from the original exemplars and retained varying levels of feature/perceptual similarity as the original. As expected, and consistent with extendability, novel variants that showed high similarity to the original exemplar were more likely to be incorporated immediately (without instruction) into the equivalence class than variants with fewer physical similarities. What is still unclear, and is most relevant to language, are the most salient physical bases on which extension occurs. The equivalence framework and its related methods, however, provide a means of exploring the separate and combined effects of different possible bases for extension.

## Object Scope

The third and final principle in the first tier is *object scope*, which has two components: "First . . . words label objects. Second . . . words refer to the whole object as opposed to its parts or attributes" (Golinkoff et al., 1994, p. 136). This principle begins to address Quine's (1960) dilemma, which asks how a language learner can decipher a word's meaning given the multiple logical possibilities. For example, picture a mother and her child in a park. The mother points to an animal sitting at the edge of a pond nibbling on clover and says "bunny." There is no logical basis for assuming that the word refers to the whole animal and not to its ear or whiskers, to "animal-on-water's-edge," to "animal-nibbling-clover" (or to the clover, for that matter), or so on. Object scope proposes a heuristic that may guide children in this task. The critical importance of object scope in word learning receives support not only from behavior analysis but also from related research in experimental psychology.

***Typical Development: Compound versus Component Responding*** An extensive literature describes children's learning about stimuli with multiple components. The research has found that typically developing young children tend to treat multicomponent stimuli as compounds (i.e., integrated wholes) rather than as stimuli composed of separable features and dimensions (House, 1989; Shepp, Barrett, & Kolbet, 1987; Tighe & Tighe, 1978; Zeaman & House, 1974). Young children's bias (for whatever reason) to respond to wholes instead of components or features seems consonant with the principle of object scope. Notably, children's tendencies to respond to compounds are most pronounced during the same period in which they are learning their first words. It would seem reasonable, therefore, that this bias would also be expressed in their word learning.

***Stimulus Overselectivity and Object Scope*** Clinical behavior analysts have reported a phenomenon termed *stimulus overselectivity* (Lovaas, Schreibman, Koegel, & Rehm, 1971) that appears to be the opposite of the "wholism" described above. Individuals who are overselective apparently focus on a single aspect of a stimulus, seemingly ignoring other potentially important features (including that of compound "wholeness"). In a dramatic example, one overselective child with autism recognized his father only when the father wore eyeglasses (Schreibman & Koegel, 1982). Many studies have reported examples of overselectivity in laboratory as well as education settings (Burke, 1991; Koegel & Rincover, 1974; Lovaas et al., 1971; Rincover, 1978; Stromer, McIlvane, Dube, & Mackay, 1993). Although overselectivity is frequently associated with autism, it is also reported with children with mental retardation who are not autistic (Wilhelm & Lovaas, 1976) and for typically developing young children (Eimas, 1969).

The relevance of overselectivity for the principle of object scope should not be underestimated (cf. Burke, 1991). Recall that appropriate stimulus control in learning conditional relations may be critical to the processes of reference. Similarly, the ability to detect the compound aspects of a stimulus is critical for developing and applying object scope. A language learner who focuses only on the specific features of a particular rabbit's ear when hearing the word "bunny" will have difficulty learning more sophisticated language. He or she would fail to generate appropriate classes because such classes require broader observations. As with reference, therefore, the existence of disruptions of object scope provides an opportunity to explore processes that are at the root of this principle.

## TIER 2: LATER-DEVELOPING PRINCIPLES

### Categorical Scope

The principle of *categorical scope* states that "the extension of novel object words occurs mainly on the basis of basic level category membership" (Golinkoff et al., 1994, p. 139) and serves to further constrain the basis for extension. Basic-level category membership has been widely discussed and debated (e.g., Lakoff, 1987; Rosch, Mervis, Gray, Johnson, & Boyes-Braem, 1976). Based on a review of several authors, including Rosch et al. (1976), Lakoff (1987) described the basic level as the "level at which categorization is determined by overall gestalt perception (without distinctive feature analysis)" (p. 46), a determination based on similarities such as overall shape or the types of motor actions typically associated with category members, as well as usage patterns such as rate of identification of category members, common usage of category labels, or short word length for category labels (i.e., "dog," "tree"). For our purposes, categorical scope has important corollaries. The principle refines the bases for extension in two ways: First, it emphasizes extension that does not necessarily require perceptual or situational similarities among exemplars, and second, it permits emergent relations between perceptually distinct exemplars as they enter into category membership.

***Equivalence Within and Among Category Members*** Earlier we argued that the equivalence paradigm provides a means to distinguish between mere paired associates and true referential relations. The equivalence paradigm also provides a means for evaluating how nonperceptually based categories evolve and how new members can be integrated into extant categories. In this area, the emergent relations described in reference are also critical for analyzing processes of category learning and expansion. A new referent entering into an equivalence relation with one class member should enter into equivalence relations with all members without further instruction. For example, consider the English-language class *dog* and the higher-order class *animal.* All exemplars of dogs are substitutable for each other in the context of animal (e.g., a poodle is an animal, a retriever is an animal). By virtue of learning that a new referent, Lhasa apso, is a dog, that creature will also be classified as an animal via the established equivalence relations.

As Sidman (1993) pointed out, equivalence classes are defined by context. Although all exemplars of dog are equivalent in the context of animal, clearly they are not in other contexts, for example, size (Pekinese versus Saint Bernard) or likely suitability as attack dog (Doberman versus Cocker Spaniel). Additionally, not all relations are equivalence relations (Sidman, 1993). In some contexts, for example, dogs and animals can be in an equivalence class (e.g., with respect to being animate, as compared to furniture). In other contexts, however, the relation between the class *dogs* and the class *animals* is not necessarily one of equivalence. Rather, the relationship is hierarchical; all dogs are animals but not all animals are dogs.

It is also important to understand that the equivalence analysis does not imply that the members of a given class cannot be distinguished from one another. Although within-class items may be functionally or otherwise substitutable for one another, the items are not necessarily the same as each other. In the example of the class containing the spoken word "cookie," the written counterpart *cookie*, and the relevant treat, the theory does not assume that a child might mistake the written word *cookie* for the treat and misguidedly try to eat it. One example of within-class discriminations derives from the so-called nodal distance phenomenon (Fields, Adams, Verhave, & Newman, 1990). To demonstrate the nodal distance effect experimentally, one might first take five different stimuli, notated here as A, B, C, D, and E. Training could then establish matching-to-sample relations AB (A goes with B), BC, CD, and DE, with a resulting five-member equivalence class, A→B→C→D→E (the arrows indicate the points of connection during teaching and thus suggest a "distance" relationship). Next, one might present test trials that, for example, present A as the sample and C and E as the comparison stimuli. Because both comparison stimuli (C and E) are members of the same class, an equivalence analysis does not predict a consistent preference of one over the other. In empirical studies, however, it has been shown that subjects tend to prefer C, perhaps because C and A are closer in the teaching sequence than E and A. Whatever its basis, the nodal distance effect demonstrates discrimination in one context of stimuli that are equivalent in others.

To summarize, the equivalence framework provides the means to explore two aspects of language: 1) generative referential relations, and 2) category formation and expansion. The next section presents two instances in which the equivalence work with individuals with mental retardation relates to broader issues in category learning.

***Bases for Category Formation: Language and Cognition*** One longstanding debate in psycholinguistics concerns the relation between linguistic categories and cognitive categories (e.g., Bowerman, 1989). Some researchers (Clark, 1973, 1977; Cromer, 1974; Rosch & Mervis, 1977) proposed that most early language categories map onto extant cognitive categories. Others (Schlesinger, 1982) argued a modified version of the perspective often associated with Whorf (1956), which suggests that at least some of our cognitive categories derive from the structures of our language. A third position, termed the *interaction perspective* (Bowerman, 1976, 1989; Cromer, 1988; Rice &

Kemper, 1984), states that both directions of influence are possible; cognition drives language, and language in turn acts as a "lure" to cognition (Bowerman, 1976).

Notably, this debate has parallels in the stimulus equivalence literature. Some researchers have argued that equivalence classes may provide the basis for linguistic categories (McIlvane, 1992; Sidman, 1993), while others have suggested that acquired linguistic "frames" provide children with the prerequisites for equivalence (Dugdale & Lowe, 1990; Hayes, 1991). Evidence from nonspeaking individuals with severe mental retardation may help to answer questions in both disciplines. For example, our research group has observed formation of equivalence classes even in individuals with severe cognitive impairments and very limited receptive or expressive language skills (Dube, McIlvane, Mackay, & Stoddard, 1987). Furthermore, formation of equivalence classes can be observed even when the classes contain only visual stimuli, suggesting that mediation by names is not necessary for class formation (Sidman, Willson-Morris, & Kirk, 1986; Stromer & Osborne, 1982). Taken together, these findings suggest that category formation can occur without the direct involvement of language.

***Words as Unique Auditory Stimuli in Category Formation*** Golinkoff and colleagues (1994) speculated that if the principle of reference is operative, words should serve as unique auditory stimuli in learning "because if words bear a 'stands for' rather than a 'goes with' relationship to referents, they should make referents more distinct and promote categorical thinking" (p. 133). However, as they pointed out, the data are inconclusive. Granting that the equivalence paradigm permits study of "stands for" relations and category formation, there is some evidence that including a word within an equivalence class facilitates formation and long-term retention of the class (Green, 1990; G. Green, personal communication, July, 1994; Sidman et al., 1986; Spradlin, Saunders, & Saunders, 1992). These studies compared equivalence class formation by subjects with mental retardation under two conditions: 1) All three members of the class were visual stimuli, and 2) two members were visual stimuli and one was a dictated word. The studies showed a reliable advantage in equivalence class formation when the class included a word. This finding may provide indirect support that a word can promote categorical thinking.

***Summary: Implications of Equivalence for Category Formation*** To summarize, two likely possibilities emerge: 1) Names are not necessary for equivalence class formation, and 2) words may promote acquisition and retention of classes. Together, these findings seem consistent with the interaction perspective in psycholinguistics. That is, although words may not be a prerequisite for category formation, they do appear to serve as a lure that facilitates the development and retention of categories. This analysis illustrates the utility of the equivalence paradigm and the research on processes in mental retardation for theories of the development of intellectual functioning.

### Novel Name–Nameless Category

N3C is one of several mechanisms that have been proposed (Clark, 1983; Golinkoff, Hirsh-Pasek, Bailey, & Wenger, 1992; Golinkoff et al., 1994; Markman, 1989) to account for the observed phenomenon of fast mapping (Carey & Bartlett, 1978; Mervis & Bertrand, 1993a). Through fast mapping, children learn new word–referent relations without explicit instruction. For example, suppose a child has several toys and has learned labels for all but one. If a communication partner speaks a novel word, the child may assume that word refers to the unlabeled toy. This assumption is made routinely by typically developing children in the second (or early third) year of life (e.g., Merriman, 1991; Merriman & Bowman, 1989; Mervis & Bertrand, 1993a; Woodward & Markman, 1991).

To account for the fast-mapping phenomenon, Golinkoff and colleagues (1994) argued that "novel terms map to previously unnamed objects" (p. 143). This N3C principle proposes that hearing a new word sets the occasion for children to search for a novel object (category) referent. N3C states, therefore, that the basis for mapping is a shared feature of novelty (or "undefined-ness") between the word and the referent. (See Golinkoff et al., 1994, for further discussion.)

N3C has frequently been contrasted with ME (mutual exclusivity) (Markman, 1989), which proposes that a child assumes that a single referent cannot have more than one name. ME predicts that children reject a named object as the referent for a new label and assign the new label to an available unnamed object. Differentiating the ME and N3C proposals is difficult empirically, as Golinkoff et al. (1992) discussed. Behavior-analytic studies of children with mental retardation can potentially contribute methods for exploring the distinctions.

***The Exclusion Phenomenon: Distinguishing N3C and ME*** Fast-mapping research has methodological and theoretical links with behavior-analytic research on exclusion (Dixon, 1977; McIlvane & Stoddard, 1981, 1985). Perhaps as a consequence, this area has received ample cross-disciplinary attention (Huntley & Ghezzi, 1993; McIlvane, Kledaras, Lowry, & Stoddard, 1992; Wilkinson & McIlvane, 1994; Wilkinson et al., 1996). Analyses of convergences in research questions, research methods, and behavioral outcomes suggest that both programs are evaluating the same learning process(es) (see Wilkinson & McIlvane, 1994; Wilkinson et al., 1996). One notable convergence concerns the distinctions between N3C (mapping based on selecting unnamed referents) and ME (mapping based on rejecting named referents).

Parallel to the N3C and ME distinction, behavior analysis has identified two possible bases for mapping. One basis, termed *S+ control*, proposes that selection is based on a relation involving the sample word and the S+ (correct) comparison. In psycholinguistic terms, the child selects unnamed "correct" comparisons when presented with new words because both are novel (or undefined; see McIlvane et al., 1987; McIlvane et al., 1992) in the mapping context. Thus, both N3C and S+ control suggest that mapping occurs without a "process of elimination" (e.g., Dixon, Dixon, & Spradlin, 1983; Mervis & Bertrand, 1993a,b).

The alternative basis, termed *S−control* (McIlvane, Munson, & Stoddard, 1988; McIlvane et al., 1992; Stromer & Osborne, 1982), proposes that selection is based on a relation involving the sample and the incorrect (S−) items. In psycholinguistic terms, the child rejects previously named comparisons in the presence of the novel word and thereby selects the "correct" unnamed one. Thus, both ME and S− control suggest that mapping occurs via a process of elimination.

Research has begun to explore ways to differentiate empirically between S+ and S− control. One method uses what has been termed a *blank comparison* procedure (see McIlvane et al., 1987, for a procedure description and McIlvane et al., 1992, for an example of use). This procedure enables the subject to respond *neither* or *none of the above* when presented with a word and several pictures. Via a programmed teaching method (see McIlvane et al., 1987, 1992), subjects are taught to touch a blank comparison key (a gray square) when none of the available choices appears correct. For example, the *neither* key would be appropriate when the choices are pictures of a tree and a house and the sample word is *dog*. When the subject responds reliably to several different trials of this type (i.e., baseline trials), the procedure can be used to evaluate selection in various mapping probes.

The blank comparison procedure was used in a study of mapping by three individuals with severe mental retardation (McIlvane et al., 1992). The subjects readily learned to select the *neither* option when appropriate on baseline trials. Then, four types of test trials were presented (see Figure 1). CONTROL trials presented a known word with its corresponding picture, a novel picture, and the *neither* option. All subjects selected the known picture in these trials. TEST-1 trials presented a novel name with an unnamed picture, a named picture, and the *neither* option. All three subjects selected the unnamed picture reliably, two immediately and one after some initial variability. TEST-2 trials presented a novel name with two defined pictures and the *neither* option. All three subjects selected *neither,* again two immediately and one after initial variability. The TEST-3 trials presented subjects with a novel name, two novel pictures, and the *neither* option. The subjects tended to select the novel pictures.

Taken together, these data suggest that both sample/S+ and sample/S− control may be operative in subjects with severe mental retardation. The TEST-1 trial findings appeared to indicate S+ control; if subjects were merely rejecting the known comparison, then they would have no reason to favor the unnamed picture over the *neither* option (unless, of course, the selection of a form over a blank key is a preferred response whenever possible). TEST-2 trials demonstrated that subjects can and will reject known pictures in the pres-

CONTROL trials

Sample | Comparison Array

"dog"

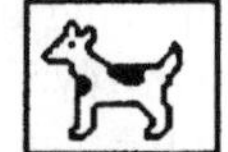
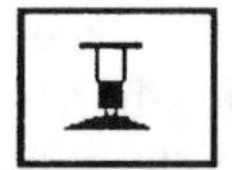
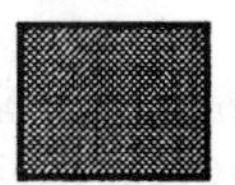

TEST-1 trials

Sample | Comparison Array

"pafe"

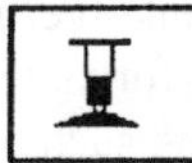
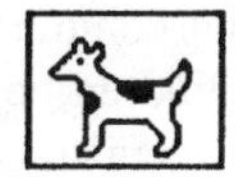
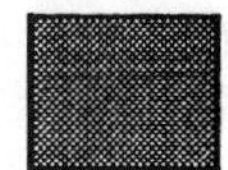

TEST-2 trials

Sample | Comparison Array

"kice"

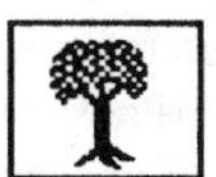
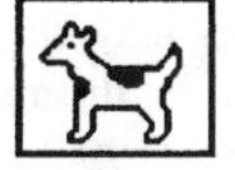
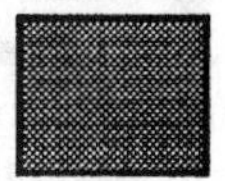

TEST-3 trials

Sample | Comparison Array

"shede"

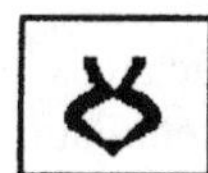
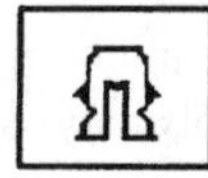
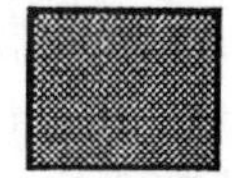

Figure 1. Blank comparison trial types.

ence of a novel word. Thus, *neither* is an option that subjects will take when appropriate. TEST-3 trials suggested that subjects indeed preferred to select a form over the *neither* key when a novel word was the sample. In psycholinguistic terms, they may be biased to assume that a new word should have a new referent (S+ control/N3C).

Although this methodology is still being developed, it does suggest a means for describing the basic processes involved in establishing fast maps between novel names and referents. Use of the blank comparison procedure converts the experimental methodology from a forced choice to one where subjects can reject other choices in favor of *neither.* Further refinement of these methods should permit exploration in more detail of the processes involved in fast mapping.

### Conventionality

The last principle, *conventionality,* is derived from Clark (1983) and states that "speakers expect certain meanings to be expressed by conventional forms within their language community" (Golinkoff et al., 1994, p. 148). On the basis of this principle, children begin to use forms that are conventionally understood in the larger linguistic community; such use often requires them to replace or preempt idiosyncratic phonetic forms. As Golinkoff and colleagues (1994) noted, "without this principle, once children had filled a lexical gap, there would be no reason for them ever to adjust their solution in the direction of the adult model" (p. 149).

A critical aspect of this principle is that children are able to add to or replace idiosyncratic forms as they adopt more conventional ones. The equivalence paradigm also may provide insight into the process(es) underlying conventionality. Via formation of equivalence relations, both idiosyncratic and conventional forms may share the same referent, with productive use determined by context (i.e., the audience). This possibility is exemplified by Golinkoff and colleagues' (1994) description of one child who used an idiosyncratic label for "pacifier" with family members and the conventional label with other listeners. The equivalence paradigm explicitly acknowledges that a single relation can be influenced by the context within which it is considered. This approach therefore allows for an analysis of changeability both within children's basic categorical structures (categorical scope) as well as within their expression of these structures (conventionality).

## CONCLUSION

This chapter has illustrated several specific areas in which research and theory from stimulus control analysis in mental retardation may contribute to theories of normal language acquisition. For instance, we argued that the equivalence paradigm may provide a means of approaching three of the operating principles within the lexical principles framework. We illustrated how the operational definition of equivalence relations, compared to mere conditional relations, might be one means for approaching the traditionally elusive distinction between paired associates and referential symbols (reference). In addition, we illustrated how the systematic analysis of emergent equivalence relations among the members of a category and among categories themselves relates to the principle of categorical scope. Finally, we raised the possibility that the emphasis on the changeability of category membership as a function of contextual control may be one means of approaching questions concerning the principle of conventionality.

In addition to these three principles, we discussed specific research from other areas of stimulus control relevant to the processes of development within the three remaining principles. Studies of equivalence class expansion were described as a means of exploring how we might analyze the bases for children's early extensions of word meanings (extendability). The implications of research on overselectivity in children, particularly those with autism, were discussed for the principle of object scope and all further lexical development. Finally, the parallels between stimulus control research on exclusion and psycholinguistic studies of fast mapping (the N3C principle) were discussed.

The analyses presented in this chapter are intended to demonstrate the potential utility of studies of stimulus control with individuals with mental retardation and other developmental disabilities for research and theory on processes of typical language development. As with psycholinguistics, research on stimulus control continues to evolve to answer increasingly sophisticated questions. For example, studies have begun to explore how generalized learning can result even from very brief (i.e., single exposure) experience (e.g., Dube, McIlvane, & Green, 1992), a topic that is relevant to the fast-mapping phenomenon. Research has also begun to develop an account of the emergence of novel behavior that cannot be traced to direct conditioning experiences (e.g., McIlvane, 1992; Sidman, 1993). We have argued that adaptations from stimulus control research could be productive for studying not only disordered but also normative lexical development. Specifically, a process-level analysis of learning can help to reveal the specific factors contributing to learning breakdowns. These breakdowns highlight the points of vulnerability and modifiability within atypical lexical development. Also highlighted are the significant milestones of lexical development, or "cusps," that all typical children must master to become fluent communicators (L. McLean, personal communication, October, 1995). The process-level analysis can therefore contribute to our understanding of normative development and the variations in development that lead to language delay or disorder.

## REFERENCES

Adamson, L.B. (1992). Variations in the early use of language. In L.T. Winegar & J. Valsiner (Eds.), *Children's development within social context* (pp. 123–141). Hillsdale, NJ: Lawrence Erlbaum Associates.

Bates, E. (1979). *The emergence of symbols: Cognition and communication in infancy.* New York: Academic Press.
Bates, E., & MacWhinney, B. (1987). Competition, variation, and language learning. In B. MacWhinney (Ed.), *Mechanisms of language development* (pp. 157–193). Hillsdale, NJ: Lawrence Erlbaum Associates.
Bowerman, M. (1976). Semantic factors in the acquisition of rules for word use and sentence construction. In D.M. Morehead & A.E. Morehead (Eds.), *Normal and deficient child language* (pp. 99–179). Baltimore: University Park Press.
Bowerman, M. (1989). Learning a semantic system: What role do cognitive predispositions play? In M.L. Rice & R.L. Schiefelbusch (Eds.), *The teachability of language* (pp. 133–169). Baltimore: Paul H. Brookes Publishing Co.
Bruner, J. (1974/1975). From communication to language: A psychological perspective. *Cognition, 3,* 255–287.
Bruner, J. (1983). *Child's talk.* New York: Norton.
Burke, J.C. (1991). Some developmental implications of a disturbance in responding to complex stimuli. *American Journal on Mental Retardation, 96,* 37–52.
Carey, S., & Bartlett, E. (1978). Acquiring a single new word. *Papers and Reports on Child Language Development, 15,* 17–29.
Clark, E.V. (1973). What's in a word? On the child's acquisition of semantics in his first language. In T.E. Moore (Ed.), *Cognitive development and the acquisition of language* (pp. 65–110). New York: Academic Press.
Clark, E.V. (1983). Meanings and concepts. In P.H. Mussen (Series Ed.), J.H. Flavell, & E.M. Markman (Vol. Eds.), *Handbook of child psychology: Vol. 3. Cognitive development* (pp. 787–840). New York: John Wiley & Sons.
Clark, R. (1977). What's the use of imitation? *Journal of Child Language, 4,* 341–358.
Corrigan, R. (1980). Use of repetition to facilitate spontaneous language acquisition. *Journal of Psycholinguistic Research, 9,* 231–241.
Cromer, R.F. (1974). The development of language and cognition: The cognition hypothesis. In B. Foss (Ed.), *New perspectives in child development* (pp. 184–252). London: Penguin Press.
Cromer, R.F. (1988). The cognition hypothesis revisited. In F. Kessel (Ed.), *The development of language and language researchers: Essays in honor of Roger Brown* (pp. 223–248). Hillsdale, NJ: Lawrence Erlbaum Associates.
Dixon, L.S. (1977). The nature of control by spoken words over visual stimulus selection. *Journal of the Experimental Analysis of Behavior, 27,* 433–442.
Dixon, M.H., Dixon, L.S., & Spradlin, J.E. (1983). Analysis of individual differences of stimulus control among developmentally disabled children. In K.D. Gadow & I. Bialer (Eds.), *Advances in learning and behavioral disabilities* (Vol. 2, pp. 85–100). Greenwich, CT: JAI Press.
Dromi, E. (1987). *Early lexical development.* New York: Cambridge University Press.
Dube, W.V., McIlvane, W.J., & Green, G. (1992). An analysis of generalized identity matching test procedures. *The Psychological Record, 42,* 17–28.
Dube, W.V., McIlvane, W.J., Mackay, H.A., & Stoddard, L.T. (1987). Stimulus class membership established via stimulus–reinforcer relations. *Journal of the Experimental Analysis of Behavior, 47,* 159–175.
Dugdale, N., & Lowe, C.F. (1990). Naming and stimulus equivalence. In D.E. Blackman & H. Lejeune (Eds.), *Behavior analysis in theory and practice: Contributions and controversies* (pp. 115–138). Hillsdale, NJ: Lawrence Erlbaum Associates.
Dunham, P.J., Dunham, F., & Curwin, A. (1993). Joint-attentional states and lexical acquisition at 18 months. *Developmental Psychology, 29,* 827–831.
Eimas, P.D. (1969). Multiple-cue discrimination learning in children. *The Psychological Record, 19,* 417–424.

Epstein, R., Lanza, R.P., & Skinner, B.F. (1980). Symbolic communication between two pigeons (*Columba livia domestica*). *Science, 207*, 543–545.

Fields, L., Adams, B.J., Verhave, T., & Newman, S. (1990). The effects of nodality on the formation of equivalence classes. *Journal of the Experimental Analysis of Behavior, 53*, 345–358.

Fields, L., Reeve, K.F., Adams, B.J., & Verhave, T. (1991). Stimulus generalization and equivalence classes: A model for natural categories. *Journal of the Experimental Analysis of Behavior, 55*, 305–312.

Gauker, C. (1990). How to learn language like a chimpanzee. *Philosophical Psychology, 3*, 31–53.

Golinkoff, R.M., Hirsh-Pasek, K., Bailey, L.M., & Wenger, N.R. (1992). Young children and adults use lexical principles to learn new nouns. *Development Psychology, 28*, 99–108.

Golinkoff, R.M., Mervis, C.B., & Hirsh-Pasek, K. (1994). Early object labels: The case for a developmental lexical principles framework. *Journal of Child Language, 21*, 125–155.

Green, G. (1990). Differences in development of visual and auditory-visual equivalence relations. *American Journal on Mental Retardation, 95*, 260–270.

Guttman, N., & Kalish, H.I. (1956). Discriminability and stimulus generalization. *Journal of Experimental Psychology, 51*, 79–88.

Hayes, S.C. (1991). A relational control theory of stimulus equivalence. In L.J. Hayes & P.N. Chase (Eds.), *Dialogues on verbal behavior* (pp. 19–40). Reno, NV: Context Press.

House, B.J. (1989). Some current issues in children's selective attention. In H.W. Reese (Ed.), *Advances in child development and behavior* (pp. 91–120). New York: Academic Press.

Huntley, K.R., & Ghezzi, P.M. (1993). Mutual exclusivity and exclusion: Converging evidence from two contrasting traditions. *The Analysis of Verbal Behavior, 11*, 63–76.

Kessel, F. (Ed.). (1988). *The development of language and language researchers: Essays in honor of Roger Brown*. Hillsdale, NJ: Lawrence Erlbaum Associates.

Koegel, R.L., & Rincover, A. (1974). Treatment of psychotic children in a classroom environment (I): Learning in a large group. *Journal of Applied Behavior Analysis, 7*, 45–59.

Lakoff, G. (1987). *Women, fire, and dangerous things: What categories reveal about the mind*. Chicago: University of Chicago Press.

Lipkens, R., Hayes, S.C., & Hayes, L.J. (1993). Longitudinal study of the development of derived relations in an infant. *Journal of Experimental Child Psychology, 56*, 201–239.

Lovaas, O.I. (1977). *The autistic child: Language development through behavior modification*. New York: Irvington.

Lovaas, O.I., Schreibman, L., Koegel, R.L., & Rehm, R. (1971). Selective responding by autistic children to multiple sensory input. *Journal of Abnormal Psychology, 77*, 211–222.

MacDonald, R.P.F., Dixon, L.S., & LeBlanc, J.M. (1986). Stimulus class formation following observational learning. *Analysis and Intervention in Developmental Disabilities, 6*, 73–87.

Mackay, H.A., & Sidman, M. (1984). Teaching new behavior via equivalence relations. In P.H. Brooks, R. Sperber, & C. MacCauley (Eds.), *Learning and cognition in the mentally retarded* (pp. 493–513). Hillsdale, NJ: Lawrence Erlbaum Associates.

Macnamara, J. (1982). *Names for things*. Cambridge: MIT Press.

Markman, E.M. (1989). *Categorization and naming in children*. Cambridge: MIT Press.

McIlvane, W.J. (1992). Stimulus control analysis and nonverbal instructional technology for people with mental handicaps. In N.R. Bray (Ed.), *International review of research in mental retardation* (Vol. 18, pp. 55–109). New York: Academic Press.
McIlvane, W.J., Dube, W.V., Green, G., & Serna, R.W. (1993). Programming conceptual and communication skill development: A methodological stimulus-class analysis. In A.P. Kaiser & D.B. Gray (Eds.), *Communication and language intervention series: Vol. 2. Enhancing children's communication: Research foundations for intervention* (pp. 243–285). Baltimore: Paul H. Brookes Publishing Co.
McIlvane, W.J., Kledaras, J.B., Lowry, M.J., & Stoddard, L.T. (1992). Studies of exclusion in individuals with severe mental retardation. *Research in Developmental Disabilities, 13*, 509–532.
McIlvane, W.J., Kledaras, J.B., Munson, L.C., King, K.A., deRose, J.C., & Stoddard, L.T. (1987). Controlling relations in conditional discrimination and matching by exclusion. *Journal of the Experimental Analysis of Behavior, 48*, 187–208.
McIlvane, W.J., Munson, L.C., & Stoddard, L.T. (1988). Some observations on control by spoken words in children's conditional discrimination and matching by exclusion. *Journal of Experimental Child Psychology, 45*, 472–495.
McIlvane, W.J., & Stoddard, L.T. (1981). Acquisition of matching-to-sample performances in severe mental retardation: Learning by exclusion. *Journal of Mental Deficiency Research, 25*, 33–48.
McIlvane, W.J., & Stoddard, L.T. (1985). Complex stimulus relations and exclusion in mental retardation. *Analysis and Intervention in Developmental Disabilities, 5*, 307–321.
McLean, J.E., McLean, L.K.S., Brady, N.C., & Etter, R. (1991). Communication profiles of two types of gesture using nonverbal persons with severe to profound mental retardation. *Journal of Speech and Hearing Research, 34*, 294–308.
Merriman, W.E. (1991). The mutual exclusivity bias in children's word learning: A reply to Woodward & Markman. *Developmental Review, 11*, 164–191.
Merriman, W.E., & Bowman, L. (1989). The mutual exclusivity bias in children's word learning (Serial No. 220). *Monographs of the Society for Research in Child Development, 54*.
Mervis, C.B., & Bertrand, J. (1993a). Acquisition of early object labels: The roles of operating principles and input. In A.P. Kaiser & D.B. Gray (Eds.), *Communication and language intervention series: Vol. 2. Enhancing children's communication: Research foundations for intervention* (pp. 287–316). Baltimore: Paul H. Brookes Publishing Co.
Mervis, C.B., & Bertrand, J. (1993b, March). *General and specific relations between early language and early cognitive development.* Paper presented at the 26th Annual Gatlinburg Conference on Research and Theory in Mental Retardation and Developmental Disabilities, Gatlinburg, TN.
Nelson, K. (1981). Individual differences in language development: Implications for development and language. *Developmental Psychology, 17*, 170–187.
Nelson, K. (1986). *Event knowledge: Structure and function in development.* Hillsdale, NJ: Lawrence Erlbaum Associates.
Nelson, K. (1988). Constraints on word learning? *Cognitive Development, 3*, 221–246.
Quine, W.V.O. (1960). *Word and object.* Cambridge, England: Cambridge University Press.
Rice, M., & Kemper, S. (1984). *Child language and cognition.* Baltimore: University Park Press.
Rincover, A. (1978). Variables affecting stimulus fading and discriminative responding in psychotic children. *Journal of Abnormal Child Psychology, 87*, 541–553.

Rincover, A., & Koegel, R.L. (1975). Setting generality and stimulus control in autistic children. *Journal of Applied Behavior Analysis, 8*, 235–246.
Rosch, E., & Mervis, C. (1977). Children's sorting: A reinterpretation based on the nature of abstraction in natural categories. In R.C. Smart & M.S. Smart (Eds.), *Readings in child development and relationships* (2nd ed., pp. 140–148). New York: Macmillan.
Rosch, E., Mervis, C., Gray, W., Johnson, D., & Boyes-Braem, P. (1976). Basic objects in natural categories. *Cognitive Psychology, 8*, 382–439.
Savage-Rumbaugh, E.S. (1984). Verbal behavior at a procedural level in the chimpanzee. *Journal of the Experimental Analysis of Behavior, 41*, 223–250.
Savage-Rumbaugh, E.S. (1986). *Ape language: From conditioned response to symbol.* New York: Columbia University Press.
Schlesinger, I.M. (1982). *Steps to language.* Hillsdale, NJ: Lawrence Erlbaum Associates.
Schreibman, L., & Koegel, O. (1982). Multiple-cue responding in autistic children. In J. Steffen & P. Karoly (Eds.), *Advances in child behavioral analysis and therapy: Vol. II. Autism and severe psychopathology* (pp. 81–89). Lexington, MA: D.C. Heath.
Schreibman, L., & Lovaas, O.I. (1973). Overselective responding to social stimuli by autistic children. *Journal of Abnormal Child Psychology, 1*, 152–168.
Schusterman, R.J., & Kastak, D. (1993). A California sea lion (*Zalophus californianus*) is capable of forming equivalence relations. *Psychological Record, 43*, 823–839.
Shepp, B.E., Barrett, S.E., & Kolbet, L.L. (1987). The development of selective attention: Holistic perception versus resource allocation. *Journal of Experimental Child Psychology, 43*, 159–180.
Sidman, M. (1979). Remarks. *Behaviorism, 5*, 123–126.
Sidman, M. (1986). Functional analysis of emergent verbal classes. In T. Thompson & M.D. Zeiler (Eds.), *Analysis and integration of behavioral units* (pp. 213–245). Hillsdale, NJ: Lawrence Erlbaum Associates.
Sidman, M. (1993). Stimulus equivalence in and out of the laboratory. In A. Brekstad & G. Svedsater (Eds.), *Proceedings from the 21st Annual Congress of the European Association for Behavior Therapy*, Oslo, Norway.
Sidman, M., Rauzin, R., Lazar, R., Cunningham, S., Tailby,W., & Carrigan, P. (1982). A search for symmetry in the conditional discrimination of rhesus monkeys, baboons, and children. *Journal of the Experimental Analysis of Behavior, 37*, 23–44.
Sidman, M., & Tailby, W. (1982). Conditional discrimination vs. matching-to-sample: An expansion of the testing paradigm. *Journal of the Experimental Analysis of Behavior, 37*, 5–22.
Sidman, M., Willson-Morris, M., & Kirk, B. (1986). Matching-to-sample procedures and the development of equivalence relations: The role of naming. *Analysis and Intervention in Developmental Disabilities, 6*, 1–19.
Skinner, B.F. (1969). *Contingencies of reinforcement: A theoretical analysis.* New York: Appleton-Century-Crofts.
Slobin, D.I. (Ed.). (1985). *The crosslinguistic study of language acquisition.* Hillsdale, NJ: Lawrence Erlbaum Associates.
Snow, C.E. (1981). The uses of imitation. *Journal of Child Language, 8*, 205–212.
Spradlin, J.E., Saunders, K.J., & Saunders, R.R. (1992). The stability of equivalence classes. In S.C. Hayes & L.J. Hayes (Eds.), *Understanding verbal relations* (pp. 29–42). Reno, NV: Context Press.
Stoddard, L.T., & McIlvane, W.J. (1989). Establishing auditory stimulus control in profoundly retarded individuals. *Research in Developmental Disabilities, 10,* 141–151.

Stokes, T., & Baer, D.M. (1977). An implicit technology of generalization. *Journal of Applied Behavior Analysis, 10*, 349–367.
Stromer, R., McIlvane, W.J., Dube, W.V., & Mackay, H.A. (1993). Assessing control by elements of complex stimuli in delayed matching to sample. *Journal of the Experimental Analysis of Behavior, 59*, 83–102.
Stromer, R., & Osborne, J.G. (1982). Control of adolescents' arbitrary matching-to-sample relations. *Journal of the Experimental Analysis of Behavior, 37*, 329–348.
Terrace, H.S. (1985). In the beginning was the "name." *American Psychologist, 40*, 1011–1028.
Tighe, T.H., & Tighe, L.S. (1978). A perceptual view of conceptual development. In R.D. Walk & H.L. Pick, Jr. (Eds.), *Perception and experience* (pp. 387–416). New York: Plenum.
Tomasello, M. (1988). The role of joint attentional processes in early language development. *Language Sciences, 10*, 69–88.
Trevarthen, C. (1980). The foundations of intersubjectivity: Development of interpersonal cooperative understanding in infants. In D. Olson (Ed.), *The social foundations of language and thought* (pp. 316–342). New York: Norton.
Whitehurst, G.J. (1978). Observational learning. In A.C. Catania & T.A. Brigham (Eds.), *Handbook of applied behavior analysis: Social and instructional processes* (pp. 142–178). New York: Irvington.
Whorf, B.L. (1956). In J.B. Carroll (Ed.), *Language, thought and reality.* Cambridge, MA: MIT Press.
Wilhelm, H., & Lovaas, O.I. (1976). Stimulus overselectivity: A common feature in autism and mental retardation. *American Journal of Mental Deficiency, 81*, 26–31.
Wilkinson, K.M., Dube, W.V., & McIlvane, W.J. (1996). A crossdisciplinary perspective on studies of rapid word mapping in psycholinguistics and behavior analysis. *Developmental Review, 16*, 125–148.
Wilkinson, K.M., & McIlvane, W.J. (1994). Stimulus organization and learning by exclusion: A preliminary experimental analysis. *Experimental Analysis of Human Behavior Bulletin, 12*, 21–25.
Woodward, A.L., & Markman, E.M. (1991). Constraints on learning as default assumptions: Comments on Merriman and Bowman's "The mutual exclusivity bias in children's word learning." *Developmental Review, 11*, 137–163.
Zeaman, D., & House, B.J. (1974). Interpretations of developmental trends in discriminative transfer effects. In A.D. Pick (Ed.), *Minnesota symposium on child psychology* (Vol. 8, pp. 144–186). Minneapolis: University of Minnesota Press.

# 3

# When *N*s Do Not Justify Means

## Small Samples and Scientific Conclusions

Roger Bakeman and Byron F. Robinson

Research in the field of language disorders has often focused on the study of relatively small samples of individuals with unique profiles of language abilities. For instance, in Chapter 4, Mervis and Bertrand examine individuals with Williams syndrome in an attempt to explicate relations between linguistic variables and other aspects of development. Williams syndrome, a genetic disorder in which individuals display unique cognitive and linguistic profiles, has an incidence of only 1 in 20,000 live births (Morris, Demsey, Leonard, Dilts, & Blackburn, 1988). Despite Herculean efforts designed to locate individuals with this rare genetic disorder, sample sizes for individual studies have often been limited to only a few subjects.

Similarly, Romski and Sevcik examined the communication of young nonspeaking individuals with mental retardation whom they provided with special computers that augmented their extant communication abilities (Romski, Sevcik, Robinson, & Bakeman, 1994; see also Chapter 8). Romski and Sevcik's research program spanned 2 years of intensive observation as the subjects gained experience with the computers. The expense of providing dedicated computers as communication devices to the subjects and the many hours of labor required to retrain teachers and parents as well as collect the data precluded the possibility of obtaining a large sample. This scenario is common in research with language disorders. Yet it is often the uniqueness of disorders and intervention strategies that simultaneously provides interesting test cases for normative theory while making research and analysis difficult and costly. Furthermore, statistical approaches that have proved useful throughout the social sciences often elude the researcher with small samples (but see Bates & Applebaum, 1994).

Thus, whenever subjects are rare or very difficult to locate and time consuming to study, investigators who turn to colleagues and consultants traditionally trained in quantitative social science for advice often are disappointed. Too often we are told that what we want to do cannot be done. Part of the problem may be the way we express what we think we need to do. The language most of us learned to speak when describing results is based on standard parametric techniques such as analysis of variance models. Perhaps as a result, too often we think the only legitimate results are those couched in terms of group differences and inferential statistics. The danger of relying solely on traditional large sample statistics is twofold. First, the researcher possessing an interesting data set obtained from a small number of subjects may feel forced to use traditional statistical analyses even when some assumptions are unmet, thereby rendering results suspect. Second, researchers armed only with a basic ANOVA toolkit may avoid the most interesting questions associated with their field of study. Although traditionally research in language disorders has centered on mean differences in communicative functioning between a target population and some comparison group—usually a typically developing MA (mental age)-matched sample—many of the most interesting aspects of research in language disorders are concerned with the universality of developmental pathways in language development, alternate pathways to linguistic competence, and the identification of unique profiles of language skills in rare populations.

In this chapter we emphasize two approaches that permit rigorous scientific scrutiny of data collected from few subjects (for a survey of other approaches see Kratochwill & Levin, 1992) and facilitate the examination of research questions beyond the scope of simple mean difference tests. Indeed, small *N* studies sometimes provide the opportunity to apply analytic techniques that would prove unwieldy were a larger number of subjects involved.

The first approach presented in this chapter, graphic presentation of data, requires little more than drawing clear figures, whereas the second approach, permutation tests, allows significance statements tailored to specific circumstances unfettered by the usual (and usually unmet) assumptions required for parametric tests. Both of these approaches are presented within the context of example studies. We demonstrate that useful information can be extracted from few subjects observed in naturalistic and sometimes difficult environments using quite simple techniques. This should be of interest to investigators in the field of language disorders, as well as others interested primarily in normative theory, who are faced with the problem of communicating results from similar studies to others.

## GRAPHIC PRESENTATION OF DATA

Displaying data graphically is hardly new, yet a quick perusal of journals shows that the art, if not moribund, is insufficiently practiced. Yet guidance and general principles are available. Tukey's (1977) *Exploratory Data Analysis* provides an excellent foundation. Tufte's (1983) *The Visual Display of Quantitative Information* gives elegant advice and examples, while Wainer (1984) provides cautions against the use of poor graphing techniques. The essential, overarching principle is straightforward: The data—all the data, in all their messy variability—should be displayed to facilitate direct and immediate comprehension. A corollary requires that data be expressed in units that make as much intuitive sense as possible. However, graphing does not preclude statistical testing (although sometimes examination of graphs may prevent us from performing inappropriate tests). Still, it is good practice to apply Ockham's razor to both graph and test: Do both accomplish the task in as simple a way as possible?

### Example 1: The !Kung Infant Object Study Revisited

As an example of both graphing and permutation tests, we revisit a study by Bakeman, Adamson, Konner, and Barr (1990) and demonstrate how the same data could be displayed in a manner we now regard as more illuminating and informative (although the general thrust of the conclusions remains the same). Reexamining the !Kung data in the context of this chapter provides the opportunity to highlight some of the pitfalls (and their solutions) prevalent in developmental research resulting in data sets collected under less than ideal, but not uncommon, conditions. After a brief introduction to the study, we discuss the selection of appropriate summary measures, graphical techniques, and hypothesis testing with data that do not always meet the assumptions required for traditional statistical tests.

In the early 1970s, Konner collected detailed records of the behavior of !Kung infants. (At that time, the !Kung were living largely traditional hunter–gatherer lives in Botswana.) There were 68 observations in all, of infants ranging from several days to almost 2 years old. Ideally, each observation comprised six 15-minute sessions, all completed within a few days of each other. The pool of infants was limited; thus, some infants were observed more than once, but at different ages. This could raise concerns for statistical purists. After all, some infants were observed more than once, so if a multiple regression design is imposed on these data, surely the assumption of independence of sampling units is violated. Is this not an impure, and unanalyzable, design comprising repeated measures for some subjects but not all and not consistently? Even on traditional statistical grounds, we would argue no or at least not necessarily. Even when infants were observed more than once, they were observed at different ages. Because the intent was to sample different age infants, we could view this as a simple case of sampling with replacement.

Sometimes samples consist only of a single subject. For the !Kung study, several infants were observed. But given other constraints, contexts, or research questions, a single infant (or child, or dyad, etc.) might have been observed repeatedly over time. As a result, comments and analyses presented here could apply to single-subject studies as well. Even so, 68 observations may seem like a relatively large number. Most of the analyses reported here, however, focus on the 36 observations made when infants were at least 8 months of age. In general, the graphing and analytic techniques used in this chapter should apply whenever observations are made for a single subject, or several subjects, over time, and change or developmental issues are of concern.

Recording procedures vary in complexity, but Konner's were simple and straightforward. He used lined paper and a simple electronic device that delivered a beep in his ear every 5 seconds. Each 5 seconds he moved to a new line, recording the codable behaviors that occurred during that interval (such data are called interval sequential; Bakeman & Quera, 1992, 1995a). Influenced by human ethologists such as Blurton Jones (1972) and developmentalists such as Tulkin and Kagan (1972), Konner developed an ethogram, an exhaustive list of some 100 infant behaviors, but we focus on just a few behaviors, some of which result from lumping together more molecular codes.

Using electronic equipment that has become inexpensive and widely available during the mid-1990s (e.g., video recorders that record and display time to the nearest second or better), investigators might record onsets and offsets of key behaviors instead, resulting in what we call timed event sequential data (Bakeman & Quera, 1992). In either case, some simple statistic is needed for the first level of description, and the obvious one is proportion of time a particular behavior was observed. Given timed event data, such proportions (or percents) will be reasonably accurate, whereas percents of intervals checked for a particular behavior will probably somewhat overestimate proportion of time. Nonetheless, graphic presentation and analysis of such percents is essentially the same. Thus, comments made here apply whenever various behaviors are observed and their rate or duration recorded.

***Simple Probabilities and Line Graphs*** Graphing data for analysis and presentation is one approach that offers studies with only a few subjects some advantage over larger studies where investigators must often resort to aggregate measures or complex graphical techniques to represent data in a comprehensible form. Aggregate measures necessarily require the loss of some information contained in the data set, while complex graphs may prove tiresome or incomprehensible to the reader. With the small *N* study, however, the selection of an appropriate measure and scale applied to familiar graphs, such as the simple line graph, may provide the most efficient avenue for displaying data.

With respect to the !Kung infant object study, five behavioral categories were of particular interest to us. One was quite global and involved any social acts directed to infants by others (including touching, talking, entertaining, caregiving, singing, encouraging, and vigorous physical stimulation). Others involved the infant and were less global (including infant playing with objects, vocalizing, smiling, and offering objects to others). These categories were motivated by our interest in shared object involvement. In particular, we wondered whether the !Kung socialize object play, as middle-class Americans typically do, or whether offering would stand as a separate, and uniquely social, way of relating objects and others (see Bakeman et al., 1990).

As a first step, it makes sense simply to graph these data (Figures 1–6). Regression lines (best-fit lines as determined by a least-squares criterion)—in this case, based on the 36 observations made when infants were between 8 and 23 months because at younger ages offers to others did not occur and object play was both less and of a different nature—provide a sense of the average and whether there is a developmental trend, whereas separate data points portray the variability and range of individual scores.

Consider how informative these simple line graphs are. Object play occurs seldom in the first several months of life, becomes more frequent after 4 months of age, and stabilizes around 31% (of 5-second intervals) beginning at 8 months. Others engage infants at somewhat higher and more variable levels in the first several months of life compared with later, but at 8 months the rate stabilizes around 21% and becomes less variable. Vocalizing and smiling are both relatively rare for the first 2 months of life but become more frequent about 3–4 months of age when, according to most developmental accounts, exogenous smiling makes its appearance. From 8 months on, averages are 20% for vocalizing and 5% for smiling. The regression line declines slightly for vocalization and increases somewhat for smiling, but neither is statistically significant.

The most common summary statistic is the mean, but sometimes it can be misleading, and perusal of line graphs can alert us to such cases. As an example, consider offering. Infants offering objects to others was the least frequent of the behaviors studied (see Figures 5 and 6). Before 8 months of age, only one infant was observed offering. Thereafter, their offering increased from an average of 0.48% to 1.52% (based on the best-fit line for the 8- to 23-month observations, where percents refer to 5-second intervals). These numbers are so low (no offering was observed during 3 of the 36 observations; the number of offers was 5 or greater for only 24 of the observations) that average percents are not very meaningful. In this case, rates are probably more informative; thus, we would report that, on average, offers increased from 5 to 16 per 90-minute observation period, or from 3.33 to 10.67 per hour, assuming, as seems likely, that a 5-second interval coded for infant offering indicates a single offer. However, with interval data, computed rates may underestimate actual rates somewhat if intervals contain more than one occurrence of the behavior studied (see Quera, 1990; Suen & Ary, 1989).

Even when means are appropriate and informative, the range and variability of scores are important and can be seen immediately by a glance at the graph. But comparisons between figures need to be made cautiously whenever scores are constrained, as here. Probabilities cannot be less than zero, by defi-

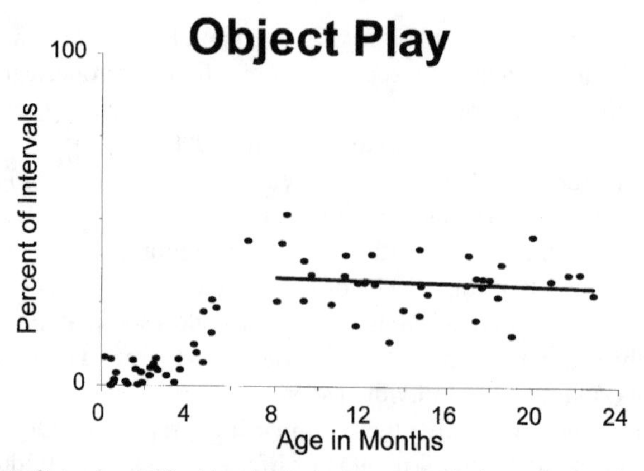


Figure 1. Percent of intervals coded for object play. Scores shown are for 68 observations, based on 70,200 5-second intervals. The least-squares best-fit line is for 36 observations of infants ages 8 through 23 months.

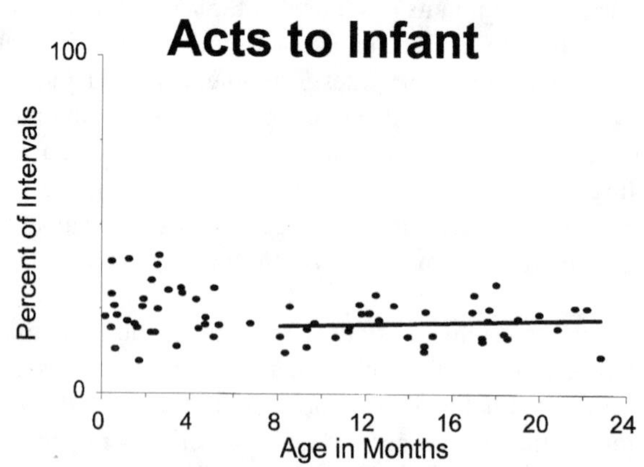


Figure 2. Percent of intervals coded for acts to infant (scale same as object play).

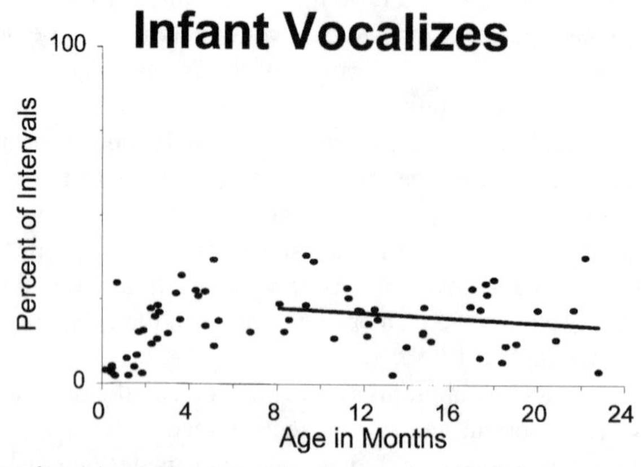


Figure 3. Percent of intervals coded for infant vocalizes (scale same as object play).

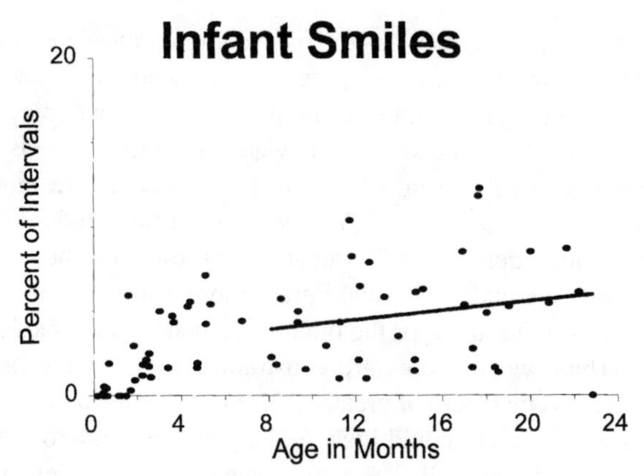


Figure 4. Percent of intervals coded for infant smiles (scale extends just to 20%).

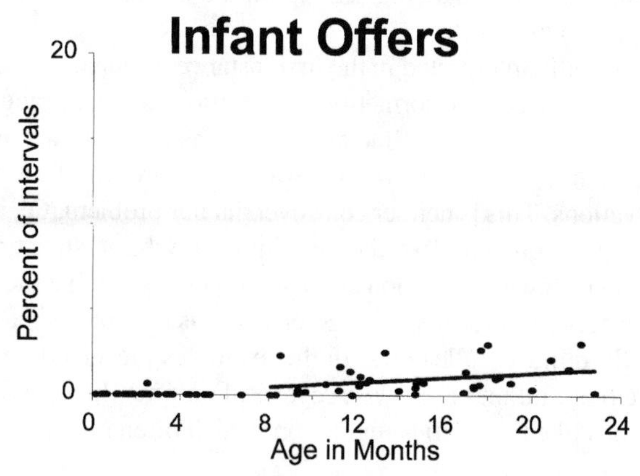


Figure 5. Percent of intervals coded for infant offers (scale same as infant smiles).

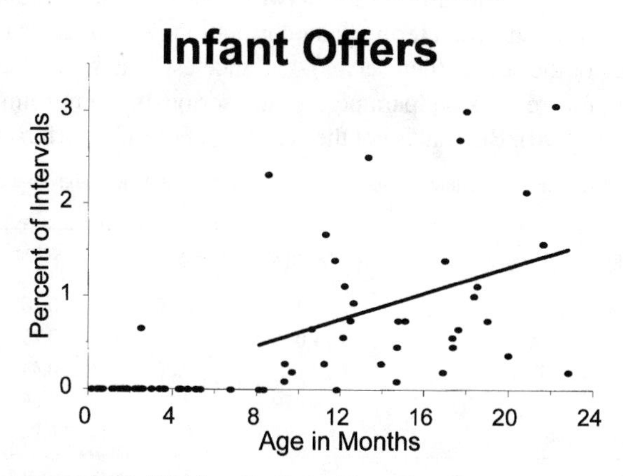


Figure 6. Percent of intervals coded for infant offers (scale extends just to 3%).

nition. Thus, the standard deviation (the most common measure of variability) is limited by the mean. In such cases, the ratio of standard deviation to mean should be used for comparisons. For example, consider object play and acts to infants (Figures 1 and 2). The standard deviations confirm our visual impression: Compared with acts to infant, object play percents are more variable (*SD*=8.16 versus 5.27; see Table 1). Yet the ratios of the standard deviation to the mean are almost identical (0.26 versus 0.25); thus, by the ratio measure these two scores are equally variable. Furthermore, ratios for object play and acts to infant are smaller than for the other three behaviors considered (again, see Table 1). Thus, when scores are constrained (like simple probabilities, which cannot be less than zero or greater than 1), and comparisons are desired, basic descriptive statistics should include not just the standard deviation and the mean but their ratio as well. The appearance of greater or lesser variability is easily manipulated by changing scaling on the ordinate as Figures 5 and 6 (and also Figure 4) demonstrate.

Change, usually interpreted in the first instance as linear trend, constitutes another important piece of information (in addition to mean, range, and variability) effectively conveyed by line graphs such as those shown in Figures 1–6. To portray change, a least-squares line was fit to scores for the 8- through 23-month observations. This is neither controversial nor problematic; it is only descriptive (computations are described in almost any basic statistics text, e.g., Bakeman, 1992). However, as soon as we attempt to assert that the slope of the best-fit line differs significantly from zero, a chorus of protests may arise from our statistically minded colleagues. In the examples presented here, a dependent measure (e.g., infant offers) was regressed on time (here, age of observation). This looks like time-series regression, which often raises concerns about serial independence.

When errors (i.e., the differences between observed and predicted scores) are serially correlated (often termed autocorrelation, which refers to the errors or residuals, not the scores themselves), variance estimates, and hence tests of significance, for regression parameters are seriously compromised (Hays, 1963; Ostrom, 1990). But that is not the case here. For infant offers, the correla-

Table 1. Means, standard deviations, and their ratios for major behavioral categories

| Category | Mean | *SD* | *SD/M* |
|---|---|---|---|
| Object play | 31.4 | 8.16 | 0.26 |
| Acts to infants | 21.0 | 5.27 | 0.25 |
| Infant vocalizes | 20.1 | 8.88 | 0.44 |
| Infant smiles | 4.87 | 3.19 | 0.66 |
| Infant offers | 0.95 | 0.89 | 0.93 |

Means are percents of 5-second intervals coded for the category, *SD* is standard deviation, and *SD/M* is the ratio of *SD* to mean. Statistics are based on 36 observations of infants ages 8–23 months.

tion between errors at time *t* and *t*-1 is .04 and the Durban-Watson *d*-statistic is 2.01 (values near 1 or 4 suggest serious autocorrelation, values near 2 suggest none; see Ostrom, 1990). Thus, we are justified in claiming that the rate of infant offers increases significantly ($R^2=.11$, $F[2,34]=4.33$, $p<.05$). None of the other slopes shown in Figures 1–4 differed significantly from zero; had they, we would also have verified that errors were serially independent before claiming statistical significance. However, this is a parametric test, which requires assumptions about population parameters and distributions. We discuss tests that do not require such assumptions in a following section.

***Conditional Probabilities and Yule's Q*** Simple probabilities and their change over time are informative but often not sufficient to address questions of interest. Often we want to know not just how much a single behavior occurs and how it changes (or not), but how two behaviors are related. For example, with respect to the !Kung infant object study, we wanted to know not just how often infants played with objects, but how often during that time they were engaged with others as well. Conditional probabilities are the ideal statistic for such questions. Thus, to continue our example, we would compute the probability that others were engaging an infant *given* that the infant was playing with objects.

For the !Kung study, six conditional probabilities were of particular interest. First, we wanted to describe the association between social behavior directed toward infants and the infants' behavior at the time, so we computed the probability that others would act (i.e., engage the infant) given that the infant was playing with objects, vocalizing, smiling, and offering, respectively. These are symbolized as *p*(Act|Object Play), *p*(Act|Vocalize), *p*(Act|Smile), and *p*(Act|Offer), where *p* represents probability and the vertical bar is read as *given*. Second, we wanted to describe the association between infants' social signals and offering, so we computed *p*(Vocalize|Offer) and *p*(Smile|Offer).

The usual descriptive statistics for these conditional probabilities are given in Table 2. Conditional probabilities were computed for an observation only if both behaviors occurred at least five times during it; any fewer and we would have had little confidence in the values computed. The mean values do

Table 2. Means, standard deviations, and their ratios for selected conditional probabilities

| Conditional probability | Mean | *SD* | *SD/M* | *N* |
|---|---|---|---|---|
| *p*(Act\|Object Play) | 0.129 | 0.048 | 0.37 | 36 |
| *p*(Act\|Vocalize) | 0.287 | 0.105 | 0.37 | 36 |
| *p*(Act\|Smile) | 0.492 | 0.169 | 0.34 | 35 |
| *p*(Act\|Infant Offer) | 0.384 | 0.224 | 0.58 | 24 |
| *p*(Vocalize\|Offer) | 0.428 | 0.225 | 0.53 | 24 |
| *p*(Smile\|Infant Offer) | 0.152 | 0.175 | 1.16 | 24 |

Conditional probabilities were computed only if both behaviors occurred at least five times during the observation. *SD* is standard deviation and *SD/M* is the ratio of *SD* to mean. Statistics are based on number of observations (*N*) shown.

not indicate linear trend, of course, but are nonetheless suggestive. In particular, relative to the simple probability for others acting (.21), the conditional probability for others acting was depressed when infants were playing with objects (.13) and elevated when infants were offering objects (.38). Infants played with objects often (31%), but during these times others seemed less likely to engage infants than at other times. In contrast, and not surprisingly, others seemed particularly likely to engage infants when infants offered them objects.

These last few statements are only impressionistic. We can see that some simple probabilities are greater (or less) than a particular associated conditional probability. Yet we need some measure of the extent to which a conditional probability differs from its expected simple probability and whether that difference is statistically significant. Statistical significance is relatively easy to determine for an individual observation. For example, the 1,080 intervals for the 90-minute observation of one 8.5-month-old infant were cross-classified as follows:

| | Act | No-Act | |
|---|---|---|---|
| Offer | 17 | 8 | 25 |
| No-Offer | 263 | 783 | 1055 |
| | 280 | 800 | 1080 |

As is easily verified, for this observation $p(\text{Act})$ was 0.30, $p(\text{Act}|\text{Offer})$ was 0.68, and the chi-square for the table (23.6) is clearly significant.

Yet the chi-square, which (granted assumptions) assesses statistical significance, is not a good measure of the size of the effect (or strength of association). It is affected by the number of tallies, thus, for example, if the effect stayed the same but the number of tallies was doubled, chi-square would increase. To gauge the magnitude of the effect, a measure of association that remains unaffected by the number of counts is needed. Several have been proposed for 2 × 2 tables and have been discussed extensively in the literature (for reviews see Bakeman, McArthur, & Quera, 1996; Bakeman & Quera, 1995b; Conger & Ward, 1984; Reynolds, 1984), but one we recommend, Yule's Q, is a simple transformation of the familiar odds ratio. Conventionally, cells of 2 × 2 tables are labeled as follows:

| | |
|---|---|
| $a$ | $b$ |
| $c$ | $d$ |

where $a$, $b$, $c$, and $d$ represent observed counts or frequencies. Then the odds ratio is

$$\text{odds ratio} = \frac{a/b}{c/d}$$

However, it ranges from zero (perfect negative association), to 1 (no association), to infinity (perfect positive association). Subtracting *c/d* from the numerator, adding *a/b* to the denominator, and simplifying, this becomes

$$\text{Yule's Q} = \frac{ad - bc}{ad + bc}$$

an index that, like the familiar correlation coefficient, ranges from $-1$ (perfect negative association), to zero (no association), to $+1$ (perfect positive association). For the example just given, the odds ratio is 6.40 and Yule's Q is 0.73, indicating a relatively strong association between infants offering and others acting.

Thus, when comparing simple with conditional probabilities, Yule's Q can be used to indicate the size of the effect. Like any other simple summary score, it can (and often will) be used for subsequent analyses. For the present example, six line graphs corresponding to the six conditional probabilities of interest were prepared (Figures 7–12). Like the figures for simple probabilities already discussed, these are quite informative. Consider Figure 7. From it we learn that for *all* 36 observations, $p(\text{Act}|\text{Object})$ was less than $p(\text{Act})$ (i.e., all values for Yule's Q were negative). This is a considerably stronger statement than simply noting that the average value of Yule's Q was $-0.39$ ($SD = 0.13$) and that it differed significantly from zero but exhibited no linear trend.

It is a stronger statement because it takes all data points into account and tells us not just what the average pattern is, but how many observations actually exemplify the average pattern. None are swept into an all-encompassing mean as can happen with the analyses of variance. By their nature, figures like those used here display all the data in all of their untidy variability and individuality, which is perhaps one of the stronger arguments for routinely including such figures in research reports.

The remaining figures are equally informative. The !Kung infants' partners were less likely to engage infants when the infants were engaged with objects, but more likely to engage infants when the infants were vocalizing, smiling, and offering (Yule's Q was above zero for 29 of 36, 34 of 35, and 18 of 24 observations, respectively; see Figures 8–10). Furthermore, as age of infant increased, the association between others acting and infants vocalizing became stronger ($R^2 = .13$, $F[1,34] = 5.25$, $p < .05$). Compared with other times, infants were more likely to vocalize when offering (Yule's Q was above zero for 22 of 24 observations, Figure 11) but not necessarily more likely to smile (Yule's Q was above zero for 14 of 24, Figure 12). As Figure 12 shows, observations were of two kinds. During the observations, $p(\text{Smile}|\text{Offer})$ was either greater than $p(\text{Smile})$ (positive values for Yule's Q) or zero ($-1$ values for Yule's Q). In other words, when offering, infants either smiled more than expected (14) or did not smile at all (10). Thus, the distribution of scores for $p(\text{Smile}|\text{Offer})$ and their associated Yule's Qs suggests a binary outcome, and for that reason no

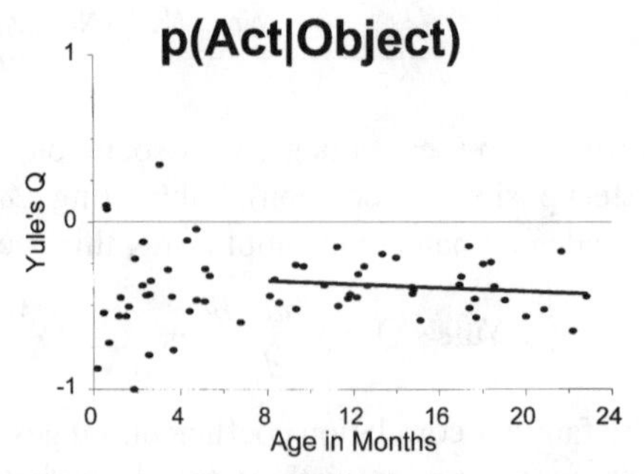


Figure 7. Yule's Q associated with the probability of other acting given infant engaged in object play.

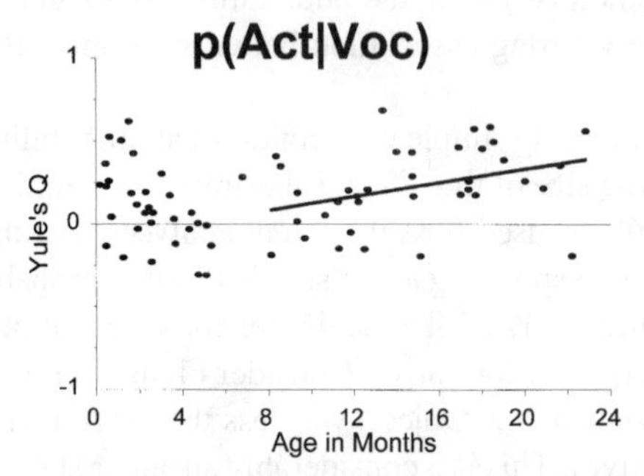


Figure 8. Yule's Q associated with the probability of other acting given infant vocalizing.

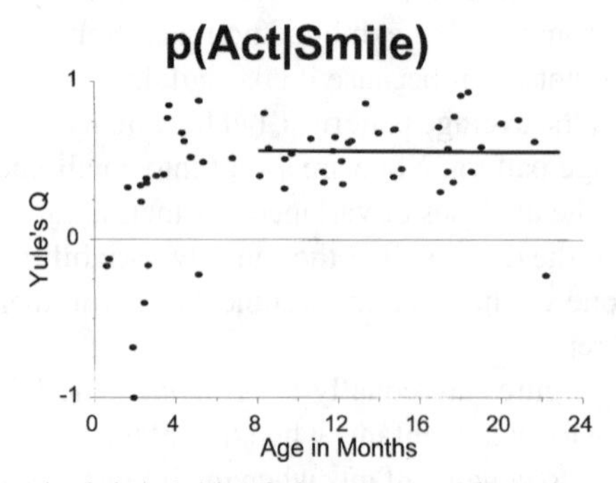


Figure 9. Yule's Q associated with the probability of other acting given infant smiling.

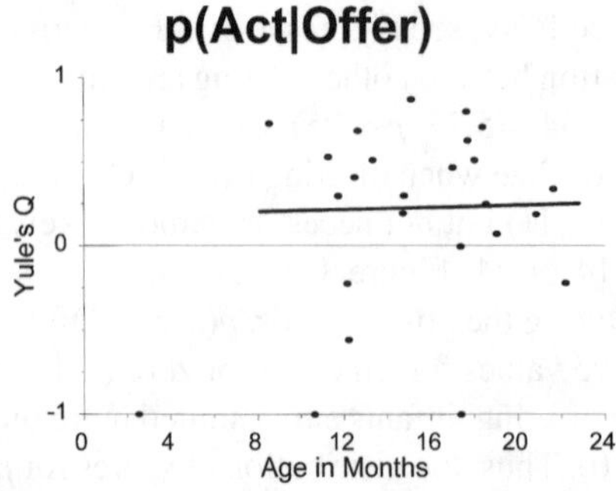


Figure 10. Yule's Q associated with the probability of other acting given infant offering object to others.

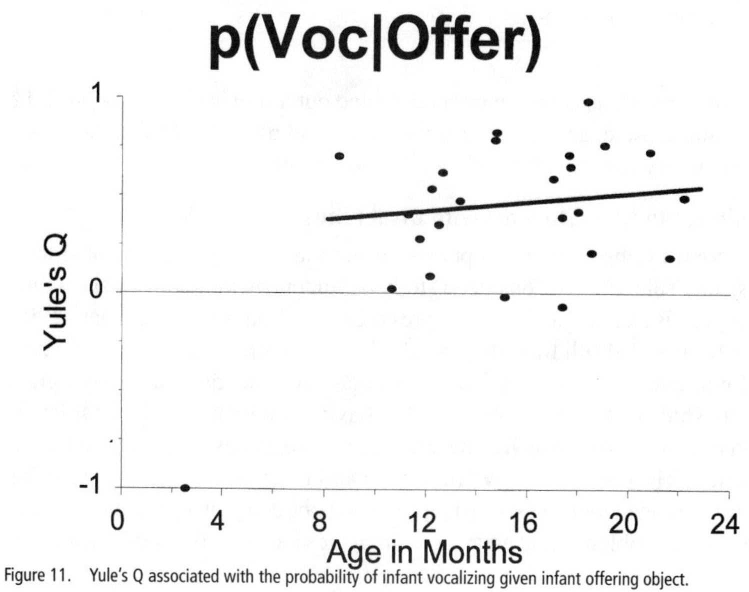

Figure 11. Yule's Q associated with the probability of infant vocalizing given infant offering object.

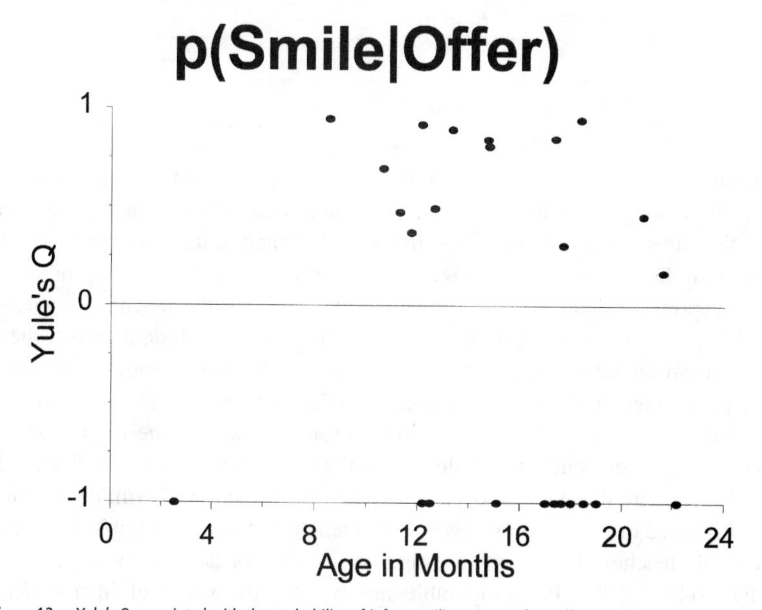

Figure 12. Yule's Q associated with the probability of infant smiling given infant offering object.

best-fit line (which assumes an interval-scaled outcome) is shown in Figure 12. Once again, close examination of figures can lead us to emphasize the appropriate summary statistic and avoid a misleading one.

### Example 2: Studying Students with Disabilities

As a second example, again emphasizing individual subjects, graphical techniques, and Yule's Q, we consider a study of students with intellectual disabilities (Logan, Bakeman, & Keefe, in press; Logan, Rankin, & Bakeman, 1994) who were included full time in general education elementary classes (i.e., not in self-contained classrooms). Twenty students in kindergarten through grade five were studied. Most were classified as having moderate mental retardation, but three were classified as having severe and two as having profound mental retardation. The distribution by grade level and level of retardation was as follows, where each letter (m, s, or p) represents a child, a plus sign indicates hand or fine motor problems, and an asterisk indicates a lack of functional hand use:

| Grade | Moderate | Severe | Profound |
|---|---|---|---|
| Kindergarten | m,m,m,m, m+,m+ | | |
| 1 | m,m+,m* | s | |
| 2 | | | |
| 3 | m,m,m | s+ | *p** |
| 4 | m | | *p** |
| 5 | m,m | s* | |

Of primary interest was students' engaged (i.e., actively on-task) behavior. Indeed, the study was undertaken to understand such behavior better with the hope that subsequent interventions might be designed to increase the time students with disabilities spent engaged, as opposed to merely attending or some other response. Logan and his colleagues thought that the teachers' focus—whether solely on the student, on a group that included the student, or on others in the classroom not including the student with disabilities—might affect these students' engaged behavior. He also thought that their engaged behavior might be affected by the kind of instructional group—whether one-to-one, small group, independent study, or whole class—the students were in when observed.

To evaluate these ideas, occasions when the 20 students with disabilities were involved or might be involved with a teacher were time sampled. For the study of teacher focus an average of 1,393 occasions was sampled (range = 649–2,780); the comparable number for the study of instructional group was 1,300 (range = 641–2,564). For each time sample, the student's behavior was coded as engaged or not engaged; the teacher's focus as solely on the student with disabilities, on that student and others, or on other students not including the student with disabilities; and the student's current instructional group as one-to-one, small group, independent work, or whole class. Then, for each student, the time sampled data were tallied in a $3 \times 2$ and a $4 \times 2$ contingency table for teacher's focus and student's group, respectively.

Yule's Q, which was introduced in the context of $2 \times 2$ tables earlier, at first might not seem appropriate for these tables, but it turns out to be quite useful. The $3 \times 2$ table is associated with 2 degrees of freedom and can be decomposed into two $2 \times 2$ tables, each with a single degree of freedom. Similarly, the $4 \times 2$ table with its 3 degrees of freedom can be decomposed into three $2 \times 2$ tables. For example, recognizing that Yule's Q is simply a transformation of the odds ratio (Bakeman, McArthur, & Quera, 1996), and following Reynold's (1984) suggestions for decomposing the odds ratio in tables larger than $2 \times 2$, the $3 \times 2$ table for teacher focus

| Focus: | Engaged | Not Engaged |
|---|---|---|
| Student only | *a* | *b* |
| Others included | *c* | *d* |
| Others only | *e* | *f* |

can be decomposed into the following two tables:

| Focus: | Engaged | Not Engaged |
|---|---|---|
| Student only | *a* | *b* |
| Others only | *e* | *f* |

| Focus: | Engaged | Not Engaged |
|---|---|---|
| Others included | *c* | *d* |
| Others only | *e* | *f* |

and a Yule's Q computed for each. The bottom row of the full table, which appears in both decomposed tables, serves as a sort of baseline, and the two Yule's Qs are equivalent to two repeated measures for each student. The Yule's Q for the first table measures the extent to which the odds for engaged behavior are increased (or decreased) when teachers focus solely on the student with disabilities versus attending to other students (not including the student with disabilities) and for the second, when teachers focus on a group that includes the student with disabilities versus attending to other students.

Similarly, for instructional group, the three decomposed tables are:

| Group: | Engaged | Not Engaged |
|---|---|---|
| 1:1 | $a$ | $b$ |
| Whole | $g$ | $h$ |

| | | |
|---|---|---|
| Small | $c$ | $d$ |
| Whole | $g$ | $h$ |

| | | |
|---|---|---|
| Indep. | $e$ | $f$ |
| Whole | $g$ | $h$ |

The first measures the extent to which the odds for engaged behavior are increased (or decreased) when in one-to-one as opposed to whole-class instruction, the second when in small group versus whole-class instruction, and the third when in independent work versus whole-class instruction.

The values for Yule's Q for the study of teacher focus are shown in Figure 13, separately for each student; students with greater disability are shown first, on the left, and those with lesser disability and higher grade levels on the right. A traditional analysis of variance (for repeated measures) would note that the mean Yule's Q for sole focus and others included ($M = .25$ & $-.13$, $SD = .25$ & 27) differed significantly ($F[1,19] = 23.8$, $p < .001$). But the figure tells us more. The positive mean Yule's Q suggests a beneficial effect of sole focus (i.e., greater engaged behavior), but from the figure we learn that the benefit occurred for 17 of the 20 students ($p < .01$, two-tailed sign test). Similarly, the negative mean Yule's Q suggests that the beneficial effect does not occur when teachers focus on a group that includes the student with disabilities. From the figure we learn that for 13 of the 20 children, engaged behavior was actually less when the teacher focused on a group that included them compared with when her focus was not on them at all. However, 13 does not differ significantly from the 10 we would expect by chance; thus, the negative effect (indicated by the negative mean Yule's Q) is not pervasive.

In addition, the figure identifies how individual students are affected by teacher focus, which could provide useful information to those familiar with each student's individual circumstances. Also, a teacher who knows the students might explain why the three students whose sole focus Yule's Q was negative did not fit the usual positive pattern. There is even a suggestion that students with more severe disabilities may be aided more by a sole focus (larger values of Yule's Q seem to occur more on the left than the right of the sole focus

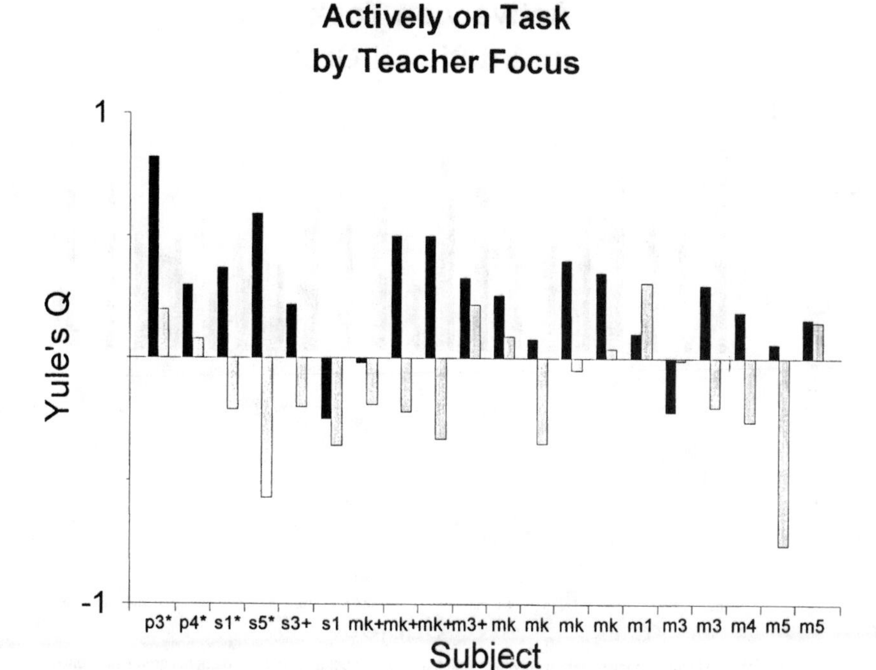


Figure 13. Yule's Q indicating association between students' engaged behavior and teacher's focus. (■ = sole focus; ■ = includes others.)

figure). This impression is not supported by statistical test, at least with the relatively small number of students included here, but might be worth pursuing in future studies.

The values for Yule's Q for the study of instructional group are shown in Figure 14, again separately for each student. The mean Yule's Q for the three instructional group comparisons (one-to-one, small group, and independent work with whole class; $M = .49, .44, \& .51$; $SD = .23, .25, \& .39$) did not differ significantly ($F[2,38] < 1$). However, all means (with the exception of a student with profound mental retardation who was never observed engaged when in independent work) were positive ($p < .01$, two-tailed sign test). Thus, compared with whole class, all instructional groups had a beneficial effect on engaged behavior, no one more than the others. Moreover, inspection of Figure 14 does not suggest that these effects were related to students' level of disability or grade level.

No matter the particular results, this example demonstrates again the utility of simple statistics like Yule's Q coupled with simple graphical presentations and simple statistical tests such as the sign test. Such techniques are always appropriate, but they are especially useful when subjects are few, as this second example demonstrates.

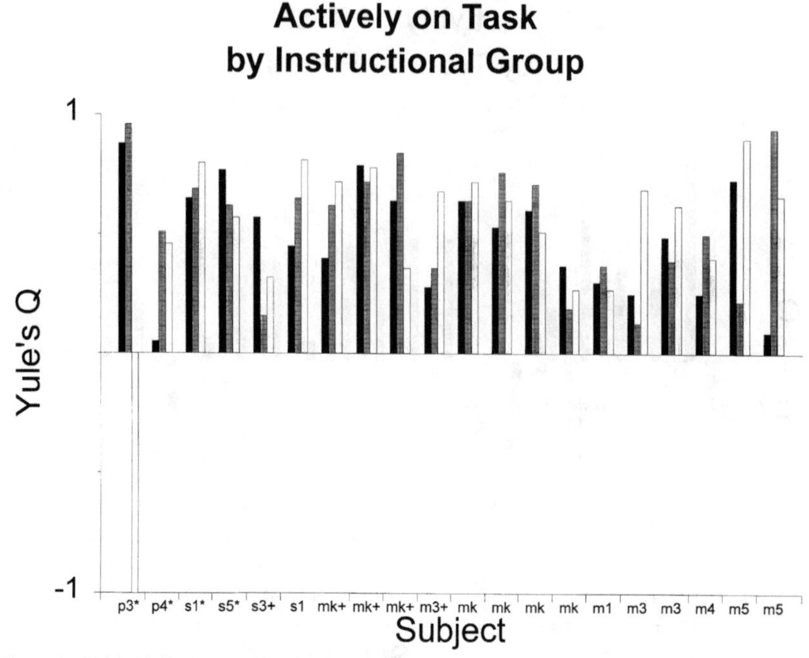


Figure 14. Yule's Q indicating association between students' engaged behavior and instructional group. (■ = one-to-one; ▒ = small group; □ = individual work.)

## PERMUTATION TESTS

With respect to the !Kung infant and students with disabilities studies, statements such as those made earlier (e.g., the probability of another acting, given that the !Kung infant was offering, was greater than expected for 18 of 24 observations) seem eminently amenable to statistical testing. Most social science investigators have been exposed to (or have used) the binomial or sign test in such situations. What many of us fail to appreciate, however—because we were never taught it—is that the sign test is one of the simplest examples of a kind of test that we probably should use in preference to all others, yet almost never do.

Often the term *exact tests* is used to designate these procedures, although they might better be called tests that yield exact, as opposed to approximate, $p$ values. They are also called randomization tests (e.g., Bradley, 1968), although at least some experts (e.g., Edgington, 1987) reserve that term for tests involving data that resulted from random assignment (either of experimental units to treatments or treatment times). *Permutation test* seems the more descriptive and more general term (Edgington, 1987; Good, 1994) and is the term we use here. There are two kinds, exact (or systematic) and sampled, both of which we will describe, but permutation tests are different from both parametric and most nonparametric tests. Like nonparametric tests, and unlike the common parametric $t$ and $F$ tests, their derivation and application do not involve explicit assumptions about population distributions and parameters (Hays, 1963). And unlike the usual applications of nonparametric tests such as those based on $\chi^2$, they do not rely on asymptotic theory that is valid only if sample sizes are reasonably large and well balanced (Mehta & Patel, 1992).

### Example 1: An Exact Permutation Test

Consider the logic of the sign test, which is an example of an exact permutation test. Given $N$ observations (or trials), and assuming a binary outcome for each (in this case, the observed conditional probability is, or is not, greater than expected), then there are $2^N$ different sets of results possible, or $2^N$ different ways that the study might have turned out. Each of the possible results can be categorized by the value of $r$ associated with it, where $r$ symbolizes the number of observations with the first binary outcome (in this case, the number of conditional probabilities greater than expected). The value of $r$ can vary from 0 to $N$, and the number of different possible results for each value of $r$ is

$$\binom{N}{r} = \frac{N!}{r!\,(N-r)!}$$

which is the binary coefficient. For the present example ($N=24$), only 1 possible result has all 24 conditional probabilities greater than expected, 24 possible results have 23 greater than expected, 276 have 22 greater than expected, 2,024 have 21 greater than expected, and so forth.

In any given study, we are concerned with only one of the many possible results—the one that actually happened. For example, in the context of the !Kung infant study, we noted that for 18 of 24 observations, $p(\text{Act}|\text{Offer})$ was greater than expected. Now we are in a position to compute the exact probability for this result. The probability of a result this extreme or more so (assume a one-tailed test) is the number of possible results for which $r$ is 18 or greater divided by $2^{24}$, the total number of possible results. This probability, rounded to three significant digits, is 0.0113 (which you can and should verify). Such exact probabilities are somewhat tedious to compute in practice but relatively easy to understand in principle.

Other permutation tests are available and a permutated version can be constructed for any statistical test, whether initially parametric or nonparametric. Rarely in psychology and almost never when special populations are studied are the usual parametric assumptions warranted, beginning with, but hardly limited to, the assumption of random sampling. This is sometimes noted in statistical texts (e.g., Keppel, 1991), but then the limitations imposed are often ignored in practice. Furthermore, when samples are relatively small or unbalanced across levels of factors, nonparametric asymptotic methods may yield inaccurate results. Given the possibility of permutation tests, or even asymptotic nonparametric ones, why did social scientists embrace parametric ones so wholeheartedly, especially as the requisite assumptions are so seldom met?

Part of the answer is technical. Exact tests, although they appeared early in the development of statistics (e.g., Fisher's exact test), can be extremely tedious and computationally intensive. Had computers been available from the beginning, it seems quite likely that exact tests would be the rule. But before computers, when computations were tedious and error-prone, the simplifications of the approximate parametric methods must have seemed worth the imposition of assumptions—and then a comforting body of literature arose, and was quickly embraced, that suggested that at least some violations did not matter that much after all. (For a review, see Keppel, 1991.)

There is much to recommend embracing permutation tests for all our work. This approach is more concrete and readily understandable than traditional parametric or asymptotic nonparametric approaches. It does not require assumptions that are rarely justified, and, as a consequence, it gives us far greater confidence in the $p$ values we report. When using traditional methods, we may miss detecting real effects. For example, Mehta and Patel (1992) gave an example of a sparse $3 \times 9$ contingency table:

| | | | | | | | | |
|---|---|---|---|---|---|---|---|---|
| 0 | 7 | 0 | 0 | 0 | 0 | 0 | 1 | 1 |
| 1 | 1 | 1 | 1 | 1 | 1 | 1 | 0 | 0 |
| 0 | 8 | 0 | 0 | 0 | 0 | 0 | 1 | 0 |

Using standard methods (if we did not abandon the enterprise at the outset, worried about the empty cells and low counts that are a problem for asymptotic methods), we would compute a Pearson chi-square statistic of 22.29, whose asymptotic $p$ value with 16 degrees of freedom is 0.1342. Yet exact methods yield a $p$ of 0.0013.

## Example 2: A Sampled Permutation Test for Slope

Earlier we asserted that a permutated version can be constructed for any statistical test. How is this so? Permutation tests rely on the *reference set*—the set of all possible results given initial constraints, like the $2^N$ possibilities given $N$ binary trials. The reference set for the sign test seems easy enough to understand and construct, and this could even be said for Fisher's exact test for a $2 \times 2$ contingency table (e.g., Hays, 1963). But for anything much more complex, constructing an appropriate reference set quickly gets bogged down in detail and tedious computation (although the StatXact package does perform the appropriate computations for most common statistical tests; Mehta & Patel, 1992).

There is a relatively simple solution. Instead of actually constructing the complete reference set, a subsample of elements randomly selected from the full set can be formed instead. Assembling the subsample, which does not require that the complete set already be constructed, relies on random or Monte Carlo procedures. StatXact (Mehta & Patel, 1992) routinely uses Monte Carlo estimates for exact $p$ values when a data set is too large for exact algorithms (i.e., those based on exact or systematic permutation). But sampled permutation can be used generally. Edgington (1987) noted the following:

> It serves the same function as systematic data permutation with a substantial reduction in the number of permutations that need to be considered. Instead of requiring millions or billions of data permutations, as would be required for the systematic data permutation method for many applications of randomization tests, the random data permutation method may be effective with as few as 1,000 data permutations. (p. 43)

To clarify how sampled permutation works and how exact probabilities can be estimated using it, we return to the slopes portrayed in Figures 1–12. As an example, consider the values of Yule's Q associated with $p(\text{Act}|\text{Voc})$ shown in Figure 8. Earlier, using standard parametric tests, we noted that this regression line was significantly different from zero. Its slope is .0209 (i.e., Yule's Q increases .0209 for each additional month of age, on average), the $F$ ratio associated with the slope is 5.25 (many computer programs list $t$, which is the square root of $F$), and its $p$ value is .0282. But to be accurate, this $p$ value requires that all of the required assumptions be met, which may or may not be warranted.

As shown in Figure 8, a value for Yule's Q was computed for each observation. Our research hypothesis claims that the 36 values for Yule's Q made when infants were at least 8 months of age are not ordered randomly but vary systematically—specifically, they increase with the age of the infant observed. But the null hypothesis, as usual, claims no effects—specifically, the scores bear no relation to age. To test this hypothesis using exact permutation, we would construct the reference set consisting of all permutations of the age-ordered scores (this is the permutation of 36 things taken 36 at a time, or 36!), compute a test statistic for each member of the set (i.e., for each different order of the 36 scores), and then compute how many values were as extreme or more so than the test statistic for the ordering of the scores actually observed (assuming a one-tailed test).

Sampled permutation is somewhat easier. All we need to do is shuffle (i.e., randomly order) the array of 36 values of Yule's Q repeatedly, using a reliable shuffling algorithm (not all shuffling algorithms are equally reliable; see Castellan, 1992). After each shuffle we compute some test statistic. For the present example we used the slope, but we could have used $R^2$ or its associated $F$ ratio or any other statistic associated with the slope; the results would be the same. Then, after some number of shuffles, we compute the percent of slopes that equal or exceed .0209, the value for the data actually observed. In effect, whether using exact or sampled permutation, we construct a sampling distribution for the test statistic of choice. But neither potentially untenable assumptions nor unjustified approximations are required; the result is an exact probability, or at least an estimate of one.

The exact probabilities that result from sampled permutation are estimates, and each time we run the procedure, the resulting probabilities will vary some. This is hardly problematic because, as Mehta and Patel (1992) noted, with enough runs estimates can be computed to any accuracy desired. Consider the present example. We shuffled the array of 36 Yule's Qs 1,000 times and then computed an exact probability. This procedure was replicated 10 times. Then, based on the 10 values, we computed the mean for the exact probabilities (which was 0.142) along with its 95% confidence intervals (which were .0115 and .0169). Thus, we can be quite confident that the exact probability is less than .02 (or, more exactly, .0169). This is certainly less than the traditional .05.

For this example, the exact probability turned out to be somewhat smaller than the probability based on parametric methods, but whether exact probabilities are more or less significant than other ones is not the point. Their major merit is the confidence we can place in them, free from worry as to whether assumptions are met (Bakeman, Robinson, & Quera, 1996). This seems especially important for those who study unusual populations, which are often associated with relatively small numbers of subjects, unevenly distributed with respect to research factors of interest.

## CONCLUSION

In some cases, when subjects are rare or difficult to observe, studies with small *N*s are unavoidable. Solutions to the small *N* problem do exist and should not necessarily be viewed as statistical patches. Part of the solution lies in considering analytic strategies outside the tradition of group comparisons and analysis of variance models for which small *N* studies rarely meet the required distributional assumptions. As the !Kung infant and students with disabilities studies demonstrate, many interesting questions can be answered without a single ANOVA source table. One alternative to traditional analytic strategies is graphical analysis. Clear, concise graphs allow the simultaneous presentation of information concerning the range, variability, and central tendency of a data set. Graphing only a small number of subjects is advantageous because every data point is presented in a manageable and comprehensible form. When inferential statistics are called for by the research question, we suggest the use of permutation tests. Such empirically based tests are logically appealing and do not require the often unmet distributional assumptions of traditional asymptotic statistics.

The approaches emphasized in this chapter are aimed primarily at the researcher analyzing an interesting data set obtained from a small sample of subjects with language disorders. It should also be noted, however, that a natural outcome of applying the techniques presented in this chapter is the clear and concise presentation of data and results. Such presentations will facilitate communication between researchers in the applied field of language disorders, who are concerned primarily with the description of special populations and the effects of interventions, and basic researchers, whose desire is to mine the rich field of language disorders in an effort to test and expand their theories of language development.

## REFERENCES


Bakeman, R. (1992). *Understanding social science statistics: A spreadsheet approach.* Hillsdale, NJ: Lawrence Erlbaum Associates.

Bakeman, R., Adamson, L.B., Konner, M., & Barr, R.G. (1990). !Kung infancy: The social context of object exploration. *Child Development, 61*, 794–809.

Bakeman, R., McArthur, D., & Quera, V. (1996). Detecting group differences in sequential association using sampled permutations: Log odds, kappa, and phi compared. *Behavior Research Methods, Instruments, and Computers, 28*, 446–457.

Bakeman, R., & Quera, V. (1992). SDIS: A sequential data interchange standard. *Behavior Research Methods, Instruments, and Computers, 24*, 554–559.

Bakeman, R., & Quera, V. (1995a). *Analyzing interaction: Sequential analysis with SDIS and GSEQ.* New York: Cambridge University Press.

Bakeman, R., & Quera, V. (1995b). Log-linear approaches to lag-sequential analysis when consecutive codes may and cannot repeat. *Psychological Bulletin, 118*, 272–284.

Bakeman, R., Robinson, B.F., & Quera, V. (1996). Testing sequential association: Estimating exact *p* values using sampled permutations. *Psychological Methods, 1*, 4–15.

Bates, E., & Applebaum, M. (1994). Methods of studying small samples: Issues and examples. In S.H. Broman & J. Grafman (Eds.), *Atypical cognitive deficits in developmental disorders: Implications for brain function* (pp. 245–280). Hillsdale, NJ: Lawrence Erlbaum Associates.

Blurton Jones, N. (1972). *Ethological studies of child behavior.* Cambridge, England: Cambridge University Press.

Bradley, J.V. (1968). *Distribution-free statistical tests.* Englewood Cliffs, NJ: Prentice Hall.

Castellan, N.J., Jr. (1992). Shuffling arrays: Appearances may be deceiving. *Behavior Research Methods, Instruments, and Computers, 24*, 72–77.

Conger, A.J., & Ward, D.G. (1984). Agreement among 2 × 2 agreement indices. *Educational and Psychological Measurement, 44*, 301–314.

Edgington, E.S. (1987). *Randomization tests* (2nd ed.). New York: Marcel Dekker.

Good, P. (1994). *Permutation tests: A practical guide to resampling methods for testing hypotheses.* New York: Springer-Verlag.

Hays, W.L. (1963). *Statistics.* New York: Holt, Rinehart & Winston.

Keppel, G. (1991). *Design and analysis: A researcher's handbook* (3rd ed.). Englewood Cliffs, NJ: Prentice Hall.

Kratochwill, T.R., & Levin, J.R. (Eds.). (1992). *Single-case research design and analysis: New directions for psychology and education.* Hillsdale, NJ: Lawrence Erlbaum Associates.

Logan, K.R., Bakeman, R., & Keefe, E.B. (in press). Effects of instructional variables on the engaged behavior of students with moderate, severe, and profound disabilities in general education elementary classrooms. *Exceptional Children.*

Logan, K.R., Rankin, D.H., & Bakeman, R. (1994, December). *Engagement levels of students with severe disabilities in regular education classes.* Paper presented at the 21st annual conference of The Association for Persons with Severe Handicaps, Atlanta, GA.

Mehta, C., & Patel, N. (1992). *StatXact: Statistical software for exact nonparametric inference.* Cambridge, MA: Cytel Software.

Morris, C.A., Demsey, S.A., Leonard, C.O., Dilts, C., & Blackburn, B.L. (1988). Natural history of Williams syndrome: Physical characteristics. *Journal of Pediatrics, 113*, 318–326.

Ostrom, C.W. (1990). *Time series analysis: Regression techniques* (2nd ed.). Beverly Hills: Sage Publications.

Quera, V. (1990). A generalized technique to estimate frequency and duration in time sampling. *Behavioral Assessment, 12*, 409–424.

Reynolds. H.T. (1984). *Analysis of nominal data.* Beverly Hills: Sage Publications.

Romski, M.A., Sevcik, R.A., Robinson, B.F., & Bakeman, R. (1994). Adult-directed communications of youth with mental retardation using the system for augmenting language. *Journal of Speech and Hearing Research, 37*, 617–628.

Suen, H.K., & Ary, D. (1989). *Analyzing quantitative behavioral data.* Hillsdale, NJ: Lawrence Erlbaum Associates.

Tufte, E. (1983). *The visual display of quantitative information*. Cheshire, CT: Graphics Press.

Tukey, J.W. (1977). *Exploratory data analysis*. Reading, MA: Addison-Wesley.

Tulkin, S., & Kagan, J. (1972). Mother–infant interaction in the first year of life. *Child Development, 43*, 31–42.

Wainer, H. (1984). How to display data badly. *The American Statistician, 38*, 137–147.

# II

# ATYPICAL DEVELOPMENTAL PATHS AND BASIC ISSUES

# 4

# Developmental Relations Between Cognition and Language

## Evidence from Williams Syndrome

Carolyn B. Mervis and Jacquelyn Bertrand

Some aspects of lexical development follow a universal pattern. For example, children's first object words reliably name basic-level categories, rather than categories at other hierarchical levels. That is, children initially call a Palomino horse by its basic-level name, "horse," rather than by its superordinate-level name (animal) or its subordinate-level name (Palomino). The child considers a wide variety of horses and other closely related types of animals such as donkeys or zebras to be horses. In contrast, other aspects of lexical development follow more variable patterns. One such characteristic is the size of the linguistic unit that children initially treat as a single word. Children who use an analytic strategy focus on units that adults consider single words (e.g., horsie, get). The early vocabularies of children who adopt a holistic strategy

This research was supported by Grant No. HD 29957 from the National Institute of Child Health and Human Development. Portions of this chapter were presented at the 1993 Society for Research in Child Development Conference in New Orleans, Louisiana; at the 1993 Gatlinburg Conference on Research and Theory in Mental Retardation and Developmental Disabilities in Gatlinburg, Tennessee; and at the 1994 National Williams Syndrome Association Professional Conference in La Jolla, California. The authors thank the National Williams Syndrome Association, Dr. Paul Fernhoff, Dr. Virginia Prout, and several local intervention programs for their help in identifying potential participants. The children and parents who have been involved in this project have been most generous with their time and their commitment to the research; the authors are very grateful to all of them. Sharon Armstrong, Jennifer Ayres, Claudia Cardoso-Martins, Sharon Hutchins, Bonnie Klein, Cindy Mervis, Echo Meyer, Byron Robinson, and Natasha Turner were involved in data collection, reduction, and/or analysis.

include a large proportion of phrases treated as single words (e.g., "giddyup-horsie," "I-got-it").

To determine whether a particular aspect of lexical development follows a universal pattern or instead involves alternate paths, groups of participants who vary on potentially relevant characteristics must be studied. Initial studies usually focus on monolingual middle-class children who are acquiring the majority language of the region in which the research is conducted. This initial sample often includes only firstborns. If the children in this sample show a consistent pattern of acquisition of the aspect of lexical development being investigated, then additional studies are likely to be conducted. In these studies, the developmental path(s) of laterborns, children of other social classes, and/or children acquiring a different native language may be considered. The children in all of these studies are likely to have intelligence in the normal range.

An important complementary approach to the search for universals and alternate paths in development focuses on the study of individuals who have mental retardation or learning disabilities (Hodapp & Burack, 1990). This research strategy forms the basis for the work reported in this chapter. Research on individuals with learning difficulties offers two major advantages not available in studies of typical individuals. First, the language development of people with learning problems is by definition slower than the norm. This stretching out of the acquisition process aids in identifying and sequencing the steps of language development and highlights any variability, facilitating the differentiation between universals and alternate paths to particular aspects of lexical competence. If, despite this extended acquisition period, little or no variability is found, the case for a universal path to attainment of that aspect of lexical development is much strengthened. When there is substantial variability in the nature and sequencing of steps in the attainment of a particular aspect of lexical competence, examination of the nature of this variability should facilitate the identification of alternate paths to that component of lexical competence.

The second advantage of research focusing on individuals who have mental retardation or learning disabilities stems from the dissociation between general level of nonlinguistic cognitive development and general level of language development that often occurs in these individuals. Several etiologies (e.g., Down syndrome) have been associated with relative strength in general cognitive development; one etiology (Williams syndrome) has been associated with relative strength in general language development. These differences are important for the study of language universals and alternate paths because many of the previously proposed lexical universals involve relations between specific aspects of language development and specific aspects of cognitive development. Individuals who have substantial differences between level of general language abilities and level of general cognitive abilities are much less likely to show spurious specific links between particular abilities in the two domains. Thus, these individuals provide a strong test of hypotheses involving universal specific links between language and nonlinguistic cognition. Some of these hypothetical universals involve the sequence of acquisition of particular cognitive and lexical abilities. In these cases, researchers have argued that particular cognitive abilities must be present before the acquisition of particular aspects of lexical development. Other hypothetical universals involve the simultaneous acquisition of particular cognitive and lexical abilities that are assumed to be based on the same underlying ability or realization (insight). Individuals who show a large discrepancy between general cognitive and general language abilities offer a compelling test of the universality of sequences and cross-domain relations between specific aspects of cognitive development and specific hypothetically linked aspects of lexical development. Furthermore, in cases in which the data do not support the universality of a particular link between cognitive development and lexical development, the findings could be used to identify alternate paths to that aspect of lexical acquisition.

The research program described in this chapter incorporates these unique advantages of studying individuals with mental retardation or borderline normal intelligence. The etiologies included in our research were selected because they differed in relative strength and weakness of general cognitive abilities and general language abilities, thereby providing a strong test of the generality of five putative universals of lexical development. Acquisition of these components of lexical development takes place during the first 2 years of life for children who are developing typically, yet may continue into the preschool or even the early school-age years for individuals with mild to moderate mental retardation. Individuals with severe or profound mental retardation may never acquire more advanced lexical abilities. The five putative universals are described in Table 1. All of these universals have been shown to hold for individuals who are developing typically and individuals who have Down syndrome. Thus, these universals apply both to individuals whose general levels of cognitive and language development are approximately equivalent (individuals who are developing typically) and to individuals whose general level of cognitive development exceeds their general level of language development (individuals with Down syndrome). An especially important test case remains, however: individuals whose general level of language development is greater than their general level of cognitive development. This test case is best represented by individuals with Williams syndrome. Bellugi and colleagues (e.g., Bellugi, Bihrle, Neville, & Doherty, 1992; Bellugi, Wang, & Jernigan, 1994) showed repeatedly that adolescents and young adults with Williams syndrome have higher levels of general language development than of general cognitive development.

We begin this chapter with a brief description of Williams syndrome and Down syndrome. We then consider whether the relations between general level of cognitive development and general level of language development that have been found for older children and adults in the three populations also obtain

Table 1. Five putative universal cross-domain relations between cognition and language

| Underlying ability or realization | Cognitive manifestation | Lexical manifestation | Order of acquisition |
|---|---|---|---|
| Production of deliberately rhythmic sounds | Rhythmic banging | Canonical or reduplicated babble | Onset at about the same time |
| Establishment of reference | Onset of production of referential pointing gestures | Onset of production of referential labels for objects or actions | Cognitive before lexical |
| Priority of categories based on salient form–function correlations | Initial categories are at the (child-)basic level | Initial object labels refer to (child-)basic categories | Not applicable |
| Parallel realizations:<br>1. All objects belong to a category<br>2. All objects have a name | Onset of spontaneous exhaustive sorting of objects | Onset of vocabulary spurt | Onset at about the same time |
| Parallel realizations:<br>1. All objects belong to a category<br>2. All objects have a name | Onset of spontaneous exhaustive sorting of objects | Onset of ability to fast-map novel object label to object (and other members of the same basic-level category) for which the child did not previously have a name, even when the speaker did not provide a direct connection (e.g., a pointing gesture) between word and object | Onset at about the same time |

during the period of early lexical development. Next, we address the question of whether several putative universal relations between specific aspects of early lexical development and hypothetically linked aspects of early cognitive development hold for children with Williams syndrome. Each of these potential universals was first shown to apply to children who are developing typically. Studies involving children with Down syndrome were then conducted to test the generality of these universals; studies of children with Williams syndrome provide a further test. We conclude by discussing the special contribution of studies of populations with contrasting etiologies to theories and models of lexical development.

## BACKGROUND: WILLIAMS SYNDROME AND DOWN SYNDROME

Williams syndrome is a rare (1 in 20,000 live births) genetic disorder affecting both the central nervous system and connective tissue. Williams syndrome is caused by a hemizygous submicroscopic deletion of chromosome 7q11.23, including the *elastin* gene (Ewart et al., 1993) and the *LIM-kinase* 1 gene (Frangiskakis et al., 1996). The disorder is characterized by unusual facial characteristics, specific heart defects, and mental retardation or learning disabilities (e.g., Jones & Smith, 1975; Williams, Barratt, & Lowe, 1961). Case studies and clinical descriptions of individuals with Williams syndrome (e.g., Burn, 1986; Morris, Dempsey, Leonard, Dilts, & Blackburn, 1988; Morris, Thomas, & Greenberg, 1993) often indicate that language level is higher than would be expected for the degree of mental retardation. Bellugi and colleagues (e.g., Bellugi, Marks, Bihrle, & Sabo, 1988; Bellugi et al., 1992, 1994; Rossen, Klima, Bihrle, & Bellugi, 1996) conducted a series of studies of adolescents and young adults who have Williams syndrome. The results of these studies indicate that obtained lexical and grammatical levels exceed the levels expected for the participants' MAs (mental ages). This pattern held for both comprehension and production.

Down syndrome is a much more common (1 in 800 live births) genetic disorder, resulting from a trisomy of chromosome 21. Down syndrome is characterized by a particular constellation of facial characteristics, specific heart defects, and mental retardation. One of the most robust findings of studies of the development of older children and adults with Down syndrome is their difficulty with language relative to other aspects of cognition (see Fowler, 1990; Gibson, 1978, 1991; Rosenberg & Abbeduto, 1993, for reviews). The developmental asynchrony between language and cognition is characteristic of both the lexicon and grammar, although difficulties with grammar are more extreme. Both comprehension and production are affected. These discrepancies between language and MA are apparent in most individuals with Down syndrome by 5 years of age (Lynch & Eilers, 1991; Miller, 1992a,b).

## RELATIONS BETWEEN GENERAL LEVELS OF COGNITIVE DEVELOPMENT AND LANGUAGE DEVELOPMENT

### Toddlers and Young Preschoolers with Williams Syndrome or Down Syndrome

As indicated in our brief review of the literature, contrasting patterns of level of general cognitive abilities and level of general language abilities have been identified for older children and adults with Williams syndrome or Down syndrome. For individuals with Williams syndrome, language abilities constitute a relative strength. In contrast, for individuals with Down syndrome, nonlinguistic cognitive abilities constitute a relative strength. To confirm that individuals with Williams syndrome or Down syndrome provide important test cases for the consideration of universals and alternate paths to early lexical competence, however, we must demonstrate that these same patterns of relations between general level of language development and general level of cognitive development hold for toddlers and young preschoolers (individuals who are in the early stages of acquiring a lexicon).

To determine if the mature pattern of relative strengths and weaknesses is already evident for toddlers and young preschoolers with Williams syndrome or Down syndrome, we considered children's performance on the Mental Scale of the Bayley Scales of Infant Development (BSID; Bayley, 1969). Six toddlers with Williams syndrome (five girls, one boy), six toddlers with Down syndrome (three girls, three boys), and six children who were developing typically (three girls, three boys) were followed longitudinally. Each child was tested on the BSID 3–5 times, at intervals of approximately 6 months. The parents of all of the children had completed high school; the majority of the parents of each group of children had attended at least 1 year of college. All of the families were lower-middle class to upper-middle class, except for the family of one girl with Williams syndrome whose family's income was below the U.S. government poverty line. The ranges of CAs (chronological ages) and MAs for each group of children during the period of study are indicated in Table 2.

The Mental Scale of the BSID (Bayley, 1969) is the most commonly ad-

Table 2. Participant description: Bayley study

| | Participant group | | |
|---|---|---|---|
| | Williams syndrome | Down syndrome | Typically developing |
| CA (months) | | | |
| Start range | 13–26 | 17–19 | 9 |
| End range | 36–44 | 30–40 | 24 |
| Number of months followed | 16–26 | 13–21 | 15 |
| MA (months) | | | |
| Mean | 18.71 | 18.01 | 20.81 |
| Range | 6.25–30+ | 8.10–30+ | 10.70–30+ |

ministered measure of intelligence for children whose MAs are 30 months or less. The BSID is particularly appropriate for differentiating between language and other cognitive abilities because the language items on this assessment tap specifically linguistic skills rather than cognitive and language skills simultaneously (as do most of the verbal tasks on IQ tests designed for older children or adults). Thus, MA as measured by the BSID can reasonably be divided into language and nonlanguage cognitive components. Items involving syllable production, linguistic imitation, comprehension of both single words and multiword utterances, and production of both single words and two-word utterances were considered language items. The remaining items were considered to be nonlanguage. These included measures of nonverbal reasoning (object permanence, means–ends relations), visual-motor integration (form boards, peg boards, block construction, drawing), and nonlinguistic imitation.

To compare individual children's performance on the language and nonlanguage items of the BSID, we considered all of the items from the child's basal (10 items before the first item failed) through the last item the child passed. This determination was made separately for each time the BSID was administered to the child. For each assessment, we then determined the number of language items attempted and the number of language items passed, and the number of nonlanguage items attempted and the number of nonlanguage items passed. To compare general level of language abilities to general level of nonlanguage abilities, we calculated the proportion of language items passed to language items attempted (language ratio) and the proportion of nonlanguage items passed to nonlanguage items attempted (nonlanguage ratio) for each assessment. We then determined the mean difference between language ratio and nonlanguage ratio separately for each child. Finally, we determined the mean difference across children separately for each of the three participant groups.

The results of this analysis are illustrated in Figure 1. For the toddlers and young preschoolers with Williams syndrome, the mean difference between the language and nonlanguage ratios was $+.239$, indicating that general language abilities exceeded general cognitive abilities. The toddlers and young preschoolers with Down syndrome showed the opposite pattern. For these children, the mean difference between ratios was $-.210$, indicating that general cognitive abilities exceeded general language abilities. There was no overlap in the distributions of ratios for the children with Williams syndrome and those with Down syndrome. For the toddlers who were developing typically, the mean difference between ratios was $+.005$, indicating that general cognitive abilities tended to be at about the same level as general language abilities. These results, in conjunction with previous findings regarding older children, adolescents, and young adults from the three target populations, indicate that each of the participant groups shows a different intellectual profile, which is consistent from early childhood through adulthood.

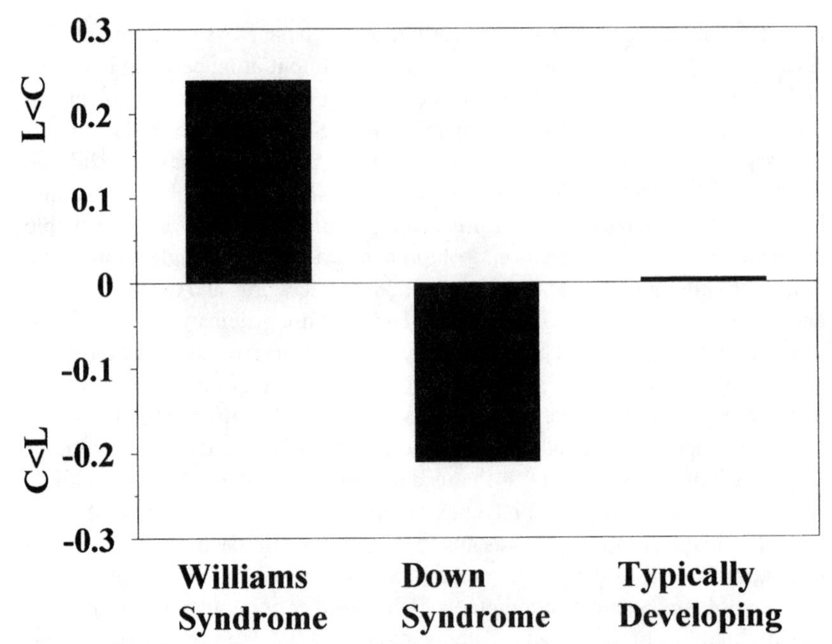


Figure 1. Relative strengths of general cognitive (C) abilities and general language (L) abilities as measured by the BSID for children with Williams syndrome, children with Down syndrome, and children who are developing typically.

## UNIVERSALS AND ALTERNATE PATHS IN EARLY LEXICAL DEVELOPMENT

The results of our analysis of children's performance on the BSID indicated that the contrasting cognitive profiles of the three groups are evident even during the early period of lexical development. For toddlers with Williams syndrome, general language abilities are better than general cognitive abilities. For toddlers with Down syndrome, general cognitive abilities are better than general language abilities. For toddlers who are developing typically, general language abilities and general cognitive abilities are at equivalent levels. Given these contrasting cognitive profiles, it is clear that young children with Williams syndrome or Down syndrome provide especially important test cases for considerations of universals and alternate paths to early lexical competence.

In particular, the typical process of early lexical development includes a number of apparently specific links between particular cognitive abilities and particular lexical abilities (refer again to Table 1). These cognitive and lexical abilities are eventually mastered by almost all children with Down syndrome or Williams syndrome. If children with Down syndrome and children with Williams syndrome evidenced the same specific links between particular aspects of cognitive development and lexical development as do children who are developing typically, then one's confidence in the universality of these links would be greatly increased. At the same time, if children with Down syndrome or Williams syndrome did not evidence these links, then examination of the development of these children could identify viable alternate paths to these aspects of early lexical development.

In this chapter, we consider five specific links between particular aspects of early cognitive development and early lexical development. Each of these links already has been shown to hold for both children who are developing typically and children with Down syndrome. To determine if these links also hold for children with Williams syndrome, we consider data from two cohorts of children who have been involved in longitudinal studies in our laboratory. The first cohort consists of the six children with Williams syndrome who were included in the Bayley analysis. The second cohort includes four younger children with Williams syndrome (one girl, three boys). Parental education levels were the same as in the first cohort: All of the parents had finished high school, and most had attended at least some college. All of the families were middle class. Summary information about each cohort, including CA range during this study, DQ/IQ range, and number of months followed for this study, is provided in Table 3.

## Basic Procedure

The basic procedure for this study was straightforward. Four of the children in the first cohort and all of the children in the second cohort were seen at least monthly. The remaining children in the first cohort were seen on an irregular schedule, but at least every 4 months. Each session included a 30-minute period in which the child and a parent played with a set of toys we provided. This play session was videotaped and later transcribed. If both parents were available, the child often participated in two play sessions, one with each parent.

In addition, parents completed two self-report measures of their child's language development: the MacArthur Communicative Development Inventories (CDI; Fenson et al., 1993) and a vocabulary checklist we developed for assessing comprehension and production of subordinate-level object names (e.g., beach ball, soccer ball, football) and the basic-level names (e.g., ball) under which the subordinate-level names were subsumed. The CDI served as a standardized measure of early language and gestural development. There are two forms of this measure. The Words and Gestures form was normed on children ages 8–16 months who were developing typically. This form includes a 396-

Table 3. Participant description: longitudinal cohorts of children with Williams syndrome

| | | CA range (months) | | | |
|---|---|---|---|---|---|
| Cohort | *N* | Start | End[a] | DQ/IQ range | Number of months followed[a] |
| 1 | 6 | 13–26 | 44–48 | <50–75 | 18–35 |
| 2 | 4 | 4–20 | 27–40 | <50–81 | 13–28 |

[a]For the data reported in this chapter, we have continued to follow five of the six children in the first cohort (current ages 5;5–7;0) and all of the children in the second cohort.

word vocabulary checklist assessing comprehension and production and also several measures of gestural development. The Words and Sentences form was normed on children ages 16–30 months who were developing typically. This form includes a 680-word vocabulary checklist assessing production and also several measures of grammatical development.

Parents were asked to complete a subset of these forms beginning when their child was 12 months old or at the start of the study if the child was already at least 12 months old. Initially, parents completed the gesture portions of the Words and Gestures form and a modified version of the 680-word vocabulary checklist included in the Words and Sentences form. Unlike the original version, the modified checklist assessed both comprehension and production. At the first session in which parents completed the modified CDI vocabulary checklist, one of the researchers explained how the checklist was to be marked. The researcher emphasized that words should be marked as comprehended only if the child appeared to understand the word in multiple situations or with regard to multiple referents. Words were to be marked as produced only if the child said the word spontaneously (not just in imitation of another person). The multiple situation/multiple referent rule also applied to production. Parents also were told that if the child did not use a particular word in a manner approximating that used by adults, the child's extension should be noted next to the relevant word on the forms. The researcher provided examples of this type of situation found in previous studies (e.g., "Coke" used to refer to all types of carbonated beverages, "soda" used to refer only to colas, "hello" used only to refer to telephones). During subsequent sessions, the researcher summarized these instructions before asking the parent to complete the vocabulary checklist. While the parent filled out the forms, one of the researchers was available to answer any questions the parent had.

Parents began to complete the subordinate vocabulary checklist when their child was between 15 and 24 months old, depending on the child's language comprehension abilities. Parents were given the same instructions for completion of this checklist as they had received for the CDI vocabulary checklist. Once the child began to combine words and/or to use morphology (e.g., plural -s, progressive -ing) productively, the parents were asked to complete the grammar sections of the Words and Sentences form of the CDI.

Some play sessions also included assessments of general development. The object permanence and means–ends subscales of the Uzgiris and Hunt (1975) measure of sensorimotor development were administered at every visit until the child had passed all items. The BSID (Bayley, 1969) was administered at the first visit and twice a year thereafter, at the visits closest to the child's birthday and half-birthday. When the second edition of the BSID (Bayley, 1993) became available, children were given both forms. Beginning at age 2½ years, children who were functioning at an appropriate developmental level were given the Differential Ability Scales (DAS; Elliott, 1990) and the Peabody Picture Vocabulary Test–Revised (PPVT–R; Dunn & Dunn, 1981) at the same visits as the BSID. In many cases, a second session was needed to complete the standardized testing. This session was scheduled as close to the initial session as possible.

### Canonical Babbling and Rhythmic Banging

The first potential universal link involves the onset of rhythmic hand banging and rhythmic (canonical or reduplicated) babbling. Researchers have argued that these two milestones should appear at about the same time because they reflect parallel manifestations of rhythmic behaviors (Cobo-Lewis, Oller, Lynch, & Levine, 1995). Rhythmic hand banging is a cognitive manifestation of rhythmic behavior, and rhythmic babbling is a linguistic manifestation. Both these behaviors appear before the onset of comprehension and production of words. The onset of rhythmic babble is considered a very important step in the language acquisition process. The rhythm of canonical babble fits the syllable patterns of mature speech. Researchers have argued that parents change the way they talk to their infants once canonical babble begins, and these changes likely facilitate the child's acquisition of an initial vocabulary.

***Background*** This relation between the onset of rhythmic babbling and rhythmic hand banging has been considered in two studies. The results of both studies are consistent with a link between the two abilities. Levine, Fishman, Oller, Lynch, and Basinger (1991) considered the development of three groups of infants: typically developing full-term, preterm, and Down syndrome. All three groups showed the same pattern of results: Rhythmic hand banging and canonical babbling emerged at about the same time. In a more extensive analysis, Cobo-Lewis et al. (1995) considered the early motor and vocal development of infants who were developing typically and infants who had Down syndrome. Once again, rhythmic hand banging and rhythmic babbling emerged at about the same time. Onsets were slightly delayed (by about 2 weeks on average) for the infants with Down syndrome.

***Infants with Williams Syndrome*** The onsets of rhythmic babble and rhythmic hand banging occur during the first year of life for both children who are developing typically and children with Down syndrome. Assuming that the onsets are within the same time frame for children with Williams syndrome, obtaining data on these milestones within a research setting will be very difficult for this population for two reasons. First, most children with Williams syndrome are not diagnosed during their first year of life. Second, the children who are diagnosed early almost always have severe heart disease, and most are too ill to participate in behavioral research projects during that first year.

Five of the six children in the first cohort were at least 11 months old when they were diagnosed with Williams syndrome. As expected, all five children were already producing both rhythmic babble and rhythmic hand banging before entry into our study. The sixth child was diagnosed with Williams syndrome at age 2 months. However, she was very ill for more than a year, and she did not enter our study until age 21 months, when she already produced both rhythmic babble and rhythmic hand banging. One child in the second cohort was not diagnosed until he was more than 1 year old. At the time he entered the study, he also had attained both rhythmic milestones. The three remaining children, who all had severe heart disease, were diagnosed at a very young age. One child entered the study at age 14 months, shortly after he had heart surgery, and at that time had demonstrated both rhythmic babble and rhythmic hand banging. The other two children were well enough to begin participation in our study shortly after diagnosis. One child entered the study at age 4 months, the other child at age 5 months. We were able to obtain data on the attainment of both rhythmic milestones for these two children.

To determine the onsets of rhythmic babble and rhythmic hand banging, we had available both observational data from our videotaped play sessions and parental report data. (Parents were asked to record any new behaviors their infants produced; these behaviors were discussed at each visit. Many parents telephoned us between visits to report new behaviors.) The data from the two sources were consistent; for both children, the parents had noted the onset of the milestone sometime during the 4-week interval between the last visit in which the milestone had not been observed on our videotapes and the first visit in which the milestone was demonstrated on our videotapes. Results indicated that for both children, the two rhythmic milestones were acquired at about the same time. Jenny demonstrated both canonical babble and rhythmic hand banging at age 7 months; Thomas demonstrated both rhythmic milestones at age 8 months. Thus, the available data for infants with Williams syndrome are consistent with the universality of a link between the onsets of rhythmic babble and rhythmic hand banging.

### Pointing and the Onset of Referential Production of Object Names

The second potential universal link between a specific aspect of cognitive development and a specific aspect of lexical development involves the acquisition of the ability to make reference. The cognitive manifestation of this ability is referential pointing; the lexical manifestation is referential productive language (e.g., "doggie," "bottle"). In this case, the link is expected to be sequential, with the attainment of the cognitive ability preceding the onset of the lexical ability.

***Background*** The sequential ordering of referential pointing and referential labeling is one of the most robust findings regarding the transition to language. Infants express communicative intentions nonverbally, by pointing, before expressing them verbally, by labeling. This apparently universal sequential relation is routinely acknowledged in textbooks on the development of communication or language (e.g., Adamson, 1995; Lane & Molyneaux, 1992; Messer, 1994). The relation presumably obtains because the cognitive manifestation of reference (pointing) provides the child with an especially useful way to determine the reference of the words he or she hears. Adults use pointing gestures to indicate the referent of object labels. Until the child is able to follow these pointing gestures, he or she will have extreme difficulty determining the intended referent of the adult's word. In addition, children use pointing gestures to elicit labels from adults for particular objects.

As indicated in Table 4, the sequential relation between the onset of pointing and the onset of referential production of words has been shown for a range of native languages, for both children who are developing typically and children with disabilities. This sequence of acquisition has been described most extensively for typically developing infants who were acquiring English as their native language. The results of these studies indicate that at about the age of 9 or 10 months, infants who are developing typically begin to comprehend simple pointing gestures, particularly pointing gestures aimed at objects that are in front of (Murphy & Messer, 1977) or near the infants (Lempers, 1976). At about 10 months, infants also begin to produce referential points (Leung & Rheingold, 1981; Murphy & Messer, 1977) and may look at their mother during or after pointing at an object (Franco & Butterworth, 1991, cited in Messer, 1994). The value of pointing for eliciting object names from adults was demonstrated in a study by Masur (1982), who found that when infants pointed at an object, mothers were very likely to respond by naming the object.

The onset of referential production of words is difficult to pinpoint based on the available literature because the first word produced by most children is nonreferential (context bound; see summary in Barrett, 1989). Thus, age at production of first word (a milestone often noted in the literature) is unlikely to be the same as age of production of first referential word. Researchers are much less likely to report age at production of first referential word. For most children, however, the onset of referential production of words occurs early in the second year of life (Adamson, 1995). Children's first referential words are almost always object names (Harris, Barrett, Jones, & Brookes, 1988).

***Children with Williams Syndrome*** To determine the onsets of referential pointing and referential object labeling, we had available both observational data from the play sessions and parental report data. Three types of ob-

Table 4. Studies documenting pointing before labeling

| Population | Native language | Source |
|---|---|---|
| Typical development | English | Messer (1994) (summary) |
| | Hebrew | Dromi (1993) |
| | Italian | Bates et al. (1975, 1979) |
| | Norwegian | Smith et al. (1988) |
| | British Sign Language | Griffith (1990) |
| Prelingually deaf | American Sign Language | Bonvillian et al. (1990) |
| | Italian Sign Language | Caselli and Volterra (1990) |
| Down syndrome | English | Greenwald and Leonard (1979) |
| | Norwegian | Smith et al. (1988) |
| Severe mental retardation | English | Koenig and Mervis (1984) |

servational data were used: 1) spontaneous production of referential object labels (or any other referential words), 2) spontaneous production of pointing gestures, and 3) comprehension of maternal pointing gestures. Parental report data were obtained from the CDI, which includes questions regarding both the production of pointing gestures and the production of words. Data were available for five of the six children in the first cohort. The remaining child had begun to produce referential language several months before the first session and was also able to produce pointing gestures. (Based on maternal report, order of onset of production of referential words and production of pointing gestures was the same as reported below for the other children with Williams syndrome.) Data also were available for three children in the second cohort.

The observational data were quite clear. The five children in the first cohort and one of the children in the second cohort produced at least one object label referentially during the first visit. None of the children produced any pointing gestures. Another child in the second cohort was 5 months old at the first visit and did not produce either pointing gestures or referential object labels at that time. However, she too began to produce referential object labels before producing pointing gestures. A third child in the second cohort had not produced either a pointing gesture or a referential object label during a laboratory visit. However, his mother reported the onset of both abilities. These data contrast strongly with those previously reported for a wide range of populations, all of whom acquired referential pointing before referential word production.

Perhaps the children with Williams syndrome were not producing pointing gestures simply because they had a specific problem with the motor component of pointing. To address this possibility, we considered whether the children were able to comprehend the pointing gestures produced by their mothers during the first play session in which the child produced a word referentially. Children were considered to comprehend a pointing gesture if they looked at the object to which their mother was pointing. During the play session, the mothers produced a mean of 8.7 pointing gestures (range: 2–21). Most of these pointing gestures (79%) were directed at objects in front of and within 2 feet of the child. This is the type of pointing gesture that should be easiest for a child to comprehend. Nevertheless, no child responded appropriately to any pointing gesture. The children either looked at the mother (if she called the child's name at the same time as she pointed) or ignored the gesture entirely. These data show that the onset of referential labeling before the onset of referential pointing could not be attributed to difficulties with the motoric component of production of pointing gestures.

Parental report data were available from the CDI for the production of both referential words and pointing gestures. For the seven children for whom we had relevant observational data, the parental report data showed exactly the same pattern. All seven children were reported to produce object words referentially before producing pointing gestures. Based on the parental report data, three children in the first cohort and one child in the second cohort either had begun to talk within the 2 months before the first visit or were not yet talking at the time of the first visit. For these four children we were able to determine the approximate interval between onset of referential production of words and onset of production of pointing gestures. For all four children, the onset of both milestones as measured by the observational data was the same as the onset as measured by parental report. The mean interval between the onset of referential production of object labels and production of pointing gestures was 6 months (range: 4–7 months).

The mother of the third child in the second cohort reported that her child has attained both reference-making abilities. According to maternal report, this child began to produce referential pointing gestures a few weeks before producing his first referential word. This order of acquisition is consistent with the putative universal, but the time interval between the onsets of the two abilities was much smaller than has been found in previous studies of children who did not have Williams syndrome.

In summary, most children with Williams syndrome show the opposite pattern from all of the other groups of children who have been studied, with regard to the relation between the onset of referential pointing and the onset of referential word production. Children with Williams syndrome reliably produce referential words before either producing or comprehending pointing gestures. Apparently, referential pointing skills are not necessary for the onset of referential language development. Either the knowledge that underlies comprehension and production of pointing gestures is not necessary for the onset of referential production of words, or there must be an alternate path to this knowledge. These possibilities are considered further at the end of this chapter.

### Priority of Basic-Level Categories: Labels and Play Patterns

The third potential universal link between a specific aspect of cognitive development and a specific aspect of lexical development concerns children's early categories. Objects can be categorized at a variety of hierarchical levels. For example, the same object can be a whiffle ball (subordinate-level category), a ball (basic level), or a toy (superordinate level). The basic level is more fundamental (cognitively efficient) than the others (Rosch, Mervis, Gray, Johnson, & Boyes-Braem, 1976). The basic level is the most general level at which category members have similar overall shapes and at which a person uses similar motor actions for interacting with category members. Although categories at every hierarchical level are based on form–function correlations, these correlations are most apparent at the basic level. Thus, basic-level categories are the categories most differentiated from each other. Because of the salience of basic-level categories, children's first object categories should be basic-level categories. The third potentially universal link involves this relation. In particular, children's initial functional play patterns (cognitive manifestation of categorization) and the initial extensions of the object labels that they comprehend and produce (linguistic manifestation of categorization) should converge at the basic level.

***Background*** The hierarchical levels of children's early functional play patterns and early object labels have been considered in a longitudinal investigation of the early lexical development of children who were developing typically and children with Down syndrome (Mervis, 1984, 1987, 1988, 1990). In this study, play patterns and labels were considered for two types of objects for which play patterns could be characterized relatively straightforwardly: balls and other spherical objects, and cars and other vehicles with four or more wheels. Results indicated that both groups of children played with all the spherical objects (e.g., balls, spherical banks, sleigh bells) in the same manner, by rolling them. Similarly, both groups of children initially treated all vehicles with four or more wheels equivalently, by pushing them along, often accompanied by engine noises. Thus, these were child-basic (cognitive) categories. The children's initial labeling patterns matched their play patterns. "Car" was initially comprehended and produced in relation to cars, trucks, and buses. "Ball" was initially comprehended and produced in relation to spherical objects, whether or not adults would consider them to be balls.

For many categories, nonverbal play patterns are difficult to observe or evaluate, especially in the laboratory. However, the prediction that basic-level categories should be acquired before categories at other hierarchical levels may still be addressed by considering the lexical manifestation of categorization, object labels. The results of a large number of diary studies of children's early vocabularies indicate that almost all of the labels produced by typically developing children age 24 months or less were names for basic-level categories (see summary in Mervis, 1983). These children were acquiring a variety of native languages, including English, German, French, and Russian. Gillham (1979) presented early vocabulary lists for four children with Down syndrome who were acquiring English as their native language. All of the object labels produced by these children were names for basic-level categories.

In these diary studies, the extension of the children's words was not reported. Thus, it is an assumption that terms used by adults as basic-level labels also were used by children in that manner. Mervis (1984, 1987) tested the extensions of the names of the toys included in the play sessions in her longitudinal study of the early lexical development of children who were developing typically and children with Down syndrome. Results of both comprehension and production tests indicated that object labels that were basic level for adults were also (child-) basic level for the children. Furthermore, in all cases, children acquired the basic-level name for a play session toy before acquiring a name for it at either the subordinate or the superordinate level.

***Children with Williams Syndrome*** To determine if the early play patterns and early object labels produced by children with Williams syndrome converged at the basic level, we had available both observational data and parental report data. Observational data included the videotapes of the play sessions and notes made regarding the child's independent play or play with a researcher while the parent completed the CDI and subordinate checklist or talked with another researcher. Parental report data included responses to the CDI and the subordinate checklist. Parents were asked to note their child's extension next to any word on either the CDI or the subordinate checklist that the child used in a manner substantially different from the way an adult would. Data were available from all of the children in both cohorts.

We were able to compare play and labeling patterns for the same two types of objects that Mervis (1984, 1987, 1988, 1990) had considered for toddlers who were developing typically and toddlers with Down syndrome: balls and other spherical objects, and cars and other vehicles with four or more wheels. All 10 children with Williams syndrome played with the spherical objects (e.g., balls, spherical candles, sleigh bells) in the same manner, by rolling them. The children did not try to roll any of the nonspherical toys. Thus, these children's play patterns indicated that they had formed a child-basic ball category. The children's lexical behavior also indicated that they had formed a child-basic ball category. All of the children comprehended "ball" in reference to a variety of spherical objects, whether or not adults would have considered these objects to be balls, but did not comprehend "ball" in reference to objects of other shapes. Eight of the ten children produced the word "ball." These children showed the same extension pattern in production as they had in comprehension.

The results for the four-wheeled vehicles were similar. All 10 children treated the four-wheeled vehicles (e.g., car, truck) equivalently, by pushing them along, often accompanied by engine noises. The children did not interact in this manner with any of the other available toys. These play patterns indicated the formation of a child-basic car category. The children's lexical behavior was consistent. The nine children (six from the first cohort and three from the second) who comprehended "car" did so in relation to a variety of four-wheeled vehicles, whether or not adults would have considered them to be cars, but did not comprehend the word in relation to other types of objects. Seven of the nine children produced the word "car." These children showed the same extension pattern in production as in comprehension. These findings indicate that for both ball and car, functional play patterns and object labels converge at the child-basic level of categorization.

We were not able to study functional play patterns for other types of objects. However, we were able to address the question of the hierarchical level of children's early object labels for a very wide range of objects. To determine if the children with Williams syndrome comprehended the basic-level name for an object before comprehending its subordinate-level name, we compiled a list of all the subordinate-level labels that a particular child comprehended. If a parent indicated that the child's extension for a particular word was different from adults', the hierarchical level we assigned to that word was based on the level appropriate for the set of referents the parent indicated. All of the children in the first cohort and two of the children in the second cohort comprehended at least one subordinate-level name.

To determine if children with Williams syndrome comprehended the basic-level names of objects before comprehending their subordinate-level name, we compared the dates of first comprehension of each subordinate label and the corresponding basic-level label. Word pairs were divided into three types: 1) basic-level label comprehended before subordinate-level label, 2) subordinate label comprehended before basic-level label, and 3) order of acquisition unclear (basic and subordinate labels acquired in the same month). The proportions of basic–subordinate label pairs of each of the three types are indicated in Figure 2. As shown in this figure, children almost always comprehended the basic-level name for an object before comprehending its subordinate-level name. In all cases in which a child comprehended the subordinate label before the basic label, the subordinate category was atypical of its basic-level category. Two subordinate categories were involved: toothbrush and school bus.

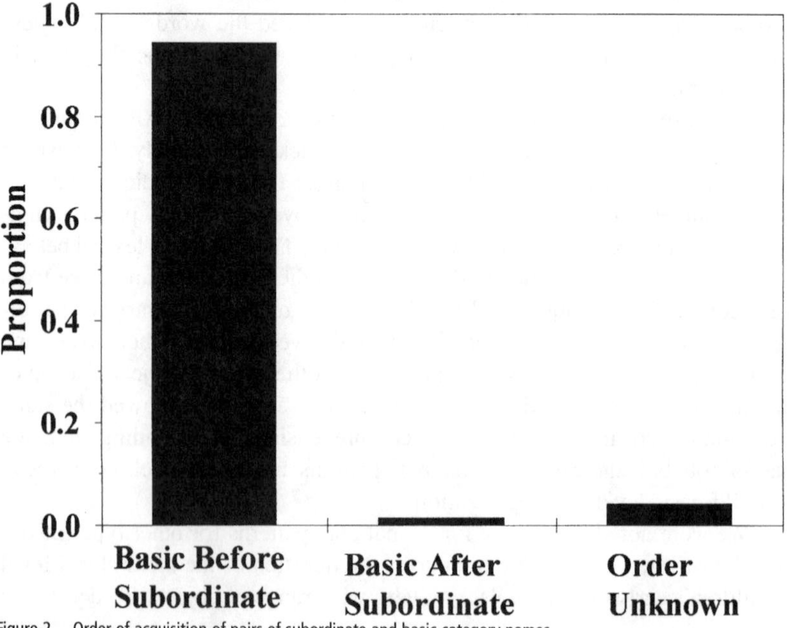


Figure 2. Order of acquisition of pairs of subordinate and basic category names.

Several superordinate category labels were included on either the CDI or the subordinate checklist. All six children in the first cohort and one of the children in the second cohort comprehended at least one superordinate-level label. To determine the order of acquisition of basic and superordinate labels, we compared the dates of first comprehension of each superordinate-level label and the first basic-level label comprehended for a member of that superordinate category. For example, if the first type of animal for which a child comprehended a basic-level label was a dog, then the date of first comprehension of "animal" would be compared with the date of first comprehension of "dog." In all cases, the superordinate-level label was not comprehended until after the child had comprehended at least one basic-level label for a category subsumed by that superordinate. In summary, the nonverbal play patterns and object label comprehension patterns of the children with Williams syndrome indicated the same priority of basic-level categories for these children as for children who were developing typically and children with Down syndrome.

### Spontaneous Exhaustive Sorting and the Vocabulary Spurt

The fourth potential universal link between a specific aspect of cognitive development and a specific aspect of lexical development involves the relation between the onset of spontaneous exhaustive sorting of objects and the onset of the vocabulary spurt. Gopnik and Meltzoff (1987, 1992) argued that these two onsets should occur at about the same time because they express parallel insights. The cognitive insight is that all objects belong to some category; the parallel linguistic insight is that all objects have a name.

***Background*** There has been little research addressing the proposed specific link between spontaneous exhaustive sorting and the vocabulary spurt. Nevertheless, this relation has been found to hold both for children who were developing typically and children with Down syndrome. The availability of the cognitive insight is assessed by an object sorting task. Eight objects (four from each of two basic-level categories, for example, four dogs, four blocks) are arranged randomly in front of the child. The experimenter then places his or her open hands in front of the child and tells the child, "Put them where they go. Fix them up." Gopnik and Meltzoff (1987, 1992) documented three developmental levels of categorization in children's responses to this task. Level 3, the most advanced level, is characterized by exhaustive sorting, the deliberate and spontaneous separation of the two types of objects into two groups. Children who demonstrate this spontaneous exhaustive categorization are considered to have the insight that all objects belong to some category (Gopnik & Meltzoff, 1987, 1992).

Gopnik and Meltzoff (1987, 1992) argued that the onset of the vocabulary spurt signifies that the child has acquired the insight that all objects have a name. When children first begin to talk, rate of acquisition of new words is very slow, perhaps one or two words every month or so (Adamson, 1995). Rate of acquisition of new words initially increases gradually. Eventually, however, rate of acquisition appears to shift dramatically, signaling the onset of the vocabulary spurt. Criteria for this onset are generally expressed in terms of number of new words produced in a given time period. For example, Gopnik and Meltzoff (1987) considered children to have attained a vocabulary spurt if they acquired 10 new object words in a 3-week period. Goldfield and Reznick (1990) used a criterion of 10 new words in a 2½-week period. Mervis and Bertrand (1994) used a criterion of 10 new words, including at least 5 object labels, in a 2-week period. For children who are developing typically, rate of vocabulary acquisition once the spurt begins is so rapid that the amount of time between when a child meets the most liberal criterion for the spurt and when he or she meets the most conservative criterion is likely to be no more than a few weeks (Robinson, 1995). Children with Down syndrome also evidence this pattern of slow initial rate of acquisition followed by a sharp increase in rate of new words acquired (Miller 1992a,b).

To test their prediction that the onsets of spontaneous exhaustive sorting and the vocabulary spurt would occur at about the same time, Gopnik and Meltzoff conducted two studies of typically developing toddlers acquiring English as their native language, one longitudinal (1987) and one cross-sectional (1992). As they expected, there was a close temporal relation between the onsets. This relation could not be attributed simply to general relations regarding age or cognitive level. In particular, there was no relation between the onset of Piagetian Stage 6 means–ends skills (as assessed by the Uzgiris & Hunt, 1975, scales) and either the onset of spontaneous exhaustive categorization or the onset of the vocabulary spurt. The relation between the onset of the vocabulary spurt and attainment of advanced Piagetian Stage 6 object permanence skills was less strong than that between the onset of the vocabulary spurt and the onset of spontaneous exhaustive categorization in the longitudinal study and was nonsignificant in the cross-sectional study. The same pattern of results was found in a study of typically developing toddlers acquiring Korean as their native language (Gopnik & Meltzoff, 1993).

Mervis and Bertrand (1994) replicated Gopnik and Meltzoff's (1987, 1992, 1993) findings in two studies of typically developing children between the ages of 16 and 20 months who were acquiring English as their native language. Again, a close temporal relation between the onset of spontaneous exhaustive sorting and the onset of the vocabulary spurt was found. The children who had not yet had a vocabulary spurt (as assessed by vocabulary size on the CDI and parental report of a dramatic increase in rate of new word learning) were followed longitudinally until they did evidence a spurt. At that time, the sorting task was repeated. Almost all of the children demonstrated Level 3 categorization. Mervis and Bertrand (1995) replicated the cross-sectional part of this study with a group of children with Down syndrome between the ages of 29 and 42 months who were acquiring English as their native language. All but one of the children with Down syndrome fit one of two patterns: Either the children had had a vocabulary spurt and were able to spontaneously sort exhaustively, or they had not had a vocabulary spurt and were not able to sort exhaustively.

***Children with Williams Syndrome*** To determine if this close temporal relation between the onset of the vocabulary spurt and the onset of spontaneous exhaustive sorting also held for young children with Williams syndrome, we identified the onsets of each of these abilities for the children in our longitudinal study. Spontaneous exhaustive sorting was assessed regularly, beginning with the visit during which the child produced his or her first referential word. Gopnik and Meltzoff's (1987) task was used. Onset of the vocabulary spurt was assessed based on parental responses to the CDI. During this period, many of the children were seen every 2 weeks. For these children, the same criteria were used for the onset of the vocabulary spurt as in the Mervis and Bertrand (1994) study. For children who were seen less frequently, the Mervis and Bertrand (1994) criteria were adapted to take into account the longer time period. The parents of all of the children who evidenced a vocabulary spurt commented spontaneously that their child's rate of acquisition of new words had shifted dramatically. For all these children, the session at which the parent volunteered this comment was the same one in which the child met the CDI criterion for a vocabulary spurt. All six of the children in the first cohort and one child in the second cohort showed both a vocabulary spurt and spontaneous exhaustive sorting of objects.

In contrast to the children who had been studied previously, none of the children with Williams syndrome first evidenced a vocabulary spurt and spontaneous exhaustive sorting of objects at about the same age. Five of the six children in the first cohort and the child in the second cohort evidenced a vocabulary spurt before demonstrating spontaneous exhaustive sorting. The gap between the onset of the two abilities ranged from 6 months to more than 1 year. The remaining child in the first cohort evidenced spontaneous exhaustive sorting of objects 5 months before her vocabulary spurt. These data make it clear that the developmental patterns of the children with Williams syndrome do not fit the hypothesized specific temporal link between the onsets of the vocabulary spurt and of spontaneous exhaustive sorting. This relation clearly is not universal. Possible reasons for the nonuniversality of this relation are discussed later in this chapter.

### Spontaneous Exhaustive Sorting and Fast Mapping of Object Labels

The fifth potential universal link between a specific aspect of cognitive development and a specific aspect of lexical development also involves the onset of spontaneous exhaustive sorting of objects. In this case, however, the predicted link is with the onset of fast mapping of object names.

***Background*** Mervis and Bertrand (1993, 1994) and Golinkoff, Mervis, and Hirsh-Pasek (1994) used the developmental lexical principles framework to consider the question of which linguistic ability expresses the realization that all objects have a name. According to this framework, children initially must rely on other people to provide an explicit connection between a new word and its referent (e.g., by showing an object to a child and labeling it at the same time, by labeling an object to which the child already was attending). Once children acquire the N3C (Novel Name–Nameless Category) principle, however, they no longer have to depend on someone else to make an explicit connection between a label and its referent. According to the N3C principle, words map to categories for which the child does not yet have a name. Within the developmental lexical principles framework, the N3C principle has been interpreted as expressing the insight that all objects have a (basic-level) name (Golinkoff et al., 1994; Mervis & Bertrand, 1994). Once the child has this principle, the indirect connection provided by hearing an unknown word in the presence of an object for which he or she does not yet have a name is sufficient for mapping between word and referent to take place. The child is motivated to map the new word to the basic-level category to which that object belongs. For example, if at the time an adult says "zucchini" a child is looking at a basket of produce including several items for which he or she already has a name and also one (the zucchini) for which he or she does not yet have a name, then the child should correctly infer that "zucchini" is the name for the previously unknown object (and the category to which it belongs). A child who makes this mapping after hearing the new word only once has fast-mapped (cf. Carey, 1978) the new word. The ability to fast-map a new word even when a direct connection between novel object and novel word is not available has been treated as the operational definition of the availability of the N3C principle.

Mervis and Bertrand considered the availability of the N3C principle in both of their studies previously described. As they predicted, results indicated that the onset of the ability to fast-map object names occurred at about the same time as the onset of spontaneous exhaustive sorting. This pattern held for both toddlers who were developing typically (Mervis & Bertrand, 1994) and toddlers and young preschoolers with Down syndrome (Mervis & Bertrand, 1995).

***Children with Williams Syndrome*** To determine if the proposed specific temporal link between the onsets of spontaneous exhaustive sorting and fast mapping of novel object names also held for toddlers with Williams syndrome, we compared the dates of onset of the two abilities. The ability to fast-map new object names was measured in a manner similar to that used by Mervis and Bertrand (1994, 1995). The child was shown an array of five objects, including four for which he or she had a name and one for which he or she did not. The researcher then asked for either a known object (e.g., "May I have the ball?") or the unknown object (e.g., "May I have the lep?"). Unknown objects included items such as garlic presses and honey dippers. If the child chose the novel object in response to the novel label, a generalization trial was administered. The purpose of this trial was to ensure that the child had not selected the novel object simply because it was novel. The generalization trial included two novel objects (a different exemplar of the same basic-level category as the original novel object and an exemplar of a different category) and three objects for which the child already had a name. Four pairs of trials were administered. If the child responded correctly on at least two pairs, he or she was considered to have acquired the N3C principle and to be able to fast-map object names. To test for the specificity of any temporal link between the onset of spontaneous exhaustive sorting and the onset of fast mapping, we also assessed the children's object permanence and means–ends abilities using the Uzgiris and Hunt (1975) scales of sensorimotor development. All children in the first cohort and one child in the second cohort acquired all four of the target abilities.

The children's ages at the time they first demonstrated fast mapping, spontaneous exhaustive sorting, advanced Stage 6 object permanence, and Stage 6 means–ends abilities are indicated in Table 5. The onsets of the two sensorimotor landmarks reliably preceded the onset of either fast mapping or exhaustive sorting. The data presented in Table 5 strongly support the universality of a specific link between onset of the ability to fast-map novel object names and onset of spontaneous exhaustive categorization. Across the seven children, age at onset of these abilities varied by more than a year. Nevertheless, the ages at onset of the two abilities for individual children were very close. Five of the seven children first showed the two abilities at the same session. One of the remaining children demonstrated fast mapping 10 days before exhaustive categorization; the remaining child first demonstrated fast mapping in the session immediately before the one in which he first showed spontaneous exhaustive categorization.

## STUDY FINDINGS AND THEIR IMPLICATIONS FOR LEXICAL DEVELOPMENT

In the introduction to this chapter, we outlined two important ways in which knowledge gained from the study of individuals with mental retardation could

Table 5. Individual data: ages of attainment of fast mapping (FM), exhaustive categorization (EC), advanced Stage 6 object permanence (OP), and Stage 6 means–ends (ME) abilities

| Child | FM | EC | OP | ME |
|---|---|---|---|---|
| Sandra | 2;06 | 2;06[a] | 1;11 | 2;03 |
| Kirsten | 2;08 | 2;08 | 2;06 | 2;06 |
| Peggy | 3;05 | 3;05 | 2;03 | 2;00 |
| Teresa | 3;05 | 3;05 | 2;00 | 2;09 |
| James[b] | 3;08 | 3;08 | 3;08 | 3;08 |
| Nora | 3;05 | 3;05 | 2;10 | 3;03 |
| Zachary[c] | 2;10 | 3;00 | 2;03 | 2;01 |

[a]Sandra first demonstrated fast mapping 10 days before she first demonstrated exhaustive categorization.

[b]James was seen at 4-month intervals.

[c]This was the visit immediately following the one in which Zachary demonstrated fast mapping. There was a 7-week interval between the two visits.

enhance our understanding of lexical development. First, the relatively slow pace of lexical development in individuals with mental retardation facilitates the identification and sequencing of steps of lexical development and highlights any variability, making it easier to differentiate between aspects of lexical development that follow a single path and aspects for which there are alternate paths. Second, individuals with mental retardation are much more likely than individuals who are developing typically to show dissociations between general levels of language abilities and nonlinguistic cognitive abilities. The pattern of general dissociations is likely to vary as a function of etiology. Accordingly, the study of individuals from contrasting etiologies provides a strong test of the universality of specific hypothesized links between particular aspects of lexical and cognitive development. In cases in which the data are not consistent with a universal relation, the findings provide a basis for identifying alternate paths to acquisition of that component of lexical competence. The study of individuals with contrasting etiologies has greatly enhanced our knowledge of universal and alternate paths to lexical competence. In this section, we summarize our findings and consider their implications for theories and models of lexical development.

### Universal Relations Between Specific Aspects of Early Lexical and Cognitive Development

In our research, we have adopted the strategy of studying cognitive and language development in populations that differ with regard to the relation between general cognitive abilities and general language abilities. We previously have focused on children who are developing typically and children who have Down syndrome. These studies have permitted comparisons between individuals who may be expected to have equivalent levels of general cognitive and language abilities and individuals whose general level of cognitive development exceeds their general level of language development. Studies of children with Williams syndrome, whose general level of language development exceeds their general level of cognitive development, complete the set of comparisons needed for our contrasting etiology strategy. For three of the potentially universal specific links that we considered between particular aspects of cognitive and lexical development, the results of the children with Williams syndrome converged with those previously reported both for children who were developing typically and children who had Down syndrome. Based on this confluence of findings, we have considerably more confidence in the assertion that these three specific links are universal.

First, the onset of rhythmic behavior occurs at about the same time in both the linguistic and cognitive domains. In particular, canonical (or reduplicated) babbling may be expected to begin at about the same time as rhythmic hand banging. From the perspective of lexical development, the onset of vocal rhythmic behavior (canonical or reduplicated babble) signals the point at which an infant's vocalizations begin to sound like words, albeit in a language that the people interacting with the infant cannot understand. Once the infant's production of canonical babble is noticed by other people, the verbal input directed to the infant is likely to change in ways that may support the infant's acquisition of words that other people can understand.

Second, children's initial categories, whether measured by nonverbal play patterns or verbal object naming patterns, are basic-level categories. The children with Williams syndrome, the children with Down syndrome, and the children who were developing typically all interacted with objects in the same manner. The categories defined by these play patterns corresponded to child-basic categories (e.g., Mervis, 1984, 1987). In turn, the labeling patterns of the children in all three groups corresponded to the same child-basic categories. We were able to study nonverbal play patterns for two types of objects and to determine the hierarchical level for the children's early object words, based on the range of referents for which the child used or understood the relevant word. The first word that a child understood for an object almost always referred to a basic-level category. The few exceptions in the early vocabularies of the children with Williams syndrome involved labels for subordinate categories that are very atypical of their basic-level category, in particular, toothbrush and school bus. These exceptions are consistent with those reported previously for children who were developing typically (e.g., Johnson, Scott, & Mervis, in press).

Third, the onsets of spontaneous exhaustive sorting and fast mapping of new object names occur at about the same time. This result fits with our argument (Mervis & Bertrand, 1993, 1994, 1995) that the realizations that all objects belong in some category and that all objects have a name represent parallel beliefs in the cognitive and linguistic domains. The universality of this temporal concordance between the onsets of the cognitive ability of spontaneous exhaustive sorting and the lexical ability of fast mapping of object names is particularly impressive, given the large differences between children with Williams syndrome and children with Down syndrome in level of general cognitive development relative to level of language development.

### Alternate Paths to Early Lexical Competence

In this chapter, we considered five links between specific aspects of cognitive and lexical development that had appeared to be universal based on studies of both typically developing children acquiring a variety of native languages and children with Down syndrome. As described previously, three of these links also obtained for children with Williams syndrome. The remaining two links, however, did not. First, although the groups of children studied previously had begun to point referentially before beginning to produce referential labels, children with Williams syndrome began to produce referential labels before beginning to comprehend or produce referential pointing gestures. Second, although both typically developing children and children with Down syndrome demonstrated spontaneous exhaustive sorting at about the same time as the onset of their vocabulary spurt, there was no relation between the onsets of these two abilities for children with Williams syndrome.

The finding that these two specific links did not hold for children with Williams syndrome precludes the universality of these particular relations between specific aspects of cognitive and lexical development. However, the children with Williams syndrome did acquire all of the cognitive or lexical abilities involved in these no-longer-universal relations. Thus, the data from these children should provide critical information regarding alternate paths to two milestones of early lexical development: onset of referential production and onset of the vocabulary spurt.

***Onset of Referential Production*** The acquisition of referential language almost certainly requires that the child participate in episodes of joint attention. Referential pointing gestures provide an obvious way to communicate the focus of one person's attention to another person. The gesturer uses pointing to indicate his or her focus of attention and to direct the recipient's focus of attention. In turn, the recipient (assuming he or she comprehends referential pointing gestures) uses the gesturer's point to determine where attention should be focused. In positing that referential pointing should precede the onset of referential productive language, researchers likely were centering on the attention-focusing function of pointing. Pointing may have been intended as a proxy for participation in episodes of joint attention involving labeling. Pointing is in principle an excellent way to establish joint attention; however, that children with Williams syndrome begin to produce words referentially before beginning to comprehend or produce pointing gestures serves as a convincing reminder that pointing is not the only way to establish joint attention.

Examination of the videotapes of the play sessions involving children with Williams syndrome and their parents indicates three alternative ways of establishing episodes of joint attention that include object labeling. (All three of these methods also are used by parents of children who are developing typically and parents of children with Down syndrome.) The first method was child centered: The adults used the direction of the child's eye gaze to determine the child's focus of attention. They would then follow in on the child's focus of attention and label the object to which the child already was attending. This effort by the adults resulted in joint attention to the object at the time it was labeled. Research involving toddlers who are developing typically has shown that this method of establishing joint attention before labeling is especially effective in facilitating acquisition of new object labels (Dunham, Dunham, & Curwin, 1993; Tomasello & Farrar, 1986). The other methods were more adult directed. The second method involved adults picking up the object to which they wanted the child to attend, putting the object in the place where the child already was looking, and then labeling the object. Along the same lines, the adults sometimes directed the child's attention by setting in motion an object whose action (including sound) was likely to attract the child's attention. Once the child was attending to the object, the adults provided its name. The third method involved directing the child's attention to an object by tapping it. Once the child was looking at the object, the adults then labeled it.

These alternative methods of establishing joint-attention episodes involving object labeling apparently are eventually successful in inducing children to comprehend and produce object labels referentially. Children with Williams syndrome begin to produce referential labels before comprehending or producing pointing gestures. The ability to comprehend and produce pointing gestures may facilitate the onset of productive language in some children, but these abilities clearly are not necessary. What probably is necessary for the onset of referential language is the ability to participate in episodes of joint attention involving object labeling.

These findings have important implications for early intervention. When determining if a child is ready to benefit from intervention directed toward acquisition of a particular skill, most programs rely heavily on what is known about the typical sequence of development. There is an implicit assumption that the typical sequence should be universal. Based on this assumption, speech therapists often use the onset of referential pointing to determine when intervention directed toward acquisition of words (object labels) should begin. This approach may work well for most individuals with mental retardation. However, our results indicate that the sequence of acquisition of referential pointing followed by referential language production is not universal. Comprehension and production of pointing gestures is not necessary for the onset of referential labeling of objects. Thus, an inability to use or follow pointing gestures should not automatically be taken as an indication that a child is not ready to benefit from intervention intended to facilitate referential language acquisition. Conversely, that a child produces referential language should not automatically be taken to mean that the child is able to use and follow deictic gestures.

***Onset of Vocabulary Spurt*** A common explanation for the onset of the vocabulary spurt is that it is due to the child's realization that all objects have names (see Gopnik & Meltzoff, 1987). Findings from toddlers who were developing typically and toddlers and young preschoolers with Down syndrome are consistent with this explanation. For these children, the onset of the vocabulary spurt coincided with the onset of the ability to fast-map new object labels, the ability that we (Mervis & Bertrand, 1993, 1994, 1995) consider to reflect the realization that all objects have names. However, the findings from children with Williams syndrome contradict this explanation for the vocabulary spurt. For all but one of the children with Williams syndrome, the onset of the vocabulary spurt occurred at least 6 months before the onset of the ability to fast-map; for some of these children, more than a year elapsed between the onsets of the two abilities.

These findings indicate that fast-mapping abilities are not necessary for the onset of the vocabulary spurt. Some of the children with Williams syndrome established very large vocabularies (>500 words) before being able to fast-map. These data indicate the presence of a viable alternative path to rapid vocabulary acquisition. Although fast mapping does provide an excellent way to increase vocabulary rapidly, other ways must be possible. In many cases, the onset of the vocabulary spurt and subsequent rapid accumulation of new words probably result from the child's increasing efficiency at acquiring words using the same procedures used before the spurt. For individuals with Williams syndrome, an increase in auditory rote memory for words provides a particularly likely alternate path. Finegan, Smith, Meschino, Vallance, and Sitarenios (1995) found that both school-age children and adults with Williams syndrome evidenced a specific strength in auditory short-term memory for words. An analysis of data we have collected regarding the performance of children with Williams syndrome on the subscales of the DAS (Elliott, 1990) indicated that this strength in auditory short-term memory for words is present by age 2½ years (the youngest age tested). A large proportion of the children with Williams syndrome scored in the normal range on the digit recall subtest; many of them scored within one standard deviation of the normal population mean (Mervis, Morris, Bertrand, & Robinson, in press). Good auditory rote memory provides a solid basis for the long-term memory for words that is needed for vocabulary acquisition and retention. Fast mapping is a relatively sophisticated strategy for the acquisition of new words. However, it is likely that even if an individual is able to fast-map, the mundane strategy of trying to remember the word just heard to label the object or action to which he or she was explicitly attending often will be used as a basis for vocabulary expansion. That is, auditory rote memory probably plays an important role in vocabulary acquisition for most individuals, not just for young children with Williams syndrome.

## CONCLUSION

By comparing the abilities of individuals who show different patterns of relations between general levels of cognitive and language development, we have learned a great deal about specific relations between particular cognitive and lexical abilities. This information could not have been gained through the study of typically developing children alone. The involvement of carefully selected contrasting etiologies in our research has enabled us to confirm the likely universality of three specific links between particular aspects of early cognitive and lexical development. This same strategy has provided evidence that two other hypothesized specific links between early cognitive and lexical development were not universal. In these cases, the contrasting etiology strategy enriched our understanding of language development by encouraging consideration of possible alternate paths to early language competence and indicating what these paths might be. In these ways, the study of individuals with contrasting patterns of relations between general level of cognitive ability and general level of language ability has permitted substantially greater specification of the processes involved in the acquisition of lexical competence.

## REFERENCES


Adamson, L.B. (1995). *Communication development during infancy.* Madison, WI: Brown & Benchmark.

Barrett, M. (1989). Early language development. In A. Slater & G. Bremmer (Eds.), *Infant development* (pp. 211–241). Hillsdale, NJ: Lawrence Erlbaum Associates.

Bates, E., Benigni, L., Bretherton, I., Camioni, L., & Volterra, V. (1979). *The emergence of symbols: Cognition and communication in infancy.* New York: Academic Press.

Bates, E., Camioni, L., & Volterra, V. (1975). The acquisition of performatives prior to speech. *Merrill-Palmer Quarterly, 21*, 205–226.

Bayley, N. (1969). *Bayley Scales of Infant Development: Birth to two years.* New York: The Psychological Corporation.

Bayley, N. (1993). *Bayley Scales of Infant Development—Second edition manual.* San Antonio, TX: The Psychological Corporation.

Bellugi, U., Bihrle, A., Neville, H., & Doherty, S. (1992). Language, cognition, and brain organization in a neurodevelopmental disorder. In M. Gunnar & C. Nelson (Eds.), *Developmental behavioral neuroscience: The Minnesota symposium* (pp. 201–232). Hillsdale, NJ: Lawrence Erlbaum Associates.

Bellugi, U., Marks, S., Bihrle, A., & Sabo, H. (1988). Dissociation between language and cognitive functions in Williams syndrome. In D. Bishop & K. Mogford (Eds.), *Language development in exceptional circumstances* (pp. 177–189). London: Churchill Livingstone.

Bellugi, U., Wang P.P., & Jernigan, T.L. (1994). Williams syndrome: An unusual neuropsychological profile. In S.H. Broman & J. Grafman (Eds.), *Atypical cognitive deficits in developmental disorders: Implications for brain function* (pp. 23–56). Hillsdale, NJ: Lawrence Erlbaum Associates.

Bonvillian, J.D., Orlansky, M.D., & Folven, R.J. (1990). Early sign language acquisition: Implications for theories of language acquisition. In V. Volterra & C.J. Erting (Eds.), *From gesture to language in hearing and deaf children* (pp. 219–232). Berlin: Springer-Verlag.

Burn, J. (1986). Williams syndrome. *Journal of Medical Genetics, 23*, 389–395.

Carey, S. (1978). The child as word learner. In M. Halle, J. Bresnan, & G.A. Miller (Eds.), *Linguistic theory and psychological reality* (pp. 264–293). Cambridge, MA: MIT Press.

Caselli, M.C., & Volterra, V. (1990). From communication to language in hearing and deaf children. In V. Volterra & C.J. Erting (Eds.), *From gesture to language in hearing and deaf children* (pp. 263–277). Berlin: Springer-Verlag.

Cobo-Lewis, A.B., Oller, D.K., Lynch, M.P., & Levine, S.L. (1995, March). *Relationships among motor and vocal milestones in normally developing infants and infants with Down syndrome.* Paper presented at the Gatlinburg Conference on Research and Theory in Mental Retardation and Developmental Disabilities, Gatlinburg, TN.

Dromi, E. (1993). The development of prelinguistic communication: Implications for language evaluation. In N.J. Anastasiow & S. Harel (Eds.), *At-risk infants: Interventions, families, and research* (pp. 19–26). Baltimore: Paul H. Brookes Publishing Co.

Dunham, P.J., Dunham, F., & Curwin, A. (1993). Joint-attentional states and lexical acquisition at 18 months. *Developmental Psychology, 29*, 827–831.

Dunn, L.M., & Dunn, L.M. (1981). *Peabody Picture Vocabulary Test–Revised.* Circle Pines, MN: American Guidance Service.

Elliott, C.D. (1990). *Differential Ability Scales.* San Diego: Harcourt Brace Jovanovich.

Ewart, A.K., Morris, C.A., Atkinson, D., Jin, W., Sternes, K., Spallone, P., Stock, A.D., Leppert, M., & Keating, M.T. (1993). Hemizygosity at the elastin locus in a developmental disorder, Williams syndrome. *Nature Genetics, 5,* 11–16.

Fenson, L., Dale, P.S., Reznick, J.S., Thal, D., Bates, E., Hartung, J.P., Pethick, S., & Reilly, J.S. (1993). *MacArthur Communicative Development Inventories: User's guide and technical manual.* San Diego: Singular Publishing Group.

Finegan, J.-A., Smith, M.L., Meschino, W.S., Vallance, P.L., & Sitarenios, G. (1995, March). *Verbal memory in children with Williams syndrome.* Paper presented at the Society for Research in Child Development, Indianapolis, IN.

Fowler, A.E. (1990). Language abilities in children with Down syndrome: Evidence for a specific syntactic delay. In D. Cicchetti & M. Beeghly (Eds.), *Children with Down syndrome: A developmental perspective* (pp. 302–328). Cambridge, England: Cambridge University Press.

Frangiskakis, J.M., Ewart, A.K., Morris, C.A., Mervis, C.B., Bertrand, J., Robinson, B.F., Klein, B.P., Ensing, G.J., Everett, L.A., Green, E.D., Pröschel, C., Gutowski, N., Noble, M., Atkinson, D.L., Odelberg, S.J., & Keating, M.T. (1996). *LIM-Kinase1* hemizygosity implicated in impaired visual-spatial constructive cognition. *Cell, 86,* 59–69.

Gibson, D. (1978). *Down's syndrome: The psychology of mongolism.* Cambridge, England: Cambridge University Press.

Gibson, D. (1991). Down syndrome and cognitive enhancement: Not like the others. In K. Marfo (Ed.), *Early intervention in transition: Current perspectives on programs for handicapped children* (pp. 61–90). New York: Praeger.

Gillham, B. (1979). *The first words language programme.* London: George Allen & Unwin.

Goldfield, B.A., & Reznick, J.S. (1990). Early lexical development: Rate, content, and the vocabulary spurt. *Journal of Child Language, 17,* 171–183.

Golinkoff, R.M., Mervis, C.B., & Hirsch-Pasek, K. (1994). Early object labels: The case for a developmental lexical principles framework. *Journal of Child Language, 21,* 125–155.

Gopnik, A., & Meltzoff, A.N. (1987). The development of categorization in the second year and its relation to other cognitive and linguistic developments. *Child Development, 58,* 1523–1531.

Gopnik, A., & Meltzoff, A.N. (1992). Categorization and naming: Basic level sorting in eighteen-month-olds and its relation to language. *Child Development, 63,* 1091–1103.

Gopnik, A., & Meltzoff, A.N. (1993). Words and thoughts in infancy: The specificity hypothesis and the development of categorization and naming. In C. Rovee-Collier & L. Lipsitt (Eds.), *Advances in infancy research* (Vol. 8, pp. 223–254). Norwood, NJ: Ablex.

Greenwald, C., & Leonard, L.B. (1979). Communication and sensorimotor development of Down's syndrome children. *American Journal of Mental Deficiency, 84,* 296–303.

Griffith, P.L. (1990). Emerging of mode-findings and mode-switching in a hearing child of deaf parents. In V. Volterra & C.J. Erting (Eds.), *From gesture to language in hearing and deaf children* (pp. 233–245). Berlin: Springer-Verlag.

Harris, M., Barrett, M., Jones, D., & Brookes, S. (1988). Linguistic input and early word meaning. *Journal of Child Language, 15,* 77–94.

Hodapp, R.M., & Burack, J.A. (1990). What mental retardation teaches us about typical development: The examples of sequences, rates, and cross-domain relations. *Development and Psychopathology, 2*, 213–226.

Koenig, M.A., & Mervis, C.B. (1984). The interactive basis of severely handicapped and normal children's initial language development. *Journal of Speech and Hearing Research, 27*, 534–542.

Johnson, K.E., Scott, P., & Mervis, C.B. (in press). Development of children's understanding of basic-subordinate inclusion relations. *Developmental Psychology.*

Jones, K.L., & Smith, D.W. (1975). The Williams elfin faces syndrome: A new perspective. *Journal of Pediatrics, 86*, 718–723.

Lane, V.W., & Molyneaux, D. (1992). *The dynamics of communicative development.* Englewood Cliffs, NJ: Prentice Hall.

Lempers, J.D. (1976). *Production of pointing, comprehension of pointing and understanding of looking behavior in young children.* Unpublished doctoral dissertation, University of Minnesota.

Leung, E.H.L., & Rheingold, H.L. (1981). Development of pointing as a social gesture. *Developmental Psychology, 17*, 215–220.

Levine, S.L., Fishman, L.M., Oller, D.K., Lynch, M.P., & Basinger, D.L. (1991, May). *The relationship between infant motor development and babbling in normally developing, at risk, and handicapped infants.* Paper presented at the Gatlinburg Conference on Research and Theory in Mental Retardation and Developmental Disabilities, Gatlinburg, TN.

Lynch, M.P., & Eilers, R.E. (1991). Perspectives on early language development from typical development and Down syndrome. *International Review of Research on Mental Retardation, 17*, 55–90.

Masur, E.F. (1982). Mothers' responses to infants' object-related gestures: Influences on lexical development. *Journal of Child Language, 9*, 23–30.

Mervis, C.B. (1983). Acquisition of a lexicon. *Contemporary Educational Psychology, 8*, 210–236.

Mervis, C.B. (1984). Early lexical development: The contributions of mother and child. In C. Sophian (Ed.), *Origins of cognitive skills* (pp. 339–370). Hillsdale, NJ: Lawrence Erlbaum Associates.

Mervis, C.B. (1987). Child-basic object categories and early lexical development. In U. Neisser (Ed.), *Concepts and conceptual development: Ecological and intellectual factors in categorization* (pp. 201–233). Cambridge, England: Cambridge University Press.

Mervis, C.B. (1988). Early lexical development: Theory and application. In L. Nadel (Ed.), *The psychobiology of Down syndrome* (pp. 101–143). Cambridge, MA: MIT Press.

Mervis, C.B. (1990). Early conceptual development of children with Down syndrome. In D. Cicchetti & M. Beeghly (Eds.), *Children with Down syndrome: A developmental perspective* (pp. 252–301). Cambridge, England: Cambridge University Press.

Mervis, C.B., & Bertrand, J. (1993). Acquisition of early object labels: The roles of operating principles and input. In A.P. Kaiser & D.B. Gray (Eds.), *Communication and language intervention series: Vol. 2. Enhancing children's communication: Research foundations for intervention* (pp. 287–316). Baltimore: Paul H. Brookes Publishing Co.

Mervis, C.B., & Bertrand, J. (1994). Acquisition of the novel name-nameless category (N3C) principle. *Child Development, 65*, 1646–1662.

Mervis, C.B., & Bertrand, J. (1995). Acquisition of the novel name-nameless category

(N3C) principle by young children who have Down syndrome. *American Journal on Mental Retardation, 100*, 23–243.

Mervis, C.B., Morris, C.A., Bertrand, J., & Robinson, B.F. (in press). Williams syndrome: Findings from an integrated program of research. In H. Tager-Flusberg (Ed.), *Neurodevelopmental disorders: Contributions to a new framework from the cognitive neurosciences*. Cambridge, MA: MIT Press.

Messer, D.J. (1994). *The development of communication: From social interaction to language.* New York: John Wiley & Sons.

Miller, J.F. (1992a). Development of speech and language in children with Down syndrome. In I.T. Lott & E.E. McCoy (Eds.), *Down syndrome: Advances in medical care* (pp. 39–50). New York: Wiley-Liss.

Miller, J.F. (1992b). Lexical development in young children with Down syndrome. In R.S. Chapman (Ed.), *Processes in language acquisition and disorders* (pp. 202–216). St. Louis: C.V. Mosby.

Morris, C.A., Dempsey, S.A., Leonard, C.O., Dilts, C., & Blackburn, B.L. (1988). Natural history of Williams syndrome: Physical characteristics. *Journal of Pediatrics, 113*, 318–326.

Morris, C.A., Thomas, I.T., & Greenberg, F. (1993). Williams syndrome: Autosomal dominant inheritance. *American Journal of Medical Genetics, 47*, 478–481.

Murphy, C.M., & Messer, D.J. (1977). Mothers, infants, and pointing: A study of a gesture. In H.R. Schaffer (Ed.), *Studies in mother–infant interaction* (pp. 325–354). New York: Academic Press.

Robinson, B.F. (1995). *Explaining the vocabulary spurt.* Unpublished manuscript, Emory University, Atlanta, GA.

Rosch, E., Mervis, C.B., Gray, W.D., Johnson, D.M., & Boyes-Braem, P. (1976). Basic objects in natural categories. *Cognitive Psychology, 8*, 382–439.

Rosenberg, S., & Abbeduto, L. (1993). *Language and communication in mental retardation: Development, processes, and intervention.* Hillsdale, NJ: Lawrence Erlbaum Associates.

Rossen, M.L., Klima, E.S., Birhle, A., & Bellugi, U. (1996). Interaction between language and cognition: Evidence from Williams syndrome. In J.H. Beitchmann, N.J. Cohen, M.M. Konstantareas, & R. Tannock (Eds.), *Language, learning, and behavior disorders: Developmental, biological, and clinical perspectives* (pp. 367–392). Cambridge, MA: Cambridge University Press.

Smith, L., von Tetzchner, S., & Michalsen, B. (1988). The emergence of language skills in young children with Down syndrome. In L. Nadel (Ed.), *The psychobiology of Down syndrome* (pp. 145–165). Cambridge, MA: MIT Press.

Tomasello, M., & Farrar, M.J. (1986). Joint attention and early language. *Child Development, 57*, 1454–1463.

Uzgiris, I., & Hunt, J.M. (1975). *Assessment in infancy: Ordinal scales of psychological development.* Urbana: University of Illinois Press.

Wang, P.P., & Bellugi, U. (1994). Evidence from two genetic syndromes for a dissociation between verbal and visual-spatial short-term memory. *Journal of Clinical and Experimental Neuropsychology, 16*, 317–322.

Williams, J.C.P., Barratt, B.G., & Lowe, J.B. (1961). Supravalvular aortic stenosis. *Circulation, 24*, 1311–1318.

# 5

# A Skills Approach to Early Language Development

## Lessons from Research on Developmental Disabilities

Peter Mundy and Antoinette Gomes

> Whatever view one takes of research on language acquisition proper—however nativist or empiricist one's bias—one must still come to terms with the role or significance of the child's pre-speech communication system. (Bruner, 1975, p. 255)

With this gracefully expressed idea, Jerome Bruner began his seminal treatise on the importance of the study of prelinguistic communicative behaviors for understanding language development. To some degree, Bruner's interest in prelinguistic communication appeared to be inspired by the observation that between 8 and 12 months of age infants begin to use gestures such as pointing, eye contact, and vocal behavior with apparent communicative intent. This "illocutionary" stage of development (Bates, Benigni, Bretherton, Camaioni, & Volterra, 1977) is marked by the development of triadic or referential communication skills (Bakeman & Adamson, 1984). Infants in this period increasingly display the ability to refer to objects or events, follow the line of regard or gesture of others, and enter into episodes of shared or joint attention relative to objects or events (Rheingold, Hay, & West, 1976; Scaife & Bruner, 1975).

Since the 1960s, there has been much theory and research on the significance of the prespeech communication system (e.g., Bates, Benigni, Brether-

---

The preparation of this chapter was supported by National Institute on Deafness and Other Communication Disorders Grant #00484 and a Florida State grant to the Center for Autism and Related Disorders at the University of Miami. Appreciation is also extended to Jennifer Stella for her assistance in completing this chapter.

ton, Camaioni, & Volterra, 1979; Dore, 1974; Dunham, Dunham, & Curwin, 1993; Halliday, 1975; Mundy, Kasari, Sigman, & Ruskin, 1995; Sigman & Mundy, 1993; Sugarman, 1984; Tomasello, 1988; Trevarthen, 1979; Werner & Kaplan, 1963). Yet the question of how the advent of prelinguistic triadic or referential communication relates to the subsequent development of language in children has been, at best, only partially addressed. In addressing the complexity of this question, researchers have adopted varied, albeit complementary, approaches to yield a complete picture of how prelinguistic communication relates to language development.

One prominent approach has been to study the changes in interaction processes that occur between caregivers and infants as the latter become increasingly capable of triadic or referential communication (Adamson & Bakeman, 1985; Bakeman & Adamson, 1984; Bruner, 1975; Dunham et al., 1993; Masur, 1981; Tomasello & Farrar, 1986; Tomasello & Kruger, 1992; Werner & Kaplan, 1963). Exemplary of this approach has been work on the hypothesis that the emergence of triadic communication skills in infants may provide caregiver–infant dyads with interactive opportunities that are prepotent with regard to the stimulation of early lexical development (Bruner, 1981; Tomasello, 1988). Preverbal referential skills may enable infants and toddlers to more easily and clearly make caregivers aware of their interests in objects or events. Furthermore, lexical acquisition in toddlers may be facilitated so that caregivers respond to the child and label objects or events that the infant initiates interest in rather than directing infants' attention to objects or events and then providing the label (Tomasello, 1988; Tomasello & Farrar, 1986). Thus, the emergence of referential gestural skills in infants may contribute to a positive feedback system in which the clarity of child referential bids enables caregivers to capitalize on the manifest interest of the infant and present the linguistic stimulation at a time best assimilated by the infant. This interaction process hypothesis on the nature of the links between preverbal communication and language development has received both observational and experimental support (Dunham et al., 1993; Masur, 1981; Tomasello, 1988; Tomasello & Farrar, 1986).

Another perspective on the possible links between nonverbal and verbal communication development is provided by an approach that focuses on the assessment of individual differences among young children in the development of nonverbal gestural communication skills (e.g., Bates et al., 1979). The skills approach does not discount the importance of the child–caregiver interaction process in the relations between nonverbal communication and language development. However, rather than concentrating on child–caregiver interactions, this approach focuses on understanding the nature of the psychological processes involved in the development of nonverbal communication skills (e.g., Bates et al., 1979; Butterworth & Jarrett, 1991). It is assumed that an understanding of these processes may also contribute to an understanding of the linkage between nonverbal and linguistic communication development (Bates et al., 1979). For example, in their initial presentation of a skills approach, Bates and colleagues argued that nonverbal communication skills involved much the same mental representational processes as did sensorimotor abilities, such as in means–ends skills. They suggested that nonverbal communication skills should be linked to language development because both involve representational processes. Finally, Bates et al. (1979) provided some correlational support of the central hypothesis of the skills approach, that children's performance on measures of nonverbal communication skill development is associated with their early language development.

In the 1980s, a program of studies adopted a skills approach to the study of nonverbal communication in research on the early characteristics of children with disorders associated with developmental language delays (Mundy, et al., 1995; Mundy, Seibert, & Hogan, 1984; Mundy, Sigman, & Kasari, 1994; Mundy, Sigman, Kasari, & Yirmiya, 1988; Mundy, Sigman, Ungerer, & Sherman, 1986). The goal of developing a detailed understanding of early language development has not been a central concern of this research (Mundy & Sheinkopf, in press). Nevertheless, because it has focused on the early development of children who were likely to experience language disturbance, this research has yielded information pertinent to several hypotheses about the nature of nonverbal communication skills and the processes that may link these skills to early language acquisition. This chapter provides an overview of this information and illustrates how studies of children with disabilities can inform attempts to understand the links between the development of prelinguistic communication skills and subsequent language acquisition.

Five hypotheses provide the organizational pivots around which the following discussion revolves:

1. Functionally distinct types of nonverbal communication skills begin to develop in children after 6–8 months of age.
2. Different types of nonverbal communication skills are not only functionally distinct but also reflect different combinations and integrations of developing cognitive, self-regulatory, and affective processes.
3. The combination and application of these processes in social interactive problem solving gives rise to specific social-cognitive structures associated with nonverbal communication skills.
4. Nonverbal communication skills, and their associated social-cognitive structures, reflect a unique component of the prelinguistic psychological foundation, requisite to language development.
5. Both biological and environmental factors contribute to individual differences in the development of nonverbal communication skills and related social-cognitive structures in the second year of life.

Observations gleaned from research on children with developmental disorders have played a seminal role in stimulating the generation of these hypotheses. For example, children with developmental disorders of differing organic etiologies display different profiles of nonverbal communicative skills development (Mundy et al., 1988; Mundy et al., 1986; Wetherby, Yonclas, & Bryan, 1989). This segregation of specific types of nonverbal communication skill impairments with specific syndromes of developmental disorders suggests that certain types of nonverbal communication skills may constitute at least partially independent behavior domains in early development. Studies of children with developmental disorders that provide data suggesting that different types of nonverbal communication skills have different neurological, cognitive, and affective correlates are consistent with this view (Caplan et al., 1993; Kasari, Sigman, Mundy, & Yirmiya, 1990; McEvoy, Rogers, & Pennington, 1993).

The remainder of this chapter presents a more detailed consideration of the research and theory that give rise to these hypotheses on the relations between nonverbal communication skills and language development. An outline of the theory that has guided the skills approach used in our own research on nonverbal communication in children with developmental disabilities is provided and followed by discussions more specific to each hypothesis. The need to integrate the skills approach with the interaction process approach to obtain a better understanding of the links between nonverbal communication and early language development is also discussed.

## SKILLS THEORY

The second year of life is a significant transition period in cognitive and social development (Bates et al., 1979; Bruner, 1975; Mandler, 1988; Piaget, 1952; Werner & Kaplan, 1963). One important method of studying development in this period involves the observation and analysis of the acquisition of skills (Bates et al., 1979; Fischer, 1980; Gopnik & Meltzoff, 1986; Piaget, 1952). Skills refer to specific types of task proficiencies that are acquired or developed with experience and maturation. For example, by 18 months, toddlers may demonstrate a particular skill in coordinating motor movement and regulating attention to search strategically for an object hidden under one of several screens. The routinely engaged, organized system of mental and motor processes associated with this type of searching is a manifestation of object permanence skill (Piaget, 1952; Uzgiris & Hunt, 1975).

Ideas about skill development in the first 2 years of life have largely been built on the work of Jean Piaget (1952, 1970). In Piaget's theory of sensorimotor development (1952), the interaction of developing cognitive processes with the diverse problem-solving situations presented by the environment gave rise to the emergence of a variety of problem-solving schemes or skills in the first 2 years of life. The development of different skills in the first 2 years was thought to reflect the emergence of common processes. Most important among these was the development of the semiotic function, or the capacity for mental representation (Piaget, 1952). By the second year, the representational process common to all skills gave rise to a somewhat distinct, task-specific, epistemological or conceptual element that was associated with each skill.

The notion that early skill acquisition primarily reflected the emergence of a common cognitive process was closely linked to Piaget's (1952) stage model of early development. Furthermore, the notion that the development of different skills reflected a common cognitive process led to the hypothesis that, within a particular developmental stage, there should be evidence of pervasive associations in individual levels of achievement across varied skills. Bates, Thal, Whitesell, Fenson, and Oakes (1989) referred to this expectation for pervasive associations across skill domains in early development as "parallelism" or the notion of "deep homologies."

By the second year of life, however, there is considerable intra-individual variability in skill development. For example, some 18-month-olds display well-developed means–ends skills but less well-developed object permanence skills, while others display the reverse pattern (Gopnik & Meltzoff, 1992). This type of individual variability in achievement across sensorimotor skills appears to be common in children with atypical development (Curcio & Houlihan, 1987; Morss, 1983) as well as in children with typical development (Bates, O'Connell, & Shore, 1987; Flavell, 1977). Thus, the Piagetian prediction of deep homologies or parallelism in skill acquisition has not been supported, diminishing its role as an optimal guide in the study of early skill development. Consequently, an alternative perspective on skill acquisition appeared to be necessary for a veridical perspective on early development.

One alternative view of early skill development is espoused in the theoretical and empirical work of several authors. These include, but are not limited to, the work of Bates et al. (1977, 1979), Fischer (1980), Gopnick and Meltzoff (1986), and Siegler (1994). This view suggests that the different skills that emerge within a developmental period may reflect the culmination of the integration of a number of distinct psychological processes, rather than the result of the emergence of a single superordinate process. Consequently, different skills may provide information about different aspects of psychological development. In keeping with this hypothesis, research suggests that, in addition to reflecting representational development and the concept of object constancy, object permanence skills may also reflect the development of other processes such as memory and the executive function capacity to regulate attention and inhibit motor movements (Diamond, 1988; Welsh & Pennington, 1988).

Different skills may hold some processes in common while also reflecting unique processes. Object permanence and imitation skills, for example, may both involve related representational, memory and attention regulation, and inhibition processes (Meltzoff, 1990). However, imitation may involve the comparative processing of proprioceptive information about the spatial arrangement of the child's body and exteroceptive information concerning the spatial arrangement of another person's body (Meltzoff, 1990; Meltzoff & Gopnik,

1993). Object permanence skill would not appear to involve this capacity at all. Hence, these two skills may reflect unique, as well as related, psychological processes.

The interaction between the child and environment suggests one important reason why skills that emerge in parallel in early development may reflect unique or distinct processes in development. Simply stated, problem solving in different environmental niches affords opportunities for different combinations of mental processes (Fischer, 1980; Gibson, 1979). Accordingly, the interaction between the capacities of the child and the environment may be expected to yield the development of skills that incorporate different blends or permutations of cognitive and other mental processes.

As a general example, consider object-oriented and social-oriented skill development. Similar cognitive processes may be applied to object-related and social-related problem-solving situations in a given developmental period. However, social- and object-oriented niches of the environment may afford different opportunities for development, therefore yielding skills that reflect different combinations of mental capacities (Valenti & Good, 1991). The comparison of object permanence and imitation skill development also illustrates this point. Both could reflect a developing capacity for representational thought. However, imitation skill acquisition may afford the opportunity to integrate exteroceptive and proprioceptive information, while the stimulation leading to object permanence skill development does not afford this opportunity.

Another example of this aspect of skills perspective is provided by the following hypothesis. Compared with object problem solving, early social problem solving may elicit different combinations of cognitive and self-regulatory processes (Valenti & Good, 1991). Dawson (1991) suggested that, compared with object problem solving, early social problem solving may involve the analysis of inherently less predictable streams of information. The unpredictable nature of social interaction may require a different degree or type of self-regulation than is typically required in object problem solving. Thus, although similar cognitive processes may be applied in the development of early object-oriented or social-oriented skills, the interaction between cognition and the self-regulatory demands of social interaction may yield the development of a very different skill than is yielded in early object-oriented problem solving.

## NATURE AND ASSESSMENT OF NONVERBAL COMMUNICATION SKILLS

One important arena of skill development that emerges at the beginning of the second year of life involves the acquisition of sophisticated, nonverbal, gestural social-communication skills. The early development of nonverbal communication skills may be conceptualized in terms of three phases (Adamson & Bakeman, 1991; Bakeman & Adamson, 1984). In the birth to 5-month dyadic phase, communication often involves face-to-face exchanges of affective signals between the infant and caregiver (Trevarthen, 1979; Tronick, 1989). In contrast to the dyadic phase, interactions in the 6- to 18-month phase increasingly are characterized by triadic exchanges (Bakeman & Adamson, 1984).

Triadic nonverbal communication skills involve the child's ability to use and respond to eye contact and conventional gestures to coordinate the attention of self and another person vis-à-vis some third object or event, such as when a child points to a toy while making eye contact with a caregiver (e.g., Bates et al., 1979; Bruner & Sherwood, 1983; Leung & Rheingold, 1981; Sugarman, 1984). The intentional nature of the child's communicative acts is increasingly apparent in this phase (Bates et al., 1979; Bretherton, 1991; Flavell, 1977; Golinkoff, 1983). Perhaps the most important support for this contention is the observation that in this period children tend to repair or change nonverbal communication bids when a desired response is not forthcoming (Golinkoff, 1983). For example, a child may initially reach to a toy on an overhead shelf, but then add eye contact to the caregiver and a difficult-to-ignore vocalization if the caregiver does not respond to the initial reach signal.

The third, or locutionary, phase overlaps with the second phase (12–24 months) and involves the child's increasing utilization of verbal communication in conjunction with nonverbal signals. In this chapter, nonverbal communication skills primarily refer to those behaviors that emerge in the second triadic phase of early communication development.

When using the skills approach, it is important to distinguish one or more consistent behavior patterns that comprise different skills within a domain. In research and speculation on infants' ability to manage these triadic interactions, Bruner and colleagues (Bruner, 1975; Bruner & Sherwood, 1983; Scaife & Bruner, 1975) distinguished among different types of social-communication skills that emerged in the latter part of the first year of life. These included the ability to engage in object-oriented offering and turn-taking routines. Another important skill domain included the infant's ability to use or respond to a visual line of regard and gestures to coordinate attention to events or objects with another person (Bruner, 1975; Scaife & Bruner, 1975). This capacity to engage in joint attention routines was not clearly manifest in most infants until the 9- to 12-month period, when infants began to consistently display the ability to follow the line of regard of others (Scaife & Bruner, 1975).

In related efforts, Bates et al. (1979) emphasized that infants' capacity to direct the line of regard of a social partner to objects appeared to bifurcate with regard to function in the 9- to 12-month period. Late in the first year of life, gestural acts were used by infants for imperative or instrumental requesting functions, such as pointing to elicit aid in obtaining an object that is out of reach. However, the functional distinct use of gestures and eye contact for declarative purposes, such as showing an object to another person, could also be distinguished (Bates et al., 1979). By the end of the 1970s, research and theory had culminated in a taxonomy of different forms of nonverbal social-communication skills that typically began to emerge in the latter part of the first year of life.

The availability of this taxonomy spurred efforts to devise measures of individual differences in the development of communication skills, assuming that these measures provide important information about the early development of young children (Coggins & Carpenter, 1981; Seibert, Hogan, & Mundy, 1982; Snyder, 1978; Wetherby & Prizant, 1993b; Wetherby & Prutting, 1984). Versions of these methods include the ESCS (Early Social-Communication Scales; Mundy, Sigman, & Kasari, 1990; Seibert et al., 1982) and the CSBS (Communication and Symbolic Behavior Scales; Wetherby & Prizant, 1993a). These similar instruments use a structured, videotaped child–tester interaction designed to elicit nonverbal communicative bids. Child–tester interactions are used to minimize the possible variability that caregivers may contribute to the display of communicative skills among young children. Both the ESCS and CSBS yield frequency scores for the number of bids within a taxonomy of three categories of nonverbal communication. Bruner and Sherwood's (1983) terminology for this taxonomy is used in both assessment systems and throughout this chapter.

In these assessment systems, *social interaction skills* refer to the use of eye contact, gestures, and affective signals to elicit and maintain turn taking, such as when a toddler smiles, makes eye contact, and displays a hands-open gesture in maintaining a game of catch-the-ball with a social partner. *Behavior regulation or requesting skills* refer to the use of gestures and eye contact to direct attention and elicit aid in obtaining an object or event (e.g., giving a jar while making eye contact with an adult to elicit aid in opening the jar). Finally, *joint attention skills* are similar to requesting skills in that they are used to direct attention. However, the function of these communicative bids appears to be to share the experience of an object or an event with someone. Thus, the function is less imperative-instrumental but perhaps more social-declarative than in requesting (e.g., a child holds up a novel toy to a caregiver).

Empirical work supports the hypothesis that the functional differences among early nonverbal communication skills reflect important, and partially independent, aspects of early psychological development. This empirical support may be found in applied research on the nonverbal communication skills profiles of children with developmental disorders and in the applied literature on the cognitive and emotional correlates of nonverbal communication skills.

## NONVERBAL COMMUNICATION SKILLS AND DEVELOPMENTAL DISORDERS

Young children with distinct forms of biologically based developmental disorders display differing profiles of development across nonverbal communication skills (Mundy et al., 1995; Mundy et al., 1986; Wetherby & Prutting, 1984; Wetherby et al., 1989). Young children with autism display a profound disturbance of joint attention skill development, a moderate disturbance of social interaction skill development, and only a mild disturbance of requesting skill development (Loveland & Landry, 1986; McEvoy et al., 1993; Mundy et al., 1994; Mundy et al., 1986; Wetherby & Prutting, 1984; Wetherby et al., 1989). Alternatively, children with Down syndrome display a disturbance of nonverbal requesting skill development, a possible mild enhancement of social interaction performance, and no differences from MA (mental age)-matched controls on referential joint attention skills (Mundy et al., 1995; Mundy et al., 1988; Wetherby et al., 1989).

It is difficult to understand the contrasting pattern of nonverbal communication skill development observed across these groups in terms of environmental and caregiver effects (Kasari, Sigman, Mundy, & Yirmiya, 1988; Mundy et al., 1988). This segregation of disturbance in nonverbal communication skills across groups with organic forms of developmental disorders suggests that different nonverbal communication skills may reflect the development of at least partially independent sets of psychological processes in young children. This hypothesis receives more direct support in studies of the correlates of different nonverbal communication skills.

## Cognitive Correlates of Nonverbal Communication Skills

Theory and research have long held that the emergence of gestural communication skills is linked to development in the capacity for representational thinking (Bates et al., 1979). Theory on the dissociation between the development of joint attention skills versus requesting or social interaction skills in children with autism, however, suggests that the former may involve more sophisticated representational processes than the latter (Baron-Cohen, 1989). In attempting to understand the degree to which representational skills are involved in requesting and joint attention skill development, Mundy, Sigman, and Kasari (1993) explored the relations between functional play and symbolic play measures, and performance on the ESCS in samples of children with developmental disorders. Hypothetically, functional play reflects a less mature form of representational thinking than does symbolic play.

In the initial assessment phase of this study, the frequency of functional play acts was correlated with the frequency of joint attention and requesting bids, but not social interaction bids, in a sample of 15 preschool children with mental retardation. One year later, the frequency of joint attention bids correlated with the frequency of symbolic play acts. However, neither requesting nor social interaction was correlated with any of the play measures at that point. Firm conclusions may not be drawn from one small study; however, to the extent that play measures index representational development, these data suggest that joint attention skills may differ from requesting and social interaction skills in the degree to which they ultimately come to involve higher order, symbolic-representation processes (Werner & Kaplan, 1963).

Another study suggested that joint attention skills involve different cognitive processes than do requesting skills. McEvoy et al. (1993) explored the relation between nonverbal communication skills, as assessed by the ESCS, and putative measures of executive functions in children with autism and comparison groups of children. Executive functions refer to the regulatory processes that enable planned and flexible problem solving. Theoretically, executive functions are mediated by neurological processes associated with the frontal lobes. An example of an executive function measure used in this study was a search task where an object was alternately placed under one of two screens across several trials. The children's ability to inhibit perseveratively looking for a hidden object in the place where it was last found was assessed. The results indicated that regardless of group, performance on this task was correlated with joint attention and social interaction skills but not with requesting skills. McEvoy et al. (1993) interpreted these results as suggesting that impaired joint attention and better requesting skill development in children with autism could be explained by the different degree to which joint attention and requesting skills may reflect executive-cognitive and frontal-neurological processes.

Results that were consistent with this conclusion were reported in a study of intervention for young children with intractable seizure disorders (Caplan et al., 1993). Thirteen children were assayed with PET (positron emission tomography) before hemispherectomy for their seizure disorders. The ESCS was used as a presurgical and postsurgical measure to evaluate developmental change in these children. The data of most interest here were that the PET index of individual differences in presurgical metabolism in the frontal hemispheres was a significant predictor of joint attention skill development in these children but not of requesting or social interaction skill development. Furthermore, individual differences in metabolism in other areas of the cortex (i.e., temporal, parietal occipital) did not predict any aspects of nonverbal communication skill development. These results suggest that individual differences in the functioning of the frontal lobes, as indexed by a measure of metabolic rate, may be associated with joint attention skill development in young children.

Thus, research has begun to suggest that different types of nonverbal communication skills reflect different types of cognitive and neurological processes. In general, these studies suggest that measures of joint attention skills may be particularly sensitive indices of both cognitive-representational and frontal-neurological processes as these are applied to the domain of early social-communication development. However, in addition to cognitive and neurological processes, research also points to the importance of distinguishing joint attention skills from other forms of nonverbal communication skills.

### Affective Correlates of Nonverbal Communication Skills

Bates et al. (1979) emphasized the cognitive correlates of nonverbal communication development. However, they also observed that joint attention acts were used not only to direct the attention of the adult to an object but also for primarily social-affective sharing purposes. Bates et al. (1977) stated, "Long before he can understand the utilitarian value of sharing information, the child will engage in 'declaring' for primarily social purposes" (p. 115). Accordingly, children's declaring or joint attention acts involve the "use of an object (through pointing, showing, giving, etc.) as a means to attain adult attention" (p. 115). Moreover, the attention-getting component, as described by Bates et al. (1977), appeared to involve the conveyance or exchange of affective signals. They suggested that the development of joint attention acts marks the emergence of attempts to "seek a more subtle kind of adult response—laughter, comment, smiles, and eye contact" (p. 121) in reference to the coordinated attention to an object and event.

Other researchers have expressed similar views of joint attention development. Rheingold et al. (1976) interpreted joint attention acts as a means to share experience with others. They described this experience-sharing function as distinct from the function of imperative, requesting gestures. Bruner (1981) also perceived that there may be "some primitive mood marking procedure to distinguish indicating from commanding or requesting" among proverbial acts of communication (p. 67). These observations suggest that joint attention acts may involve the attempts of young children to convey or share their affective experience of an object with others. Alternatively, affective sharing may play a lesser role in imperative requesting acts.

The empirical literature supports and expands on this view of joint attention behaviors. Although Bates et al. (1977) suggested that joint attention bids may involve seeking an affective response from adults, research also suggests that by 10 months of age infants may also initiate positive affective exchanges in a joint attention context. In play with objects, they often first express positive affect to objects, then turn to display this affect to a social partner (Jones, Collins, & Hong, 1991). In addition, Jones and Raag (1989) presented data that suggest by 18 months the tendency of toddlers to share positive affect vis-à-vis an object is as strong with strangers as it is with familiar caregivers.

Adamson and Bakeman (1985, 1991) also noted that sharing affect may be integral to some forms of nonverbal communication skill, especially joint attention skill. In home observations of mother–child interactions, the time engaged in passive or active joint attention episodes has been observed to increase between 6 and 18 months (Bakeman & Adamson, 1984). Furthermore, throughout this period, relatively high proportions of all affective displays occur within joint attention episodes (Adamson & Bakeman, 1985). For example, Bakeman and Adamson (1984) observed 10 minutes of child–caregiver interactions when the children were 6, 9, 12, 15, and 18 months of age. The percentage of time infants and caregivers spent engaged in face-to-face interaction decreased across these ages, 11.7%, 12.2%, 7.6%, 4.6%, and 4.6%, respectively. In contrast, the percentage of time spent in active or passive joint attention routines increased, 19%, 23%, 34%, and 48%, respectively (Bakeman & Adamson, 1984). Of all the child affective expressions recorded in this 10-minute observation, relatively high percentages were observed in the face-to-face state at the respective ages: 23%, 24%, 13%, 7%, and 9%. However, the percentage of observed affect associated with joint attention routines was even higher: 33%, 36%, 35%, 48%, and 61%, respectively (Adamson & Bakeman, 1985). Thus, these data suggest that joint attention episodes may be a prepotent context in mother–infant interaction for the conveyance of affect.

Although important and informative, these studies did not attempt to directly distinguish between joint attention and other types of nonverbal communication skills in terms of the conveyance of affect. However, a direct comparison of the affective components of nonverbal joint attention and requesting was presented in an attempt to understand the disassociation between these types of acts in the development of children with autism (Kasari et al., 1990). In this study, both the nonverbal communication skills and facial affect of children with autism and comparison children were carefully observed. The MAX (maximally discriminant facial movement coding system; Izard, 1979) was used to rate facial affect, and this coding system was amalgamated with the ESCS, which was used to rate nonverbal social-communication behavior.

The results of this study indicated that children with autism displayed the same total amount of positive affect compared with MA-matched groups, but the distribution of positive affect across joint attention and requesting acts was different for the groups. The comparison children displayed much more positive affect in conjunction with joint attention bids compared with requesting bids. Alternatively, the children with autism displayed equivalent levels of affect in conjunction with both types of communicative behavior and displayed significantly less positive affect in conjunction with joint attention bids.

A related study was conducted with a sample of 32 typically developing infants (Mundy, Kasari, & Sigman, 1992). The results indicated that these infants displayed more positive affect in conjunction with each of four types of joint attention acts relative to four types of requesting acts. Positive affect was displayed between 50% and 70% of the time during joint attention acts, but for only 18%–36% of the time during requesting acts. The results of this study were interpreted to suggest that the assessment of joint attention bids on the ESCS reflects a tendency to initiate states of "affective intersubjectivity," or states of shared positive affect vis-à-vis objects or events (Mundy et al., 1992).

## NONVERBAL COMMUNICATION SKILLS AND SOCIAL COGNITION

The studies reviewed so far suggest that different nonverbal communication skills may tap different combinations of cognitive, self-regulatory, and affective processes (see Mundy, 1995). These basic processes, by themselves, may contribute to links between nonverbal communication and language development. However, if they were the sole source of the linkage between nonverbal communication and language development, then the assessment of nonverbal communication skills would not be expected to yield information beyond the information yielded by other object-oriented cognition, self-regulation, and affective measures. However, the skills approach raises another important possibility. Different types of intentional nonverbal communication skills may involve the growth and development of emerging cognitive, self-regulatory, and affective processes, as they are applied to the specific context of problems encountered in reciprocal social interaction (Adamson & Bakeman, 1985; Bruner, 1975; Mundy et al., 1992; Mundy & Sheinkopf, in press). The end product of this application of emerging psychological processes to social problem solving may be expected to be superordinate structures, specific to social-communicative functions and the developing social-cognitive system of the child (Bretherton, 1991; Mundy & Hogan, 1994; Mundy & Sheinkopf, in press; Tomasello, 1995).

The cognitive and other psychological processes involved in nonverbal communication skills development may be similar to those involved in object-oriented problem-solving skills that emerge in the same developmental period. For example, an early social-communicative capacity, such as nonverbal requesting skill, and an early object-oriented problem-solving capacity, such as means–ends skill, may involve similar cognitive processes (Bates et al., 1979). However, a basic tenet of skills theory is that the child's application of similar cognitive processes to different problem-solving contexts (e.g., social versus inanimate objects) may yield the formation of distinct skills and superordinate structures (Fischer, 1980). Thus, the study of early social-communication skill development may provide information on a different domain of early cognitive development than does the study of object-oriented problem-solving skill development.

Related to this conceptualization of nonverbal communication skills is the long-standing hypothesis that the distinct social-cognitive structures that are reflected in nonverbal communication behaviors may play an especially important role in subsequent language development (Bruner, 1975). This hypothesis is consistent with the notion that, in part, language facility does not develop in isolation but rather grows out of earlier foundations in cognitive and social development (Bruner, 1975; Piaget, 1952). These nonverbal cognitive foundations may include cognitive structures that are tapped by object-oriented measures of skills such as measures of symbolic play with objects (Ungerer & Sigman, 1984) or object categorization (Gopnik & Meltzoff, 1992). However, language is often used in the service of social communication. The skills perspective on development suggests that strong, and relatively unique, sources of variance may be shared by language and nonverbal skills that develop in the context of solving social-communication problems.

In more concrete terms, Bretherton, McNew, and Beeghly-Smith (1981) suggested that referential nonverbal communication skills reflect rudimentary aspects of a developing "theory of mind" in infants and toddlers. That is, triadic nonverbal communicative acts indicate that the child can appreciate that others have perceptions and intentions relative to objects or events and that these perceptions or intentions can be affected by the child's behavior. Subsequently, numerous researchers working on issues in typical and atypical development have expanded on the notion that referential nonverbal communication skills reflect an awareness that self and others can experience common covert psychological phenomena relative to objects and events. Two convergent examples of these elaborations may be found in somewhat divergent literatures. In an attempt to understand interpersonal development, Stern (1985) argued that the social-communication behaviors of infants between 7 and 12 months of age suggest that they have the capacity to share three aspects of mental states with others: 1) *share intentions* or a common goal orientation with regard to objects or events, 2) engage in joint attention and *share a common visual/sensory perspective* on objects or events, and 3) *share affective states* or a common emotional response to objects and events. Similarly, Wellman (1993) proposed that in the last quarter of the first year of life infants understand people in terms of three aspects of behavior: 1) *desire* or that people can seek to attain the same objects or experiences; 2) *perception* or that people can see, hear, or feel the same object or event; and 3) *emotion* or that people can have the same affective reactions to objects or events.

The aspects of social cognition described by Stern (1985) and Wellman (1993) have an apparent relation to the three categories of nonverbal communication skills described by Bates, Bruner, and others. The ability to recognize that self and others can experience intentions or goal orientations may be reflected by the capacity of the child to initiate and respond to nonverbal requests. The capacity to understand that both self and others can share a common visual perspective of an event or object may be involved in both joint attention and requesting, as these both involve coordinating attention between self and another person, vis-à-vis an object or event. Finally, both social interaction and joint attention skills may involve affective sharing. In the former, affective sharing occurs in the face-to-face enterprise of turn taking. In the latter, the tendency to share affective states may have a more sophisticated expression as the child displays affective states that are referenced to an object or event (Mundy et al., 1992).

## NONVERBAL COMMUNICATION SKILLS AND LANGUAGE DEVELOPMENT

Research with children with developmental disorders has led to an elaboration of previous conceptualizations of the nature of nonverbal communication skills and their putative association with language development. The idea that nonverbal communication skills, because of their social-cognitive substrate, may provide unique information about early language development has been implicit in the literature for some time (Bretherton et al., 1981; Bruner, 1975). Therefore, it is rather surprising that very few studies have directly examined the hypothesis that nonverbal communication skills, and their associated social-cognitive structures, contribute to language development.

Bates et al. (1979) reported significant concurrent correlations between measures of nonverbal communication skills, sensorimotor skills, and language development. However, their data were not prospective, and their study did not attempt to determine if nonverbal communication skills provided information about the early foundations of language development beyond that associated with other measures, such as measures of object-oriented sensorimotor skills. At least one study suggests that measures of nonverbal communication skills may provide a unique, predictive source of information about early language development. Olson, Bates, and Bayles (1984) examined numerous aspects of infant– and toddler–caregiver interaction measures at 6 and 13 months. They reported that frequency of positive verbal interactions, close and nurturing mother–child contact, and child–object communication showed a greater relation to measures of child cognitive and language competence at age 2 than did other measures of interaction. The child–object communication variable was a 13-month measure composed of observations of the frequency with which infants gave or offered objects, complied with requests, and pointed in infant–caregiver interaction. However, the issue of the relation of nonverbal communication to language development was not a focus for this study. Therefore, the precision of the nonverbal measure was not optimal (e.g., combining a child responding to caregiver communications with child initiation of communicative bids). Hence, limited information was available concerning the types of nonverbal communication skills that were linked to language development.

These studies notwithstanding, the potential importance of nonverbal communication skills assessment for both theoretical and applied research on language development has not been fully realized. Nevertheless, several clear, testable predictions exist about the nature of the relations between nonverbal communication skills and early language development. Let us consider two of these. First, the theoretical assumption above the unique social-cognitive nature of the processes reflected in measures of nonverbal communication skills would suggest that individual differences in nonverbal communication skills should predict early language development beyond variance associated with standard object-oriented measures of early cognitive development. Second, because nonverbal communication skills appear to reflect different basic psychological processes, different types of nonverbal communication skills may be more or less strongly associated with early language development.

To find data pertinent to these predictions, we must again consider the research with children with developmental disabilities. To our knowledge, the first demonstration that nonverbal communication skills may provide information about language development beyond that provided by object-oriented measures of cognitive development was provided by Smith and von Tetzchner (1986) in a study of children with Down syndrome. These authors reported that a measure of nonverbal requesting predicted language development in children with Down syndrome over a 1-year period beyond variance associated with performance on a standardized measure of cognitive development. These results have been replicated and extended in a study that examined the predictive relations between the ESCS and language development in samples of children with Down syndrome or typical development (Mundy et al., 1995). At the beginning of this study, these children had an estimated expressive language age of approximately 15 months based on the Revised Reynell Developmental Language Scales (Reynell, 1977). Each child was initially assessed with the ESCS, the Reynell Language Scales, and the Bayley Scales of Infant Development (BSID, Bayley, 1993). A follow-up assessment was conducted 13 months later (+/−21 days) in which each child was again presented with the Reynell Language Scales and the ESCS.

The results indicated that, after considering initial age and expressive language status, the ESCS measures of requesting and social interaction accounted for a significant portion of expressive language outcome variance among children with Down syndrome (5% and 7% of the residual outcome variance, respectively). Alternatively, the joint attention measures did not significantly relate to outcome variance in expressive language among the children with Down syndrome after considering variance in initial language level. Among the children with typical development only the social interaction measure (18%) was a significant predictor of residual expressive language variance after considering variance in initial language. It should also be noted that once initial age and expressive language were considered, Bayley MA did not share a significant unique source of variance with expressive language outcome in either group. Thus, the initial measures of expressive language and general cognitive development appeared to index largely overlapping sources of variance that were associated with expressive language development in these samples. However, measures of nonverbal communication skills reflected a unique, additional source of variance related to the early phase of expressive language development in both children with Down syndrome and typical development.

A different profile of associations between nonverbal communication and receptive language development was observed in this study. None of the nonverbal communication variables was significantly associated with receptive language development among children with Down syndrome after considering initial variance in receptive language skills. However, after considering initial expressive language and MA, a measure of responding to joint attention or following the gaze and direction of pointing by a tester was a significant predictor of receptive language test performance (18%) among the children with typical development.

The data from this study corroborate Smith and von Tetzchner's (1986) observation that early expressive language difficulties of children with Down syndrome may be linked with nonverbal communication development, especially that of nonverbal requesting skills. It is also important to note that children with Down syndrome display stronger delays in the development of nonverbal requesting skills than in joint attention or social interaction skill development (Mundy et al., 1988, 1995; Wetherby et al., 1989). In a more general vein, though, the results of this study are important because they support the skills theory hypothesis that individual differences in nonverbal communication skills would predict early language development beyond variance associated with other measures of early cognitive and communicative development.

The data from this study also suggest two other points of interest. First, different types of nonverbal communication skills may be more or less strongly related to language development in different groups of children. Several studies suggest that nonverbal requesting may be a correlate of expressive language development among children with Down syndrome (Mundy et al., 1988, 1995; Smith & von Tetzchner, 1986). However, in studies of children with other developmental disorders such as autism, or among children with typical development, the limited extant data suggest that measures of joint attention or social interaction but not nonverbal requesting are correlates of language development (Loveland & Landry, 1986; Mundy et al., 1988, 1990, 1995). Clear contrasts among these data sets are difficult because the groups of children involved tend to be at different levels of language development, which may affect comparative profiles of correlations with nonverbal communication skills (e.g., Mundy et al., 1995). The possibility that different groups of children may display different profiles of relations between nonverbal communication and language development, however, may be important to explore in developing a deeper understanding of the links between nonverbal communication and language development.

The Mundy et al. (1995) study of children with Down syndrome also raises two potentially important methodological issues. First is the prospect that different types of nonverbal communication skills may be more or less strongly correlated with different aspects of language development. In this particular study, for example, responding to joint attention appeared to have a relatively strong relation to receptive language, while social interaction skills had a relatively strong relation with expressive language development. Other research has suggested that receptive and expressive language proceed along partially independent paths of development in toddlers (Bates et al., 1989). Therefore, it may be judicious for researchers at least to distinguish between receptive and expressive language development, or to make even finer distinctions in language outcome measures (e.g., Tomasello & Kruger, 1992), in studying the links between nonverbal communication and language development.

The second issue is that, in interpreting the data from any one study, we must remind ourselves of the possibility that the pattern of correlations observed between nonverbal communication and language may be specific to the developmental level of children in a particular study. For example, the pattern of correlations observed in Mundy et al. (1995) may be specific to toddlers between 12 and 18 months of age. An illustration of the potential importance of considering age-specific associations in work on nonverbal communication and language development was presented in a study by Mundy and Gomes (1994), who examined the profiles of concurrent correlations observed between nonverbal communication measures and language measures at different ages to determine if these changed over time. As part of this study, 20 14- to 18-month-olds and twenty-eight 19- to 24-month-olds were assessed with the BSID, the ESCS, and the Reynell Language Scales. The results of this study indicated that significant correlations between nonverbal communication and language development were observed at each age. However, the nonverbal communication variables involved in these correlations changed over age.

In the 14- to 18-month-olds, responding to joint attention skill was correlated with expressive language age estimates for the Reynell Language Scales ($r = .44$, $p < .05$). No other correlations between nonverbal communication and language development were significant at this age. In particular, it is important to note that a measure of initiating joint attention skill, or the frequency with which toddlers directed the attention of the tester for a nonrequesting function by pointing or showing, was not correlated with expressive language ($r = -.04$).

In contrast, among the 19- to 24-month-olds, initiating joint attention was significantly correlated with expressive language development ($r = .41$, $p < .05$). No other correlations between nonverbal communication, including the correlation between expressive language and responding to joint attention ($r = .31$), were significant. However, the BSID MA was also a significant correlate of expressive language in this age group ($r = .74$). Nevertheless, even after taking variance shared with MA into account, initiating joint attention skill was still correlated with a significant 13% of the residual variance in expressive language in this sample ($p < .05$).

We regard these results as preliminary and are engaged in a larger-scale replication. However, it may be useful to consider the possibilities the results raise about the nature of the relations between nonverbal communication skills and language development. First, these data again suggest different types of nonverbal communication skills may have different relations with language development. Joint attention skill measures of the ESCS yielded significant correlations with language beyond variance associated with general cognitive level. Alternatively, other referential, nonverbal communication skills with similar behavior topography but different function, such as pointing or giving for nonverbal requesting, may not be as closely related to language development. This difference may reflect the greater degree to which joint attention skills appear to involve the application and integration of representational, frontal self-regulatory, and affective processes in early social-communicative interactions (Caplan et al., 1993; McEvoy et al., 1993; Mundy, 1995; Mundy et al., 1992, 1993). However, the data in this study did not address directly the issue of why certain nonverbal communication skills appear to be more closely related to language development than do others.

A second possibility raised by the data in this study is that the types of nonverbal communication skill most closely related to an aspect of language development may change with age. In Mundy and Gomes (1994), responding to joint attention was correlated with expressive language in 14- to 18-month-olds, while initiating joint attention skill was correlated with expressive language in 19- to 24-month-olds. How is this shifting pattern in correlations to be explained? Although there was some difference in the mean percent correct scores on responding to joint attention across these two age groups (75%, $SD=22$; 88%, $SD=12$), this difference was not significant. For initiating joint attention, there was very little difference in the mean scores across ages (3.52, $SD=3.4$; 3.45, $SD=2.9$). Thus, it was not obvious whether this shifting pattern could be explained in terms of changes in means, distributions, or other psychometric characteristics of these variables.

Yet it may be that initial acquisition of a lexicon is facilitated by the capacity of the child to attend to a referent selected by a caregiver. However, once the toddler has some practice and begins to conceptually understand the connection between words and objects or events, lexical acquisition is best facilitated in the context of the child's tendency to initiate joint attention with a caregiver relative to an object or event. This is a restatement of the hypothesis that caregiver responsiveness to opportunities to label objects and events that a toddler is attending to facilitates lexical development (Tomasello & Farrar, 1986). However, the results observed by Mundy and Gomes (1994), albeit preliminary, provide an example of how the skills approach may complement the interaction process approach to understanding the relations between nonverbal communication and language development. Relative to Tomasello and Farrar's hypothesis, these results suggest that the toddler's tendency to initiate joint attention bids, as well as the caregiver's skill at recognizing and responding to the child's focus, may be related to early aspects of expressive language development. However, at early periods in the second year, the toddler's ability to recognize the caregiver's focus of attention and to process information relative to that focus may also be related to early aspects of expressive language development.

## CONCLUSION

Much of our work since 1980 has focused on using measures of nonverbal communication skills to help uncover the early cognitive and social characteristics of children with different types of developmental disorders. An important byproduct of this research has been the emergence of a network of general assumptions and hypotheses regarding the links between nonverbal communication skills and language development. We have come to regard nonverbal communication as characterized by the development of various skills that may be distinguished not only on the basis of communicative function, such as requesting versus joint attention functions, but also on the degree to which they involve and integrate various cognitive, self-regulatory, and emotional processes.

This perspective may have important ramifications. It suggests that researchers should resist the tendency to regard nonverbal communication as a monolithic domain of development. For example, there may be significant differences in the psychological processes involved in early referential acts for requesting versus referential acts for joint attention. These differences may need to be considered when speculating on the nature of triadic communicative development or on the nature and importance of one particular type of nonverbal communication (Bakeman & Adamson, 1984; Barresi & Moore, 1996; Mundy, 1995; Tomasello, 1995). Furthermore, even within a class of behaviors, there may be important differences associated with whether the child initiates, or responds to, a particular type of nonverbal act (e.g., the observation of an asynchrony in development, with young children with autism demonstrating better proficiency in responding to joint attention than initiating joint attention [Mundy et al., 1994], suggests that initiating and responding to joint attention skills may reflect somewhat different domains of early development). Observations of different profiles of correlations with language that have been observed for measures of responding to joint attention bids as opposed to initiating joint attention bids are consistent with this notion (Mundy & Gomes, 1994; Mundy et al., 1995). Thus, when studying the nature of joint attention (e.g., Butterworth & Jarrett, 1991; Moore & Corkum, 1994; Scaife & Bruner, 1975; Tomasello, 1995), it may be important to recognize the potential for differences in the processes involved in initiating versus responding to joint attention bids. A skills approach suggests that we must be careful to understand the differences among types of nonverbal communication behaviors to better interpret and integrate the burgeoning data available on development in this domain.

Another byproduct of the skills approach is that it suggests important hypotheses about the nature of the links between nonverbal communication and language development. In particular, measures of nonverbal communication tap unique information about individual differences in early development that are related to language development. Although some evidence in support of this contention is available (Mundy et al., 1995), more rigorous examinations of this hypothesis would be useful. One approach would be to study the different linkages that may exist between early language development and nonverbal measures of object-oriented skills versus social-communication skills.

For example, Gopnik and Meltzoff (1992) suggested that certain types of skills have specific relations to early language development. In exploring their specificity hypothesis, they provided evidence that object categorization skill appears to have a specific relation to early lexical development. The skills model outlined in this chapter raises the possibility that nonverbal communication skills and object categorization skills would reflect at least partially independent sources of variance associated with language development. The examination of this prediction may yield a better understanding of the network of skill development that may support the early phases of language development.

Another set of issues concerns the relations between caregiver interaction style, nonverbal communication skills, and language development. A central question is to what degree does the development of different nonverbal communication skills reflect differences that are inherent to the child or the effects of the caregiver environment? This issue invokes the need to integrate the skills approach with the interaction process approach in studying the relations between nonverbal communication and language development. In this regard, it may be useful to adopt a moderate nativist perspective and suggest that, although nonverbal communication skills development is undoubtedly affected by the caregiver environment, a substantial portion of the variance in these skills reflects inherent aspects of development. This nativist perspective may be supported by the observation that children with different, presumably organically based, developmental disorders display different profiles of nonverbal communication skills development (Mundy et al., 1986, 1988). A nativist model of a portion of the variance in individual differences in nonverbal communication skills development may also be supported by data suggesting that frontal-neurological processes predicted joint attention development in a group of infants and toddlers whose capacity to respond to the environment was severely compromised by intractable seizure disorders (Caplan et al., 1993).

This perspective leads to a consideration of hypotheses for future research. First, measures of nonverbal communication skills may be expected to contribute an independent source of information to the prediction of individual differences in early language development, beyond the information provided by measures of caregiver style of interaction. Second, nonverbal communication skills development and caregiver style may interact in the prediction of early language development. For example, the tendency of caregivers to follow the direction of attention of toddlers and label objects or events that the toddlers are focused on appears to be related to early lexical development (Masur, 1981; Tomasello, 1988). Caregivers may display marked individual differences in this tendency. However, toddlers may also display marked individual differences in how frequently or clearly they refer to objects or events with joint attention or requesting bids. These individual differences in child nonverbal communication skills may interact with caregiver style so that we might expect optimal language learning in situations where the toddler has well-developed skill in initiating communicative bids and the caregiver is adept at following and remarking on the focus of the child's interest. In contrast, children with poorly developed tendencies to initiate referential bids may not profit as readily from this caregiver style of interaction. Similarly, the child with relatively well-developed referential skills may not suffer as much from a caregiver who redirects attention frequently as may a child with poorly developed joint attention skills.

In closing, we return to the opening statement of this chapter: "Whatever view one takes of research on language acquisition proper—however nativist or empiricist one's bias—one must still come to terms with the role or significance of the child's pre-speech communication system" (1975, p. 255). In part, Bruner appears to have made this statement in response to what he perceived to be a resurgence of a nativist bias in research and theory on language development that led to a disregard for the prelinguistic social and cognitive foundations for language development (Bruner, 1975, p. 256). Bruner emphasized the need to explore the environmental and transactional processes that supported the infants' capacity to acquire language. Much of the interactive process work has followed Bruner's lead and emphasized the exploration of potential environmental effects, especially caregiver effects, in the study of nonverbal communication and its links with language development (Dunham et al., 1993; Moore & Corkum, 1994; Tomasello, 1988). Thus, it is with some irony that we observe that one marker of the progress made since 1975 on the significance of the child's prespeech communication system is that the field is now sufficiently rich to consider nativist as well as empiricist biases in formulating hypotheses about the links between nonverbal communication and language. However, we note that these biases need not nor should not be inculcated into schools of research and thought that are viewed as in opposition. Rather, a reasonable expectation is that the articulation of the skills approach, with its transactional, but nativist bias, will be integrated hand-in-hand with the more empiricist bias implicit in the interaction process approach to yield a more sophisticated understanding of the nature of the relations between the child's prespeech communication system and language development.

## REFERENCES

Adamson, L., & Bakeman, R. (1985). Affect and attention: Infants observed with mothers and peers. *Child Development, 56*, 582–593.

Adamson, L., & Bakeman, R. (1991). The development of shared attention during infancy. In R. Vasta (Ed.), *Annals of child development* (Vol. 8, pp. 1–41). London: Kingsley.

Bakeman, R., & Adamson, L. (1984). Coordinating attention to people and objects in mother–infant and peer–infant interaction. *Child Development, 55*, 1278–1289.

Baron-Cohen, S. (1989). Joint-attention deficits in autism: Towards a cognitive analysis. *Development and Psychopathology, 3*, 185–190.

Barresi, J., & Moore, C. (1996). Intentional relations and social understanding. *Behavioral and Brain Sciences, 19*, 107–154.
Bates, E., Benigni, L., Bretherton, I., Camaioni, L., & Volterra, V. (1977). From gesture to first word. In I.M. Lewis & L. Rosenblum (Eds.), *Interaction, conversation and the development of language* (pp. 247–308). New York: John Wiley & Sons.
Bates, E., Benigni, L., Bretherton, I., Camaioni, L., & Volterra, V. (1979). *The emergence of symbols: Cognition and communication in infancy.* New York: Academic Press.
Bates, E., O'Connell, B., & Shore, C. (1987). Language and communication in infancy. In J. Osofsky (Ed.), *Handbook of infant development* (2nd ed., pp. 149–203). New York: John Wiley & Sons.
Bates, E., Thal, D., Whitesell, K., Fenson, L., & Oakes, L. (1989). Integrating language and gesture in infancy. *Developmental Psychology, 25*, 1004–1019.
Bayley, N. (1993). *Bayley Scales of Infant Development—Second edition manual.* San Antonio, TX: The Psychological Corporation.
Bretherton, I. (1991). Intentional communication and the development of an understanding of mind. In D. Frye & C. Moore (Eds.), *Children's theories of mind: Mental states and social understanding* (pp. 271–289). Hillsdale, NJ: Lawrence Erlbaum Associates.
Bretherton, I., McNew, S., & Beeghly-Smith, M. (1981). Early person knowledge as expressed in verbal and gestural communication: When do infants acquire a theory of mind? In M. Lamb & L. Sherrod (Eds.), *Infant social cognition* (pp. 333–373). Hillsdale, NJ: Lawrence Erlbaum Associates.
Bruner, J. (1975). From communication to language: A psychological perspective. *Cognition, 3*, 255–287.
Bruner, J. (1981). Learning how to do things with words. In J. Bruner & A. Garton (Eds.), *Human growth and development* (pp. 62–84). London: Oxford University Press.
Bruner, J., & Sherwood, V. (1983). Thought, language and interaction in infancy. In J. Call, E. Galenson, & R. Tyson (Eds.), *Frontiers of infant psychiatry* (pp. 38–55). New York: Basic Books.
Butterworth, G., & Jarrett. N. (1991). What minds have in common is space: Spatial mechanisms serving joint visual attention in infancy. *British Journal of Developmental Psychology, 9*, 55–72.
Caplan, R., Chugani, H., Messa, C., Guthrie, D., Sigman, M., Traversay, J., Mundy, P., & Phelps, M. (1993). Hemispherectomy for early onset intractable seizures: Presurgical cerebral glucose metabolism and postsurgical nonverbal communication patterns. *Developmental Medicine and Child Neurology, 35*, 582–592.
Coggins, T., & Carpenter, R. (1981). The communicative intention inventory. A system for observing and coding children's early intentional communication. *Applied Psycholinguistics, 2*, 235–251.
Curcio, F., & Houlihan, J. (1987). Varieties of organization between domains of sensorimotor intelligence in normal and atypical populations. In I. Uzgiris & J.M. Hunt (Eds.), *Infant performance and experience: New findings with the ordinal scales* (pp. 103–131). Urbana: University of Illinois Press.
Dawson, G. (1991). A psychobiological perspective on the early socioemotional development of children with autism. In D. Cicchetti & S. Toth (Eds.), *Rochester Symposium on Developmental Psychopathology* (Vol. 3, pp. 77–111). Rochester, NY: University of Rochester Press.
Diamond, A. (1988). Abilities and neural mechanisms underlying AB performance. *Child Development, 59*, 259–285.

Dore, J. (1974). A pragmatic description of early language development. *Journal of Psycholinguistic Research, 3*, 343–350.
Dunham, P., Dunham, F., & Curwin, A. (1993). Joint-attentional states and lexical acquisition at 18 months. *Developmental Psychology, 29*, 827–831.
Fischer, K. (1980). A theory of cognitive development: The control and construction of hierarchical skill. *Psychological Review, 87*, 477–526.
Flavell, J. (1977). *Cognitive development.* Englewood Cliffs, NJ: Prentice Hall.
Gibson, J. (1979). *The ecological approach to visual perception.* Hillsdale, NJ: Lawrence Erlbaum Associates.
Golinkoff, R. (1983). The preverbal negotiation of failed messages. In R. Golinkoff (Ed.), *The transition from prelinguistic to linguistic communication* (pp. 57–78). Hillsdale, NJ: Lawrence Erlbaum Associates.
Gopnik, A., & Meltzoff, A. (1986). Relations between semantic and cognitive development at the one word stage: The specificity hypothesis. *Child Development, 57*, 1040–1057.
Gopnik, A., & Meltzoff, A. (1992). Categorization and naming: Basic-level sorting in eighteen-month-olds and its relation to language. *Child Development, 63*, 1091–1103.
Halliday, M. (1975). *Learning how to mean.* London: Edwin Arnold.
Izard, C. (1979). *The maximally discriminant facial movement coding system.* Newark: University of Delaware, Instructional Resources Center.
Jones, S., Collins, K., & Hong, H. (1991). An audience effect on smile production in 10-month-old infants. *Psychological Science, 2*, 45–49.
Jones, S., & Raag, R. (1989). Smile production in older infants: The importance of a social recipient for the facial signal. *Child Development, 60*, 811–818.
Kasari, C., Sigman, M., Mundy, P., & Yirmiya, N. (1988). Care giver interactions with autistic children. *Journal of Abnormal Child Psychology, 16*, 45–56.
Kasari, C., Sigman, M., Mundy, P., & Yirmiya, N. (1990). Affective sharing in the context of joint attention interactions of normal, autistic and mentally retarded children. *Journal of Autism and Developmental Disorders, 20*, 87–100.
Leung, H., & Rheingold, J. (1981). Development of pointing as a social gesture. *Developmental Psychology, 17*, 215–220.
Loveland, K., & Landry, S. (1986). Joint attention and language in autism and developmental language delay. *Journal of Autism and Developmental Disorders, 16*, 335–349.
Mandler, J. (1988). How to build a better baby: On the development of an accessible representational system. *Cognitive Development, 3*, 113–136.
Masur, E. (1981). Mothers' responses to infants' object related gestures. Influence on early lexical development. *Journal of Child Language, 9*, 23–30.
McEvoy, R., Rogers, S., & Pennington, R. (1993). Executive function and social communication deficits in young, autistic children. *Journal of Child Psychology and Psychiatry, 34*, 563–578.
Meltzoff, A. (1990). Towards a developmental cognitive science: The implications of cross-modal matching and imitation for the development of representation and memory in infancy. In A. Diamond (Ed.), The developmental and neural bases of higher cognitive functions. *Annals of the New York Academy of Sciences, 608*, 1–29.
Meltzoff, A., & Gopnik, A. (1993). The role of imitation in understanding persons and developing a theory of mind. In S. Baron-Cohen, H. Tager-Flusberg, & D. Cohen (Eds.), *Understanding the minds of others: Perspectives from autism* (pp. 335–366). New York: Oxford University Press.

Moore, C., & Corkum, V. (1994). Social understanding at the end of the first year of life. *Developmental Review, 14*, 349–372.

Morss, J. (1983). Cognitive development in the Down's syndrome infant: Slow or different. *British Journal of Educational Psychology, 53*, 40–47.

Mundy, P. (1995). Joint attention, social-emotional approach in children with autism. *Development and Psychopathology, 7*, 63–82.

Mundy, P., & Gomes, A. (1994, April). *Nonverbal and verbal communication in the second year.* Paper presented at the Thirteenth Biennial Conference on Human Development, Pittsburgh, PA.

Mundy, P., & Hogan, A. (1994). Intersubjectivity, joint attention and autistic developmental pathology. In D. Cicchetti & S. Toth (Eds.), *Rochester Symposium on Developmental Psychopathology: Vol. 5. The self and its disorders* (pp. 1–30). Rochester, NY: University of Rochester Press.

Mundy, P., Kasari, C., & Sigman, M. (1992). Nonverbal communication, affective sharing and intersubjectivity. *Infant Behavior and Development, 15*, 377–381.

Mundy, P., Kasari, C., Sigman, M., & Ruskin, E. (1995). Nonverbal communication and language development in children with Down syndrome and children with normal development. *Journal of Speech and Hearing Research, 38*, 1–11.

Mundy, P., Seibert, J., & Hogan, A. (1984). Relationship between sensorimotor and early communication abilities in developmentally delayed children. *Merrill-Palmer Quarterly, 30*, 33–48.

Mundy, P., & Sheinkopf, S. (in press). Early communication skill acquisition and developmental disorders. In J. Burack, R. Hodapp, & E. Zigler (Eds.), *Handbook of mental retardation and development.* New York: Cambridge University Press.

Mundy, P., Sigman, M., & Kasari, C. (1990). A longitudinal study of joint attention and language development in autistic children. *Journal of Autism and Developmental Disorders, 20*, 115–128.

Mundy, P., Sigman, M., & Kasari, C. (1993). The theory of mind and joint attention deficits in autism. In S. Baron-Cohen, H. Tager-Flusberg, & D. Cohen (Eds.), *Understanding other minds: Perspective from autism* (pp. 181–203). Oxford, England: Oxford University Press.

Mundy, P., Sigman, M., & Kasari, C. (1994). Joint attention, developmental level, and symptom presentation in young children with autism. *Development and Psychopathology, 6*, 389–401.

Mundy, P., Sigman, M., Kasari, C., & Yirmiya, N. (1988). Nonverbal communication skills in Down syndrome children. *Child Development, 59*, 235–249.

Mundy, P., Sigman, M., Ungerer, J., & Sherman, T. (1986). Defining the social deficits of autism: The contribution of nonverbal communication measures. *Journal of Child Psychology and Psychiatry, 27*, 657–669.

Olson, S., Bates, J., & Bayles, K. (1984). Mother–infant interaction and the development of individual differences in children's cognitive competence. *Developmental Psychology, 20*, 166–179.

Piaget, J. (1952). *The origins of intelligence in children.* New York: Norton.

Piaget, J. (1970). *Structuralism.* New York: Basic Books.

Reynell, J. (1977). *Reynell Developmental Language Scales.* Los Angeles: Western Psychological Corporation.

Rheingold, H., Hay, D., & West, M. (1976). Sharing in the second year of life. *Child Development, 83*, 898–913.

Scaife, M., & Bruner, J. (1975). The capacity for joint visual attention in the infant. *Nature, 253*, 265–266.

Seibert, J.M., Hogan, A.E., & Mundy, P.C. (1982). Assessing interactional competencies: The Early Social-Communication Scales. *Infant Mental Health Journal, 3*, 244–245.

Siegler, R. (1994, April). *Recent advances in understanding cognitive developmental change*. Paper presented at 13th Biennial Meeting of the Conference on Human Development, Pittsburgh, PA.

Sigman, M., & Mundy, P. (1993). Infant precursors of childhood intellectual and verbal abilities. In D. Hay & A. Angold (Eds.), *Precursors and causes in development and psychopathology* (pp. 123–143). New York: John Wiley & Sons.

Smith, L., & von Tetzchner, S. (1986). Communicative, sensorimotor, and language skills of young children with Down syndrome. *American Journal of Mental Deficiency, 91*, 57–66.

Snyder, L. (1978). Communicative and cognitive abilities in the sensorimotor period. *Merrill-Palmer Quarterly, 24*, 161–180.

Stern, D. (1985). *The interpersonal world of the infant*. New York: Basic Books.

Sugarman, S. (1984). The development of preverbal communication. In R.L. Schiefelbusch & J. Pickar (Eds.), *The acquisition of communicative competence* (pp. 23–67). Baltimore: University Park Press.

Tomasello, M. (1988). The role of joint attention in early language development. *Language Sciences, 11*, 69–88.

Tomasello, M. (1995). Joint attention as social cognition. In C. Moore & P. Dunham (Eds.), *Joint attention: Its origins and role in development* (pp. 103–130). Hillsdale, NJ: Lawrence Erlbaum Associates.

Tomasello, M., & Farrar, J. (1986). Joint attention and early language. *Child Development, 57*, 1454–1463.

Tomasello, M., & Kruger, A. (1992). Joint attention on actions: Acquiring verbs in ostensive and non-ostensive contexts. *Journal of Child Language, 19*, 311–333.

Trevarthen, C. (1979). Communication and cooperation in early infancy: A description of primary intersubjectivity. In M. Bullowa (Ed.), *Before speech: The beginning of interpersonal communication* (pp. 321–347). New York: Cambridge University Press.

Tronick, E. (1989). Emotions and emotional communication in infants. *American Psychologist, 44*, 112–119.

Tronick, E., Als, H., & Adamson, L. (1979). The communicative structure of early face-to-face interaction. In M. Bullowa (Ed.), *Before speech: The beginnings of interpersonal communication* (pp. 349–372). New York: Cambridge University Press.

Ungerer, J., & Sigman, M. (1984). The relation of play and sensorimotor behavior to language in the second year. *Child Development, 55*, 1448–1455.

Uzgiris, I., & Hunt, J.M. (1975). *Assessment in infancy: Ordinal scales of psychological development*. Urbana: University of Illinois Press.

Valenti, S., & Good, J. (1991). Social affordances and interaction I: Introduction. *Ecological Psychology, 3*, 77–98.

Wellman, H. (1993). Early understanding of the mind: The normal case. In S. Baron-Cohen, H. Tager-Flusberg, & D. Cohen (Eds.), *Understanding other minds: Perspectives from autism* (pp. 40–58). Oxford: Oxford University Press.

Welsh, M., & Pennington, B. (1988). Assessing frontal lobe functioning in children. Views from developmental psychology. *Developmental Neuropsychology, 4*, 199–230.

Werner, H., & Kaplan, S. (1963). *Symbol formation*. New York: John Wiley & Sons.

Wetherby, A., & Prizant, B. (1993a). *Communication and Symbolic Behavior Scales*. Chicago: Riverside.

Wetherby, A.M., & Prizant, B. (1993b). Profiling communication and symbolic abilities in young children. *Journal of Childhood Communication Disorders, 15*, 23–32.
Wetherby, A.M., & Prutting, C.A. (1984). Profiles of communicative and cognitive-social abilities in autistic children. *Journal of Speech and Hearing Research, 27*, 367–377.
Wetherby, A., Yonclas, D., & Bryan, A. (1989). Communication profiles of preschool children with handicaps: Implications for early identification. *Journal of Speech and Hearing Disorders, 31*, 148–158.

# 6

# Language Acquisition and Theory of Mind

## Contributions from the Study of Autism

Helen Tager-Flusberg

Since the 1980s there has been an explosion of research on children's developing theory of mind. The focus of much of this work has been on the cognitive achievements during the toddler and preschool years, as the child develops a mentalistic view of people (Lewis & Mitchell, 1994). These achievements culminate at approximately age 4, in a representational view of the mind (e.g., Perner, 1991; Wellman, 1990). At this point, the child is able to interpret human action within a causal-explanatory framework, understanding that the mind does not simply copy reality but provides a representation of the world. With this representational theory, the 4-year-old understands, for example, that beliefs do not necessarily match reality and that different people may hold different beliefs about the world. The implications of these cognitive achievements for the child's social understanding have been the subject of research in developmental psychology (e.g., Dunn, 1994; Dunn, Brown, Slomkowski, Telsa, & Youngblade, 1991; Pillow, 1991). With a more mature theory of mind, children's social relationships are transformed in important ways, and work on social cognition has been reinterpreted from a theory of mind perspective (see Perner, 1988).

These advances in theory of mind research have had less influence on the field of developmental psycholinguistics. One exception has been the investigation of children's talk about mental states, using verbs such as want, think, know, and forget (Bartsch & Wellman, 1995; Bretherton & Beeghly, 1982;

---

This chapter was written with grant support from the National Institute on Deafness and Other Communication Disorders (RO1 DC-01234).

Shatz, Wellman, & Silber, 1983). Children begin talking about desires at approximately the age 2 and cognitive mental states by the time they are 3 years old (Bartsch & Wellman, 1995). In general, this work on the content of children's language has been taken as additional evidence that reflects their growing awareness of a variety of mental states. Psycholinguistic studies are taken as demonstrations that the language of mental states is driven by conceptual developments in theory of mind.

Within the study of autism, the connections between language and theory of mind have been a more central focus of both theory and research (e.g., Happé, 1993; Tager-Flusberg, 1993). Autism is a rare neurodevelopmental disorder that involves primary impairments in social functioning, language and communication, and imaginative behavior (American Psychiatric Association, 1994; Wing & Gould, 1979). In most cases, problems are clearly evident by the end of the first year or during the second year of life, when infants, later diagnosed with autism, fail to engage in secondary intersubjectivity or joint attention (Klin & Volkmar, 1993). Language and symbolic play fail to emerge in the second year, and few attempts at communication with other people are evident. There has been considerable interest in the field of autism to understand the connections between some of these primary impairments that characterize children with this disorder. The seminal research by Baron-Cohen, Leslie, and Frith (1985), demonstrating that autism involves specific impairments in acquiring a theory of mind, paved the way for using the theory of mind hypothesis of autism to explain the social and language impairments that are at the core of the syndrome (Baron-Cohen, 1988; Frith, 1989; Happé, 1994b).

We have learned much from the study of autism about the role of theory of mind in both prelinguistic communicative developments and later-developing aspects of communicative competence. Research on autism has provided theories of language acquisition with crucial information about the significance of theory of mind in the development of language in all children. It is only through the study of these children, who are specifically impaired in this domain, that we have learned exactly what contribution is made by knowledge of other minds to the acquisition of different aspects of language. In typically developing children, developments in different cognitive domains (e.g., conceptual, theory of mind, language) all occur at similar rates and are closely correlated and integrated with one another. The study of atypical children, such as children with autism, provides us with unique opportunities to observe development when one or more cognitive domain is impaired and therefore no longer in synchrony with other domains (Tager-Flusberg, 1988). Studies of children with autism provide us with the clearest data on where the joints between two cognitive domains, language and theory of mind, can be carved.

As with the research on typically developing children, the focus of research on children with autism has been on how theory of mind influences language functioning in this population. The first part of this chapter surveys some of this evidence, demonstrating the critical role played by theory of mind in language development. Yet studies also suggest that the direction of influence may work the other way, that is, language development may, in turn, play an important role in certain developments in theory of mind, in particular facilitating the child's move from a simple mentalistic view of people to a representational theory of mind (de Villiers, 1995b; Tager-Flusberg, 1995a). The last part of this chapter explores this idea, drawing on studies of both typically developing preschoolers and individuals with autism.

## A MODEL OF LANGUAGE ACQUISITION

There has been a move away from the view, which first had its roots in the behaviorist tradition and later in the social interactionist perspective, that language acquisition is made possible by a general purpose learning mechanism that relies on language input as well as positive and negative feedback to shape the development of a linguistic system. Because of the fundamental learnability problems that this simple model is unable to handle (Pinker, 1979, 1984), a more complex view of language acquisition is now generally accepted, which holds that language acquisition is made possible by several distinct cognitive systems, each processing different types of information relevant to language and communication, interacting with the environment and with each other. John Locke (1994) has proposed a theory to explain the ontogenetic path toward spoken language called the *dual specialization hypothesis*. In it, there are two cognitive systems that are critical for language acquisition. The first, the SSC (Specialization for Social Cognition) processes information about faces and voices and is critical in the development of a theory of mind. The second, the GAM (Grammatical Analysis Module), takes inputs from the SSC and is the mechanism that makes phonological and grammatical computations possible. In Locke's theory, the SSC feeds utterance data to the GAM, and plays a central role in a variety of communicative aspects of language that do not involve computational analysis.

Our model of language acquisition shares many features with Locke's theory (Tager-Flusberg, in press); however, we posit three critical cognitive systems, each processing different categories of information. The first is a computational system, similar in function to Locke's GAM, dedicated to processing hierarchical linguistic information as in phonological and grammatical structures. The second mechanism parallels Locke's SSC, though it is more explicitly referred to as a theory of mind system that processes both visual and vocal information about people and builds conceptual representations of mental constructs and social stimuli. (See Baron-Cohen, 1995, for a detailed description of one model of the component modules that constitute a theory of mind cognitive system.) Our model differs from Locke's in that we add a third mechanism, which is amodal. This final mechanism involves general cognitive systems (i.e., not domain specific) that are critical in building conceptual structures that are the foundation for categorization and the lexical-semantic components of language (Jackendoff, 1983). Although these mechanisms are integrated and must interact to allow for normal functioning, there is evidence to suggest that they represent independent systems based on distinct neurobiological substrates (e.g., Baron-Cohen et al., 1994; Fletcher et al., 1995; Mazoyer et al., 1993; Wilkins & Wakefield, 1995).

The difference between this view and Locke's theory is that in this model it is the conceptual structure, not the SSC, that feeds utterance information to the computational system and interacts with it to create linguistic meaning. The theory of mind mechanism is not involved in feeding much of the content of language, as in Locke's model, though it does provide the critical communicative motivation for language and is involved in many aspects of pragmatic functioning. In autism, therefore, there is selective impairment to one of these three critical mechanisms, the theory of mind. We can examine prelinguistic communication and language functioning in children with autism to explore the consequences of impairment to this system for language acquisition. In turn, we can learn what role the theory of mind system plays in language acquisition in all children, where the specific contributions of each mechanism may not be so clear. Autism provides us with the opportunity to observe where the joints between these three systems may be delineated.

## IMPACT OF THEORY OF MIND IMPAIRMENTS ON LANGUAGE

### Prelinguistic Communication

By the end of the first year of life, typically developing infants begin to engage in joint attention behaviors (Corkum & Moore, 1995; Scaife & Bruner, 1975). The key components of joint attention involve the child's coordinating attention to an object and adult at the same time as the adult engages in the same coordinating behaviors. Joint attention is considered a critical achievement that marks the intersection between key cognitive developments, new forms of social engagement with others, and the onset of intentional communication (Moore & Dunham, 1995). At its core, the triadic form of joint attention demonstrates an infant's awareness of another person's mental state and is often taken as an early indicator that the infant has an incipient understanding of mentalism (e.g., Baron-Cohen, 1993; Tomasello, 1995). In joint attention, the child demonstrates an awareness of the attentional focus of the adult and that the adult behaves in an intentional way.

In autism, impairments in joint attention are among the first clear signs of social-cognitive impairment (Baron-Cohen, Allen, & Gillberg, 1992). Infants with autism fail to engage in joint attention behaviors, and even older children with autism remain significantly impaired in their capacity to engage in joint attention (Loveland & Landry, 1986; Mundy, Sigman, & Kasari, 1994). These impairments have significant implications for communicative development in autism, especially when communication serves a commenting function. Numerous scholars have identified the two primary functions of language as request and comment (Austin, 1962; Grice, 1975). Both emerge at about the same time in typically developing infants (Bates, Camaioni, & Volterra, 1975). However, it is primarily the comment functions that exploit the ability to attribute intentions to others; thus, it is not surprising that they are profoundly impaired in autism even at the earliest stages in development.

During the prelinguistic period, which may last a lifetime for some individuals with autism, impairments in joint attention are reflected in communicative impairments that entail manipulating or commenting on the object of another person's attention. Studies of children with autism have repeatedly found a dissociation between the two key communicative functions of the prelinguistic period: protoimperative and protodeclarative functions (Mundy, Sigman, Ungerer, & Sherman, 1986; Wetherby, 1986). For example, in a controlled experimental study, Baron-Cohen (1989) found that although children with autism were able to use a pointing gesture in the context of requesting an object, that is, protoimperative pointing, they were significantly impaired in using a protodeclarative point to comment on an object of interest.

Although most research has emphasized the selective impairments in protodeclarative communication in children with autism, one study suggests that there are also differences in young autistic children's use of protoimperative functions. Phillips, Gómez, Baron-Cohen, Laá, and Rivière (in press) compared a group of preschoolers with autism to CA (chronological age)- and MA (mental age)-matched children with mental retardation and MA-matched typically developing children in a context designed to elicit requests. They found that the children with autism were significantly less likely than the other two groups to use a protoimperative gesture combined with eye contact. Overall, the three groups did not differ in their ability to communicate requests; however, the form of such requesting behaviors was different in the children with autism. The authors of this study interpret their findings in terms of the inability of children with autism to understand the other person in the communicative context as a perceiving subject. The impairments found in the children with autism in combining communicative gestures with gaze contact reflect their difficulties with joint attention.

Studies of prelinguistic communication in individuals with autism suggest that one key source of their impairments lies in joint attention. In turn, these impairments reflect a fundamental deficit in early understanding of other minds. Because many children with autism do not understand even simple intentional mental states in other people, such as attention, they fail to grasp the essence of communication and language as a means of commenting on objects of interest.

## Early Language Development

As some children with autism make the transition to spoken language, they continue to demonstrate the same fundamental impairments in the use of language to make assertions, to comment on objects or events of interest, or to provide new information to their conversational partner (Tager-Flusberg, 1993). These impairments also reflect impairments in the development of a theory of mind, particularly in appreciating the use of language to influence the mental states of others, including intentions, knowledge, and beliefs. The most striking reflection of these impairments is found in the impoverished conversations that individuals with autism engage in with others. Even when children with autism have acquired both lexical and syntactic forms, they remain at very primitive levels of communicative competence, hampered by their inability to add new information and extend a conversational topic over several communicative turns (Tager-Flusberg & Anderson, 1991). They seem limited to using language for maintaining social contact and meeting their own needs and goals (Wetherby & Prutting, 1984). These conversational impairments stem from a lack of awareness that people communicate not only to achieve goals but also to exchange information, and indeed, that people may have access to different information.

Parallel impairments emerge in more detailed studies of the functions expressed by children with autism with particular syntactic forms. It has repeatedly been noted in the literature that children with autism evidence fundamental dissociations between the acquisition of form and function (Mermelstein, 1983; Paul, 1987; Tager-Flusberg, 1989a, 1994). But not all functions are impaired equally; it is only those functions that entail an understanding of other minds that are used at a significantly lower frequency among children with autism compared with typically developing children or other populations of children with developmental disorders.

One source of evidence for these specific form/function impairments comes from a longitudinal study of six children with autism (all boys) and six children with Down syndrome (four boys and two girls). We (Tager-Flusberg et al., 1990) included in this study a group of children without autism who were delayed in acquiring language, thus ensuring that any differences in developmental patterns found among the children with autism were not simply the result of later onset of language acquisition. The children were individually matched at the start of the study on age (ranging from 3 to 7 years old) and MLU (mean length of utterance), measured in morphemes (ranging from 1.17 to 3.74). The children were visited bimonthly in their homes and were videotaped while they played with their mothers. They were followed for 1 or 2 years, and the transcripts of these visits form the primary data for this study. (For more details about the subjects, methods, and procedures, see Tager-Flusberg et al., 1990.) These data were then used to study the development of different constructions, focusing within each construction on the acquisition of syntactic forms and pragmatic functions. The following sections discuss the main findings for the development of negation, questions, and modal verbs to illustrate how form and function develop in asynchronous ways in children with autism.

***Development of Negation*** One of the earliest words that children learn is "no." Within a few years they acquire the complex syntax of sentential negation, which involves mastery over the auxiliary verb system of English, and negation can be used to express a range of semantic functions, including rejection, nonexistence, and truth-functional denial (Bloom, 1970). Our analysis of the development of negation in children with autism and Down syndrome was based on transcripts taken over the course of the first year of the longitudinal project for four of the six children in each group (Tager-Flusberg & Keenan, 1987). All nonimitative utterances containing a negative morpheme were extracted from the transcripts and coded on syntactic and functional dimensions.

To explore the development of syntactic forms of negation, we drew on Klima and Bellugi's (1966) seminal work on typically developing children. Klima and Bellugi identified three periods or phases in the acquisition of the syntactic structures of negation. During the first period (A), a simple proposition is preceded or followed by a simple negative element (e.g., *No get a chip*; *No go see Ann*). In the second period (B), negative elements such as *no*, *don't*, or *can't* are usually correctly placed inside the sentence; however, the child does not yet have a fully developed auxiliary verb system (e.g., *He not little*; *I don't like a smell of fish*). By the third and final period (C), sentential negation is well formed, and the child has acquired the auxiliary verb system (e.g., *I'm not going*; *It doesn't have air in it*).

Each child's transcript was evaluated for the phase of syntactic development it exemplified, according to Klima and Bellugi's (1966) system. Table 1 shows mean age and MLU values (and ranges) for the children with autism and Down syndrome at each negation period. Compared with typically developing children, both groups lag somewhat behind, not only in CA but also in MLU levels. Only one child, an older boy with autism, had reached the final period of acquiring a productive auxiliary verb system at the end of the first year of the study. These data indicate no significant group differences in the development of syntactic aspects of negation.

Table 1. Development of syntactic forms of negation in children with autism and Down syndrome: Age and MLU values at each stage

| | | Autism[a] | | Down syndrome[b] | |
|---|---|---|---|---|---|
| | | Age | MLU | Age | MLU |
| Negation period | | | | | |
| A | *M* | 4;3 | 2.27 | 4;8 | 1.66 |
| | range | (3;4–5;8) | (1.2–3.8) | (3;3–6;11) | (1.2–2.0) |
| B | *M* | 5;6 | 3.58 | 6;7 | 3.01 |
| | range | (4;8–6;4) | (3.0–4.0) | (5;3–8;8) | (2.6–3.2) |
| C | *M* | 7;1 | 4.22 | — | — |

[a]*N*=4.
[b]*N*=4.

The set of negation utterances were then evaluated using Bloom's (1970) functional categories of nonexistence (e.g., *No more Twinkies*; *No fever for you*); rejection (e.g., *No, I don't want this; I don't want a snack*); and denial (e.g., *No, not cheese from milk* [=cheese is not made from milk]; *No, it's green* [=after mother has stated object is blue]). Table 2 presents the mean frequency per 1,000 utterances for each of these functional categories of negation at each MLU stage and the proportion of utterances at each stage within each category. During the early stages, most negation utterances for both groups of children fall into the categories of nonexistence and rejection. At later stages, the children with Down syndrome begin using negation to express denial, following the pattern reported for typically developing children. In contrast, the children with autism almost never express this function. Clearly, the primary difference in children with autism is their very rare use of denial negation. This paucity of denial reflects impairments in theory of mind: To deny the truth of another person's statement entails the understanding that the other person may hold different beliefs, or that language is itself a representation of reality, not reality itself. These aspects of mental state understanding are specifically impaired in autism.

***Development of Questions*** During the earliest stages, children depend primarily on rising intonation to convey questions. Two major question types

Table 2. Distribution of functional categories of negation in children with autism and Down syndrome

| | Autism[a] | | Down syndrome[b] | |
|---|---|---|---|---|
| | *M*[c] | %[d] | *M* | % |
| MLU Stage I | | | | |
| Nonexistence | 6.0 | 34 | 7.3 | 19 |
| Rejection | 11.6 | 66 | 31.0 | 79 |
| Denial | 0 | 0 | 1.0 | 2 |
| MLU Stage II | | | | |
| Nonexistence | 15.5 | 52 | 4.9 | 10 |
| Rejection | 13.4 | 45 | 43.8 | 89 |
| Denial | 1.0 | 3 | 0.7 | 1 |
| MLU Stage III | | | | |
| Nonexistence | 22.1 | 60 | 3.3 | 4 |
| Rejection | 12.7 | 34 | 58.5 | 73 |
| Denial | 2.2 | 6 | 17.8 | 22 |
| MLU Stage IV/V | | | | |
| Nonexistence | 4.1 | 7 | 4.5 | 7 |
| Rejection | 51.3 | 92 | 46.0 | 74 |
| Denial | 0.5 | 1 | 11.4 | 18 |

[a]*N*=4.

[b]*N*=4.

[c]Average frequency per 1,000 utterances.

[d]Percentage for each function at MLU stage.

are used: yes/no questions and wh- questions. Both require complex syntactic knowledge, including the insertion of an appropriate auxiliary verb, inverting the subject and auxiliary verb, and in the case of wh- questions, moving the wh-word (e.g., *what*, *where*, *why*) to the front of the sentence. Developments of these syntactic features of questions take place over a period of years and are not usually complete until children are about 4 or 5 years old (Stromswold, 1995). Both types of questions are used to express a range of functions, including information seeking, conversational (e.g., agreement, clarification), and directives (James & Seebach, 1982).

From our study of children with autism and Down syndrome, we selected for analysis four transcripts from each of the six children in both groups, taken across the span of 1 year (Tager-Flusberg, 1989b). All nonimitative questions were extracted from the transcripts, using context and prosodic contours to identify them. On average, the children with autism asked 34 questions per 1,000 utterances compared with 49 for the children with Down syndrome. This difference did not reach statistical significance on a two-tailed $t$-test. There were, however, significant differences in the types of questions that the two groups of children asked. Table 3 shows the mean frequency per 1,000 utterances for the two groups. Although the majority of the questions asked by the children with Down syndrome were wh- questions, the children with autism asked about equal numbers of yes/no and wh- questions. Compared with the children with Down syndrome, the children with autism asked significantly fewer wh- questions ($t\,[10]=2.47, p<.05$).

To examine the development of the syntactic form of questions, we tallied the percentage of well-formed yes/no and wh- questions. Well-formedness was defined as the correct use of the auxiliary verb in an inverted position in the sentence. The data from this analysis are presented in Table 4, showing that during later MLU stages, the children with autism tended to use more well-formed questions than the children with Down syndrome, primarily because

Table 3. Distribution of types of questions used by children with autism and Down syndrome: Average frequency per 1,000 utterances and proportion of each question type

| | Autism[a] | | Down syndrome[b] | |
|---|---|---|---|---|
| | M | % | M | % |
| Question type | | | | |
| Intonation | 15.5 | 45 | 18.8 | 37 |
| Yes/no | 9.3 | 27 | 1.3 | 3 |
| Wh- | 9.3[c] | 27 | 28.2[c] | 58 |
| Tag | 0 | 0 | 0.3 | 1 |

[a] $N=6$.
[b] $N=6$.
[c] $p<.05$.

Table 4. Percentage of well-formed questions used by children with autism and Down syndrome at each MLU stage

| | Autism[a] | | Down syndrome[b] | |
|---|---|---|---|---|
| MLU stage | Wh- | Yes/no | Wh- | Yes/no |
| Stage I | 7 | 0 | 8 | 0 |
| Stage II | 40 | 44 | 27 | 60 |
| Stage III | 89 | 4 | 55 | 11 |
| Stage IV | 100 | 57 | 82 | 25 |
| Stage V | 91 | 83 | 84 | 46 |

[a] $N=6$.
[b] $N=6$.

the latter had particular difficulty acquiring the auxiliary system (Fowler, Gelman, & Gleitman, 1994). These findings confirm that the children with autism had little difficulty acquiring the syntactic form of questions.

The semantic functions of all questions were then coded into the following mutually exclusive categories: information seeking; test (for which the child knew the correct answer); requests (for permission, for an object or activity); directing attention; and conversational (seeking agreement or clarification). Table 5 shows the distribution of questions in these functional categories (per 1,000 utterances) for the children with autism and Down syndrome. The two categories that yielded significant group differences were the information-seeking ($t=1.97$, $p<.05$) and conversational functions ($t=3.03$, $p<.01$); the children with autism asked significantly fewer questions that served these functions. It is not surprising to note that most information and conversational questions typically use wh- forms, whereas requests typically involve yes/no questions. Thus, the differences in the types of questions asked by the two groups reflect the different functions expressed by them. It is precisely those functional categories of questions that entail an understanding that another may have access to different knowledge (information seeking) or attitudes (seeking agreement or clarification) that were used significantly less frequently by the children with autism. In contrast, requests, test questions, and attention-seeking questions only entail an understanding of how language can be used to affect another person's behavior, not his or her mental states. These findings thus provide strong supporting evidence for the influence of theory of mind impairments on the functional use of questions by the children with autism in this study.

***Development of Modal Verbs*** The final construction is the development of modal verbs in children with autism and Down syndrome. Because modal verbs form part of the class of auxiliary verbs in English, their use overlaps considerably with questions and sentential negation. The set of modal verbs includes *can*, *could*, *may*, *might*, *must*, *will*, *would*, *shall*, *should*, and

Table 5. Distribution of functions of questions used by children with autism and Down syndrome

| | Autism[a] | | Down syndrome[b] | |
|---|---|---|---|---|
| | *M*[c] | %[d] | *M* | % |
| Information seeking | 10.5[e] | 40 | 19.4[e] | 45 |
| Test | 4.2 | 16 | 3.2 | 7 |
| Request | 5.4 | 20 | 2.8 | 7 |
| Attention | 1.7 | 6 | 1.6 | 4 |
| Conversational | 4.8[e] | 18 | 15.7[e] | 37 |

[a]*N*=6.

[b]*N*=6.

[c]Average frequency per 1,000 utterances.

[d]Percentage of questions in each category.

[e]$p < .05$.

*ought*. They are used to express a range of meanings such as permission, intention, or obligation as well as epistemic meanings that require the evaluation of evidence and one's own and others' knowledge (Palmer, 1979). The emergence of epistemic meanings in the use of modal verbs is closely tied to developments in theory of mind, particularly false belief (Shatz & Wilcox, 1991), but even some nonepistemic meanings entail some mentalistic understanding (e.g., intention).

Using the entire corpus from the children with autism and Down syndrome, we extracted all examples of nonimitative utterances containing modal verbs. Two primary forms, *can* and *will*, accounted for 95% of all the modal verbs used by both groups of children. The total frequency of use was almost identical: 255 from the group with autism and 256 from the group with Down syndrome. Again, the distribution between *can* and *will* was similar across both groups: About three quarters of the utterances contained *can*, one quarter, *will*. Thus, the distribution of the form of modals was the same across the two groups of children.

Utterances containing modal verbs were then coded for semantic function, borrowing from the coding system used by Shatz (1991). *Can* (and *could, may/might*) modals were used to express the following mutually exclusive functions: ability (e.g., *Can't do this*), permission (e.g., *Can I have chocolate milk?*), and possibility (e.g., *This could be a hat*). *Will* (and *would, shall/should*) modals were used to express other functions: prediction (e.g., *The house will get dirty*), volition (e.g., *My babies won't sit here*), intention (e.g., *I will dress her later*), and insistence (e.g., *I won't say it!*). The proportion of utterances in each functional category for each modal verb category is presented in Table 6.

For both groups, epistemic meanings of modals were rarely expressed; the category of possibility made up only a small percentage of utterances, and there

Table 6. Distribution of semantic functions of modal verbs in children with autism and Down syndrome: Proportion of utterances for each semantic function within each modal verb

| | Autism[a] (%) | Down syndrome[b] (%) |
|---|---|---|
| Can | | |
| Ability | 22[c] | 79[c] |
| Permission | 70[c] | 16[c] |
| Possibility | 8 | 6 |
| Will | | |
| Prediction | 85[c] | 38[c] |
| Volition | 5[c] | 29[c] |
| Intention | 8[c] | 29[c] |
| Insistence | 2 | 3 |

[a] $N=6$.
[b] $N=6$.
[c] $p<.05$.

were no examples of utterances expressing speaker uncertainty. The distribution of functional meanings for both *can* and *will* were quite different for the children with autism and Down syndrome. The children with autism used modals mostly to express prediction (i.e., future tense) and permission requests. In contrast, the children with Down syndrome made significant use of both mentalistic functions, volition and intention, and talked a lot about ability (often speaking about their inability to carry out some activity). Similar to negation and questions, we see that functional differences between the children with autism and Down syndrome emerge for precisely those categories that entail some understanding of mentalism.

In summary, when children with autism do acquire language, the main stages of syntactic and morphological development can be characterized as delayed but not significantly impaired or different. This supports the view that the computational system, which is responsible for processing hierarchical information critical in building syntactic representations, is not specifically impaired in autism. The autism-specific impairments that were highlighted in the preceding sections all involved impoverished uses of those language functions that entail some understanding of mentalism. This profile of language functioning in autism underscores the importance of a theory of mind system for language acquisition. Impairments in theory of mind are reflected in limitations in the way language is used by the child with autism.

## Later Language Development

Once children have mastered the basic phonological, lexical, and morphosyntactic components of language, they acquire other aspects of language such as narrative discourse skills, metalinguistic abilities, literacy, and nonliteral uses of language. These developments continue well into the school years for typically developing children. Although many older, high-functioning verbal individuals with autism have little trouble learning how to read and write, they do have problems with both narrative discourse and nonliteral aspects of language. These difficulties lead to poor scores on standardized assessments of reading comprehension and interpretation of written and oral discourse (Minshew, Goldstein, & Siegel, 1995). Such higher-level language impairments have also been interpreted within a theory of mind framework by numerous researchers. The following sections briefly review some of the work on these more advanced aspects of language use in older subjects with autism.

***Narrative Discourse*** Children's narratives provide rich information about their developing linguistic, cognitive, and social knowledge (e.g., Bamberg & Damrad-Frye, 1991; Britton & Pellegrini, 1990). Social-cognitive, or theory of mind, knowledge is particularly relevant for the interpretation of characters' intentions, motivations, beliefs, and reactions that must be woven into the depiction of event sequences within an overall story structure (Bruner, 1986). It is not until typically developing young children reach the age of 4 that they begin to incorporate these psychological components of human experience into their stories, coinciding with the period of major developments in theory of mind (Astington, 1990).

The first study on storytelling in individuals with autism was conducted by Baron-Cohen, Leslie, and Frith (1986). After sequencing sets of pictures depicting physical causation, behavioral, and false belief stories, subjects were asked to narrate the stories shown in the pictures. Only half the subjects with autism and Down syndrome in this study were able to tell any stories in this context. The stories that were produced were coded only for the presence of mental state language, and not surprisingly, the subjects with autism were significantly less able than the matched subjects with Down syndrome and typical development in using mental state terms to explain the false belief stories.

A more detailed study was conducted by Loveland, McEvoy, Tunali, and Kelley (1990), who asked individuals with autism and Down syndrome, matched on CA and verbal MA, to retell the story they were shown in the form of a puppet show or video sketch. Compared with the controls, the subjects with autism were more likely to exhibit pragmatic violations including bizarre or inappropriate utterances and were less able to take into consideration the listener's needs. Some of the subjects with autism in this study even failed to understand the story as a representation of meaningful events, suggesting that they lacked a cultural perspective underlying narrative (Bruner & Feldman, 1993; Loveland & Tunali, 1993). Loveland et al. (1990) concluded that the discourse problems they had identified in the narratives of the children with autism reflected their impairments in theory of mind.

Tager-Flusberg (1995b) compared the stories narrated from a wordless picture book by 10 children with autism and 10 verbal MA-matched children with mental retardation (non–Down syndrome) and typical children. Overall, the children with autism produced significantly shorter and more impoverished stories, and, as in Loveland et al.'s (1990) study, a small number of children with autism did not interpret the picture book as a narrative sequence of events and therefore failed to produce more than simple independent descriptions of each page in the book. One other significant difference was found in this study: Not one of the subjects with autism included in his or her narratives any causal explanations for the events in the stories. Not only did the subjects with autism not use mentalistic explanations, they also failed to provide even physical causal explanations, suggesting that they had quite fundamental impairments in viewing behavior and action within a causal-explanatory framework.

Only one study has directly investigated the relationship between narrative abilities and performance on a standard theory of mind (false belief) task in subjects with autism (Tager-Flusberg & Sullivan, 1995). A larger group of individuals with autism was matched on IQ and standardized measures of language production and comprehension to a group of individuals with mental retardation. Again, a wordless picture book was used to elicit a story. Subjects were later probed about the emotional states of characters in the story. As in the Tager-Flusberg (1995b) study, the subjects with autism were significantly less able to provide appropriate explanations for the emotional states of the story characters. In addition, in the group with autism, all the narrative measures (including length, number of connectives, emotion and cognition terms) were significantly correlated with performance on the false belief task. In contrast, except for the use of cognitive mental state terms, none of the narrative measures from this study was correlated significantly with false belief performance for the group with mental retardation.

The findings from this set of studies confirm that theory of mind impairments in autism are reflected in difficulties found among individuals with autism in narrating a story. Such difficulties vary widely from an inability to perceive a related sequence of pictures or events as a coherent narrative, to limitations in producing a rich and complex narrative that places the sequence of events in the story within a causal-explanatory framework.

***Nonliteral Language*** The understanding of nonliteral, or figurative, uses of language, such as metaphor, irony, or lies, involves going beneath the conventional code of language to interpret the intentions and attitudes of the speaker (Sperber & Wilson, 1986). It is not surprising, therefore, to find that individuals with autism, even those who are older and high functioning, have great difficulty in understanding metaphors and other figurative expressions (Minshew et al., 1995).

Happé (1993) explored the relationship between theory of mind abilities and understanding nonliteral uses of language from the perspective of relevance theory (Sperber & Wilson, 1986). According to relevance theory, different levels of theory of mind understanding are needed to interpret different types of nonliteral language. Similes (e.g., *He was like a lion*) can be interpreted correctly at a literal level and therefore do not entail any theory of mind understanding. In contrast, metaphors (e.g., *The dancer was so graceful, she really was a swan*) cannot be taken at a purely literal level, but the speaker's first-order intentions need to be considered to reach a meaningful interpretation. Ironic statements (e.g., *What a great route we took!* [as the car is stuck in an hour-long traffic delay]) are even more complex, as they entail understanding second-order mental states (the speaker's thoughts about a thought).

Happé (1993) tested a group of subjects with autism on a standard battery of theory of mind tasks and a set of tasks designed to test their understanding of similes, metaphors, and ironic statements. Some of the subjects with autism failed all the theory of mind tasks, some passed the first-order tasks but not the second-order tasks, and a small number passed both first- and second-order false belief tasks. The main findings were that performance on the theory of mind tasks was highly predictive of the subjects' ability to understand metaphors and ironic statements, confirming the predictions from relevance theory. None of the subjects with autism had difficulty with the similes, only those subjects who passed the first-order theory of mind battery were able to interpret the metaphors correctly, and only those subjects who passed the second-order tasks could understand irony. This study demonstrates the significance of theory of mind abilities for nonliteral communication and suggests that there is a small group of individuals with autism, who tend to be older and have relatively high levels of language, who do acquire some ability to understand complex mental states.

In another study, Happé (1994a) further explored these same subjects' understanding of everyday nonliteral language using a set of stories that contained an utterance that was not literally true (e.g., lie, joke, pretend, misunderstanding, irony, double bluff). Two control groups of subjects with mental retardation and typically developing individuals were included in this study, all of whom had passed all the theory of mind tasks. The subjects were told or read each story and were then asked to explain why the character said what he or she said. Across all stories, the number of appropriate explanations provided by the subjects with autism was highly predicted by performance on the theory of mind battery. Nevertheless, the subjects with autism, overall, had greater difficulty giving correct mentalistic explanations compared with controls.

Studies of later developments of language abilities, even in relatively high-functioning people with autism, reveal subtle impairments in mental state understanding. Research on storytelling has highlighted the limited abilities of subjects with autism to tell good stories that incorporate what Bruner (1986) called the "landscape of consciousness." And Happé's (1993, 1994a) experiments on the interpretation of nonliteral language underscore the difficulties that the majority of people with autism have in understanding a speaker's intentions. At the same time, this work on autistic language impairment demonstrates the significance of theory of mind abilities for the acquisition of language in all children. We have learned much about the role of theory of mind in typical development from the study of impairments in autism.

## ROLE OF LANGUAGE IN THE DEVELOPMENT OF A THEORY OF MIND

### Complementation and Propositional Attitudes

Thus far we have considered a unidirectional relationship from theory of mind to aspects of language, particularly functional aspects of language that entail mentalistic understanding. Yet at about the same time as typically developing children reach the watershed period of developing a representational understanding of mind (as evidenced by their ability to pass false belief tasks), they are also mastering a crucial aspect of the syntax of their language concerned with embedded clauses (Roeper & de Villiers, 1994). It has been proposed that these twin developments are not coincidental (de Villiers, 1995b; Tager-Flusberg, 1995a). From an evolutionary perspective, those parts of the grammar (complementation and control) that allow for the embedding of one propositional argument under another proposition seem to be specially designed for the expression of propositional attitudes that are at the heart of a theory of mind (Pinker & Bloom, 1990). Indeed, the two primary classes of verbs that take sentential complements (i.e., embed one sentence under a matrix clause) are verbs of mental state (e.g., *Jane* thinks *that no one read her story*) and verbs of communication (e.g., *Peter* said *that the play was terrible*).

De Villiers (1995a) argued that complementation involves special syntactic and semantic properties that are intimately linked to theory of mind developments. At the syntactic level, the subordinate clause appearing under verbs of mental state or communication is not merely an optional argument (or *adjunct*), but is selected by the verb in an obligatory fashion (or *complement*). Thus, one cannot simply state "John thinks," rather, the content of John's thought must be included, for example, "John thinks that Mary is coming to tea." Other mental state verbs could easily be inserted in this embedded sentence (e.g., *knows, believes, forgot*), illustrating the point that complementation is an important entry for the child into talk about the mental life of people. De Villiers (1995b) suggested that "command of complementation provides a means for representing someone's false belief" (p. 2). As in the above example, it may not be true that Mary is planning to go to John's for tea after all.

The remainder of this chapter reviews evidence both from typically developing preschoolers and from individuals with autism that knowledge of the syntax of complementation is closely linked to developments in a theory of mind.

### Evidence from Preschoolers

Based on an extensive series of studies, de Villiers and colleagues argued that the way children interpret complex wh- questions provides a sensitive measure of their knowledge of complementation (de Villiers, 1995b, 1996; de Villiers, Roeper, & Vainikka, 1990; Roeper & de Villiers, 1994). de Villiers and colleagues' method involves telling the child a brief story (accompanied by a series of pictures) and following the story with a wh- question. In a preliminary study, de Villiers, Sherrard, & Fretwell (1992) gave a group of 3- and 4-year-olds a series of stories of the following sort:

> This mom sneaked out late one night and bought a birthday cake for her little girl. When the girl saw the bag from the store, she asked, "What did you buy?" The mom wanted the cake to be a surprise, so she said, "Oh, just some paper towels."

The children were then asked the test wh- question: "What did the mother say she bought?" The children were also given a false belief task in which they were told a story about an unexpected change in the location of an object. The younger children who failed the false belief task also were likely to give the wrong response to the wh- stories. They typically answered "birthday cake"; that is, they answered the medial clause: *She bought . . . birthday cake.* This kind of response indicates that the child is treating the matrix and embedded clauses more like coordinates and not as a true embedding. Children who passed the false belief task were able to correctly answer the complex wh- question on the story task, suggesting that they had mastered the syntax of complementation. This preliminary evidence provides support for the idea that complementation and false belief understanding are closely associated in development.

In a related set of studies, Tager-Flusberg and colleagues (Tager-Flusberg, 1995a; Tager-Flusberg, Sullivan, Barker, & Harris, 1994) employed a similar methodology but used cognitive mental state verbs in the wh- question study instead of verbs of communication. Cognition verbs divide into two semantic classes: factive and nonfactive verbs. Factive verbs (e.g., *know, forget*) presuppose the truth of the embedded proposition, whereas nonfactive verbs do not (e.g., *think, believe*). Consider the following sentences:

(a) John knew that Mary went shopping.
(b) John did not know that Mary went shopping.
(c) John thought that Mary went shopping.
(d) John did not think that Mary went shopping.

For sentences (a) and (b) the embedded proposition *Mary went shopping* would be judged as true, whereas for sentences (c) and (d) it is unclear whether the proposition is true. This semantic property has consequences for the syntax of wh- questions containing these verbs. Contrast the following two questions:

(e) When did John think that Mary went shopping?
(f) When did John know that Mary went shopping?

The answer to (e) could be, *when he saw her carrying lots of packages*, or, *last Saturday.* That is, the wh- question could be about when John thought it, or when Mary went shopping. For (f), the answer could only be, *when he saw her carrying lots of packages*. In other words, factive verbs such as *know* do not allow the wh- question to cross clause boundaries. Our studies have examined whether children's ability to respond to questions of this type is related to their performance on false belief tasks.

In the first study, 18 preschoolers were given two trials of a standard false belief task. For example, one story was about a boy whose mother tells him she'll make hamburgers for dinner, but while he is gone she changes the menu to spaghetti. The children were then asked a knowledge question (e.g., *Does Bobby know what Mom made for dinner?*) and a belief question (e.g., *What does Bobby think Mom made for dinner?*). They also heard eight stories (four with factive verbs and four with nonfactive verbs) that ended in a wh- question. One such story was about a girl who rode her bike while carrying her radio. She rode over a stone, the radio dropped, and the girl worried that it was broken. After getting home, she plugged the radio in, but it did not work. The story, which was accompanied by a series of photographs, was then followed by the test question: *When did the girl know/think that the radio was broken?* Children's responses to the wh- question were coded as short (i.e., to the matrix verb: *when she plugged it in*), long (i.e., to the embedded clause: *when she dropped it*), or other (e.g., *last week*).

We divided the children into those who passed the false belief task ($N=10$) and those who failed ($N=8$). The responses of these two groups on the wh- movement task are presented in Table 7. The analysis of variance of these data showed that the children who failed the false belief task gave significantly fewer short responses to both the factive and nonfactive verbs ($F$ [1, 16]$=20.83$, $p<.003$) and significantly more other responses ($F$ [1, 16]$=16.35$, $p<.0009$). These other responses suggest that the children had great difficulty processing the complex wh- questions. Five of the eight who failed gave a curious error response to the complex yes/no knowledge question on the false belief task. Instead of saying either *yes* (incorrect) or *no* (correct), these five chil-

Table 7. Mean scores (and standard deviations) on the wh- movement task by preschoolers in experiment 1

| | Passed[a] | | Failed[b] | |
|---|---|---|---|---|
| | *M* | (*SD*) | *M* | (*SD*) |
| Factive verbs[c] | | | | |
| Short | 2.40 | (0.97)[d] | 0.50 | (0.93)[d] |
| Long | 1.10 | (0.88) | 0.75 | (1.04) |
| Other | 0.50 | (0.85)[d] | 2.75 | (1.83)[d] |
| Nonfactive verbs[c] | | | | |
| Short | 2.10 | (1.45)[d] | 0.25 | (0.71)[d] |
| Long | 1.80 | (1.32) | 1.00 | (1.51) |
| Other | 0.10 | (0.32)[d] | 2.75 | (1.83)[d] |

[a] $N=10$.

[b] $N=8$.

[c] Scores are averaged across four stories for each verb type.

[d] $p<.05$.

dren answered "spaghetti." In other words, they answered the medial wh- question (*Does Bobby know*) *what Mom made for dinner*, underscoring their incomplete knowledge of complementation. The relationship between false belief and understanding of complex wh- questions was assessed using a point-biserial correlation between pass/fail on the false belief task and the number of short responses on the wh- question task. This correlation was statistically significant ($r$ [16] = .72, $p < .01$), after age was partialled out.

In a follow-up study, we included a larger sample of preschoolers. This time the false belief task only included a prediction question that did not contain a cognition verb (i.e., *Where will X look for Y?*). The wh- question task was similar, though we made small modifications to the stories. Out of 41 children, 16 passed the false belief task, and 25 failed. The data for the wh- question task are presented in Table 8. As in the previous study, the analysis of variance revealed that those who failed gave significantly fewer short responses ($F$ [1, 39] = 13.0, $p < .0009$) and significantly more other responses ($F$ [1, 39] = 5.65, $p < .03$). The point-biserial correlation between pass/fail on the false belief task and the number of short responses was again highly significant even with the effects of age partialled out ($r$ [39] = .44, $p < .01$).

Across all the studies reported here similar findings were obtained: In typically developing preschoolers, there is a significant close relation between performance on false belief tasks and knowledge of syntactic complementation, as assessed by the children's ability to correctly interpret complex wh- questions. Because of the correlational nature of these studies, we do not have clear evidence about the direction of influence: Do developments in theory of mind drive the syntactic changes, or do syntactic developments lead to changes in the child's understanding of representational mental states? It is highly likely that there is a mutual influence between these two key interrelated achievements in

Table 8. Mean scores (and standard deviations) on the wh- movement task by preschoolers in experiment 2

| | Passed[a] | | Failed[b] | |
|---|---|---|---|---|
| | *M* | (*SD*) | *M* | (*SD*) |
| Factive verbs[c] | | | | |
| Short | 1.73 | (1.62)[d] | 0.61 | (0.84)[d] |
| Long | 0.60 | (0.83) | 1.13 | (0.81) |
| Other | 1.40 | (1.40)[d] | 2.26 | (1.29)[d] |
| Nonfactive verbs[c] | | | | |
| Short | 0.80 | (1.21)[d] | 0.13 | (0.46)[d] |
| Long | 1.53 | (1.35) | 1.34 | (1.23) |
| Other | 1.40 | (1.68)[d] | 2.52 | (1.41)[d] |

[a] $N = 16$.

[b] $N = 25$.

[c] Scores are averaged across four stories for each verb type.

[d] $p < .05$.

typically developing children, although recent evidence from oral deaf children who have typical intelligence but are significantly delayed in acquiring a first language suggests that with only rudimentary language abilities, theory of mind development may be significantly delayed (Gale, de Villiers, de Villiers, & Pyers, 1995).

### Evidence from People with Autism

Since the earliest studies of false belief in individuals with autism, researchers have repeatedly found a significant relation between the ability to pass theory of mind tasks and verbal MA (for review and summary, see Happé, 1995). Most of these studies have relied on standardized measures of vocabulary comprehension (e.g., PPVT–R [Peabody Picture Vocabulary Test–Revised] [Dunn & Dunn, 1981] or the British equivalent) to assess verbal MA; however, in our studies we also employed a measure of syntactic comprehension, the Sentence Structure subtest of the CELF–R (Clinical Evaluation of Language Fundamentals–Revised) (Tager-Flusberg & Sullivan, 1994, 1995). On this test almost half the items involve some form of sentence embedding. By including this syntactic measure we were able to directly investigate theory of mind performance and syntactic ability.

In our primary study, we tested subjects with autism and nonspecific mental retardation on two theory of mind tasks. The 28 subjects with autism had an average age of 16 years 11 months, and their average IQ score was 70. They all had language scores on both the PPVT–R and Sentence Structure subtest above the 4-year-old level. The 28 subjects with mental retardation had an average age of 12 years 5 months, and their average IQ score was 74. They were closely matched to the subjects with autism on IQ and the standardized language tests. The theory of mind tasks included a standard false belief task and a newly designed task called the explanation of action task that required the subjects to provide mentalistic explanations for story characters' actions (Tager-Flusberg & Sullivan, 1994).

The main findings were that for the subjects with autism, performance on the syntax test was significantly correlated with performance on the false belief task ($r$ [26] = .60, $p < .001$) and the explanation of action task ($r$ [26] = .64, $p < .001$). None of the other standardized measures was significantly correlated with these tasks. For the subjects with mental retardation, the syntax test was only related to the false belief task ($r$ [26] = .67, $p < .001$). In addition, performance IQ was also predictive of performance on this task for this group ($r$ [26] = .56, $p < .001$), which suggests that other information-processing factors are also important in mental retardation. In our work, once we had included a syntax measure, we did not find that scores on the PPVT–R were significantly correlated with theory of mind abilities. We preselected our subjects on the basis of the syntax measure, such that only individuals who passed at least some of the complex sentences were included in this study. Having ensured that all our subjects had at least partial knowledge of embeddings, in our sample almost 90% of the subjects with autism showed some knowledge of false belief. This pass rate is far higher than has been reported in any previous studies. These findings provide strong support for the idea that in autism knowledge of complex syntax is strongly linked to theory of mind abilities.

Finally, in a pilot study, we have begun to explore more directly the relationship between false belief knowledge and syntactic complementation in subjects with autism (Tager-Flusberg, 1995a). We tested 16 adolescents with autism and mental retardation, who were similar in age, IQ, and verbal ability to the subjects in the previous study, and we ensured that the groups were matched on IQ and scores on the PPVT–R and the Sentence Structure subtest of the CELF–R. In this study, subjects were given the same false belief and wh-questions tasks that we used with our second group of preschoolers. For the subjects with autism, performance on these tasks was highly correlated: $r(14) = .59$, $p < .02$. In contrast, there was no relationship between these tasks for the subjects with mental retardation ($r[14] = .12$).

These studies suggest that for individuals with autism, performance on a range of theory of mind tasks is strongly linked to syntactic knowledge. In contrast, such consistent relations were not found for the subjects with mental retardation, for whom information-processing factors may be a more significant predictor of theory of mind abilities. I suggest that some people with autism are able to exploit the parallels between syntactic complementation and the abstract structure of propositional attitudes to "bootstrap" some understanding of mental states. Thus, although the subjects with autism in our studies still have impairments in theory of mind that are quite evident in their everyday social functioning, those who have acquired advanced syntactic abilities, specifically knowledge of complementation, have been able to use that linguistic knowledge to help them figure out the logic of theory of mind tasks.

## CONCLUSION

In this chapter I have surveyed a range of studies that illustrate the relation between theory of mind and language. Much has been learned about the role of a theory of mind mechanism in the acquisition of language from studies of children with autism. It is probable that without these studies of autism, the precise role of a theory of mind would not have been so clearly delineated. We see here the important contribution made by studies of atypical populations for theories of language acquisition. The evidence presented here confirms the independent contributions made by the computational system and the theory of mind cognitive system in the acquisition of language. Thus, the evidence summarized in the first part of this chapter underscores the significant influence of a theory of mind on language functions. Much of our everyday use of language involves understanding intentions and related mental states in other people. Impairments in a theory of mind lead to a highly restricted use of language that lacks the richness for which it has been designed.

At the same time, the studies reviewed in the last part of this chapter suggest that all three cognitive systems outlined at the beginning of this chapter in our model of language acquisition interact in critical ways over the course of development. For example, these studies suggest that there are influences of the computational system, specifically the syntax of complementation, on the acquisition of a theory of mind. Both typically developing preschoolers and individuals with autism show strong relations between these domains. The data from the subjects with mental retardation underscore the connections between the general cognitive system and theory of mind. Development consists not only of maturational and developmental changes within each of these systems but also in changes in the ways these systems interact over time. Both aspects of development may be affected in different populations of neurodevelopmental disorders. Data from these populations provide unique opportunities to observe these critical aspects of development in language and other cognitive systems that are not otherwise apparent from the study of typically developing children.

Future research needs to explore further the direction of these relations. Ultimately it is hoped that one avenue for at least higher-functioning individuals with autism to understand more about the minds of others would be through syntactic training. In turn, such interventions may lead to their capacity to understand and use language in more advanced ways, enhancing their everyday conversations with other people, their narrative skills, and the ability to enjoy stories and other fictional works.

## REFERENCES

American Psychiatric Association. (1994). *Diagnostic and statistical manual of mental disorders* (4th ed.). Washington, DC: Author.

Astington, J. (1990). Narrative and the child's theory of mind. In B. Britton & A. Pellegrini (Eds.), *Narrative thought and narrative language* (pp. 151–171). Hillsdale, NJ: Lawrence Erlbaum Associates.

Austin, J.L. (1962). *How to do things with words.* Oxford, England: Blackwell.

Bamberg, M., & Damrad-Frye, R. (1991). On the ability to provide evaluative comments: Further explorations of children's narrative competencies. *Journal of Child Language, 18*, 689–710.

Baron-Cohen, S. (1988). Social and pragmatic deficits in autism: Cognitive or affective? *Journal of Autism and Developmental Disorders, 18*, 379–402.

Baron-Cohen, S. (1989). Perceptual role-taking and protodeclarative pointing in autism. *British Journal of Developmental Psychology, 7*, 113–127.

Baron-Cohen, S. (1993). From attention-goal psychology to belief-desire psychology: The development of a theory of mind and its dysfunction. In S. Baron-Cohen, H. Tager-Flusberg, & D.J. Cohen (Eds.), *Understanding other minds: Perspectives from autism* (pp. 59–82). Oxford, England: Oxford University Press.

Baron-Cohen, S. (1995). *Mindblindness.* Cambridge, MA: MIT Press.

Baron-Cohen, S., Allen, J., & Gillberg, C. (1992). Can autism be detected at 18 months?

The needle, the haystack, and the CHAT. *British Journal of Psychiatry, 161*, 839–843.
Baron-Cohen, S., Leslie, A., & Frith, U. (1985). Does the autistic child have a "theory of mind"? *Cognition, 21*, 37–46.
Baron-Cohen, S., Leslie, A.M., & Frith, U. (1986). Mechanical, behavioral and intentional understanding of picture stories in autistic children. *British Journal of Developmental Psychology, 4*, 113–125.
Baron-Cohen, S., Ring, H., Moriarty, J., Schmitz, B., Costa, D., & Ell, P. (1994). The brain basis of theory of mind: The role of the orbito-frontal region. *British Journal of Psychiatry, 165*, 640–649.
Bartsch, K., & Wellman, H. (1995). *Children talk about the mind.* New York: Oxford University Press.
Bates, E., Camaioni, L., & Volterra, V. (1975). The acquisition of performatives prior to speech. *Merrill-Palmer Quarterly, 21*, 205–226.
Bloom, L.M. (1970). *Language development: Form and function in emerging grammars.* Cambridge, MA: MIT Press.
Bretherton, I., & Beeghly, M. (1982). Talking about internal states: The acquisition of an explicit theory of mind. *Developmental Psychology, 18*, 906–921.
Britton, B.K., & Pellegrini, A.D. (Eds.) (1990). *Narrative thought and narrative language.* Hillsdale, NJ: Lawrence Erlbaum Associates.
Bruner, J. (1986). *Actual minds, possible worlds.* Cambridge, MA: Harvard University Press.
Bruner, J., & Feldman, C. (1993). Theories of mind and the problem of autism. In S. Baron-Cohen, H. Tager-Flusberg, & D.J. Cohen (Eds.), *Understanding other minds: Perspectives from autism* (pp. 267–291). Oxford, England: Oxford University Press.
Corkum, V., & Moore, C. (1995). Development of joint visual attention in infants. In C. Moore & P. Dunham (Eds.), *Joint attention: Its origins and role in development* (pp. 61–83). Hillsdale, NJ: Lawrence Erlbaum Associates.
de Villiers, J.G. (1995a). Empty categories and complex sentences: The case of wh-questions. In P. Fletcher & B. MacWhinney (Eds.), *The handbook of child language* (pp. 508–540). Oxford, England: Blackwell.
de Villiers, J.G. (1995b, March). *Steps in the mastery of sentence complements.* Paper presented at the Biennial Meeting of the Society for Research in Child Development, Indianapolis, IN.
de Villiers, J.G. (1996). Defining the open and closed program for acquisition: The case of wh- questions. In M. Rice (Ed.), *Towards a genetics of language* (pp. 145–184). Hillsdale, NJ: Lawrence Erlbaum Associates.
de Villiers, J.G., Roeper, T., & Vainikka, A. (1990). The acquisition of long-distance rules. In L. Frazier & J.G. de Villiers (Eds.), *Language processing and acquisition* (pp. 76–97). Dordrecht, the Netherlands: Kluwer.
de Villiers, J.G., Sherrard, K., & Fretwell, L. (1992). *Wh- questions and theory of mind.* Paper presented at the Second Roundtable on Wh- Questions, University of Massachusetts, Amherst.
Dunn, J. (1994). Changing minds and changing relationships. In C. Lewis & P. Mitchell (Eds.), *Children's early understanding of mind* (pp. 104–125). Hillsdale, NJ: Lawrence Erlbaum Associates.
Dunn, J., Brown, J., Slomkowski, C., Telsa, C., & Youngblade, L. (1991). Young children's understanding of other people's feelings and beliefs: Individual differences and their antecedents. *Child Development, 62*, 1352–1366.
Dunn, L.M., & Dunn, L.M. (1981). *Peabody Picture Vocabulary Test–Revised.* Circle Pines, MN: American Guidance Service.
Fletcher, P.C., Happé, F., Frith, U., Baker, S.C., Dolan, R.J., Frackowiak, R.S.J., &

Frith, C.D. (1995). Other minds in the brain: A functional imaging study of theory of mind in story comprehension. *Cognition, 57*, 109–128.

Fowler, A., Gelman, R., & Gleitman, L. (1994). The course of language learning in children with Down syndrome: Longitudinal and language level comparisons with young normally developing children. In H. Tager Flusberg (Ed.), *Constraints on language acquisition: Studies of atypical children* (pp. 91–140). Hillsdale, NJ: Lawrence Erlbaum Associates.

Frith, U. (1989). *Autism: Explaining the enigma.* Oxford, England: Blackwell.

Gale, E., de Villiers, P.A., de Villiers, J.G., & Pyers, J. (1995, November). *Language and theory of mind in oral deaf children.* Paper presented at the Boston University Conference on Language Development, Boston.

Grice, H.P. (1975). Logic and conversation. In R. Cole & J. Morgan (Eds.), *Syntax and semantics: Speech acts* (pp. 56–84). New York: Academic Press.

Happé, F. (1993). Communicative competence and theory of mind in autism: A test of relevance theory. *Cognition, 48*, 101–119.

Happé, F. (1994a). An advanced test of theory of mind: Understanding of story characters' thoughts and feelings by able autistic, mentally handicapped and normal children and adults. *Journal of Autism and Developmental Disorders, 24*, 129–154.

Happé, F. (1994b). *Autism: An introduction to psychological theory.* London: University College London Press.

Happé, F. (1995). The role of age and verbal ability in the theory of mind task performance of subjects with autism. *Child Development, 66*, 843–855.

Jackendoff, R. (1983). *Semantics and cognition.* Cambridge, MA: MIT Press.

James, S., & Seebach, M. (1982). The pragmatic functions of children's questions. *Journal of Speech and Hearing Research, 25*, 2–11.

Klima, E.S., & Bellugi, U. (1966). Syntactic regularities in the speech of children. In J. Lyons & R.J. Wales (Eds.), *Psycholinguistics papers* (pp. 183–208). Edinburgh, Scotland: Edinburgh University Press.

Klin, A., & Volkmar, F. (1993). The development of individuals with autism: Implications for the theory of mind hypothesis. In S. Baron-Cohen, H. Tager-Flusberg, & D.J. Cohen (Eds.), *Understanding other minds: Perspectives from autism* (pp. 317–331). Oxford, England: Oxford University Press.

Lewis, C., & Mitchell, P. (Eds.). (1994). *Children's early understanding of mind.* Hillsdale, NJ: Lawrence Erlbaum Associates.

Locke, J. (1994). *The child's path to spoken language.* Cambridge, MA: Harvard University Press.

Loveland, K.A., & Landry, S. (1986). Joint attention and language in autism and developmental language delay. *Journal of Autism and Developmental Disorders, 16*, 335–349.

Loveland, K.A., McEvoy, R.E., Tunali, B., & Kelley, M.L. (1990). Narrative story telling in autism and Down's syndrome. *British Journal of Developmental Psychology, 8*, 9–23.

Loveland, K., & Tunali, B. (1993). Narrative language in autism and the theory of mind hypothesis: A wider perspective. In S. Baron-Cohen, H. Tager-Flusberg, & D.J. Cohen (Eds.), *Understanding other minds: Perspectives from autism* (pp. 247–266). Oxford, England: Oxford University Press.

Mazoyer, B.M., Tzourio, N., Frak, V., Syrota, A., Murayama, N., Levrier, O., Salamon, G., Dehaene, S., Cohen, L., & Mehler, J. (1993). The cortical representation of speech. *Journal of Cognitive Neuroscience, 5*, 467–479.

Mermelstein, R. (1983, October). *The relationship between syntactic and pragmatic development in autistic, retarded, and normal children.* Paper presented at the Eighth Annual Boston University Conference on Language Development, Boston.

Minshew, N., Goldstein, G., & Siegel, D.J. (1995). Speech and language in high-functioning autistic individuals. *Neuropsychology, 9*, 255–261.

Moore, C., & Dunham, P. (Eds.). (1995). *Joint attention: Its origins and role in development.* Hillsdale, NJ: Lawrence Erlbaum Associates.

Mundy, P., Sigman, M., & Kasari, C. (1994). Joint attention, developmental level, and symptom presentation in autism. *Development and Psychopathology, 6*, 389–401.

Mundy, P., Sigman, M., Ungerer, J., & Sherman, T. (1986). Defining the social deficits in autism: The contribution of nonverbal communication measures. *Journal of Child Psychology and Psychiatry, 27*, 657–669.

Palmer, F.R. (1979). *Modality and the English modals.* London: Longman Group.

Paul, R. (1987). Communication. In D.J. Cohen & A.M. Donnellan (Eds.), *Handbook of autism and pervasive developmental disorders* (pp. 61–84). New York: John Wiley & Sons.

Perner, J. (1988). Higher-order beliefs and intentions in children's understanding of social interaction. In J.W. Astington, P.L. Harris, & D.R. Olson (Eds.), *Developing theories of mind* (pp. 217–239). New York: Cambridge University Press.

Perner, J. (1991). *Understanding the representational mind.* Cambridge, MA: MIT Press.

Phillips, W., Gómez, J.C., Baron-Cohen, S., Laá, V., & Rivière, A. (in press). Treating people as objects, agents, or "subjects": How young children with and without autism make requests. *Journal of Child Psychology and Psychiatry.*

Pillow, B. (1991). Children's understanding of biased social cognition. *Developmental Psychology, 27*, 539–551.

Pinker, S. (1979). Formal models of language learning. *Cognition, 1*, 217–283.

Pinker, S. (1984). *Language learnability and language development.* Cambridge, MA: Harvard University Press.

Pinker, S., & Bloom, P. (1990). Natural language and natural selection. *Behavioral and Brain Sciences, 13*, 707–784.

Roeper, T., & de Villiers, J.G. (1994). Lexical links in the wh- chain. In B. Lust, G. Hermon, & J. Kornfilt (Eds.), *Syntactic theory and first language acquisition: Cross linguistic perspective: Vol. 2. Binding dependencies and learnability* (pp. 63–96). Hillsdale, NJ: Lawrence Erlbaum Associates.

Scaife, M., & Bruner, J.S. (1975). The capacity for joint visual attention in the infant. *Nature, 253*, 265–266.

Shatz, M. (1991). Using cross-cultural research to inform us about the role of language in development: Comparisons of Japanese, Korean, and English, and of German, American English, and British English. In M. Bornstein (Ed.), *Cultural approaches to parenting* (pp. 217–254). Hillsdale, NJ: Lawrence Erlbaum Associates.

Shatz, M., Wellman, H., & Silber, S. (1983). The acquisition of mental verbs: A systematic investigation of first references to mental state. *Cognition, 14*, 301–321.

Shatz, M., & Wilcox, S.A. (1991). Constraints on the acquisition of English modals. In S.A. Gelman & J.P. Byrnes (Eds.), *Perspectives on language and thought: Interrelations in development* (pp. 319–353). Cambridge, England: Cambridge University Press.

Sperber, D., & Wilson, D. (1986). *Relevance: Communication and cognition.* Cambridge, MA: Harvard University Press.

Stromswold, K. (1995). The acquisition of subject and object wh- questions. *Language Acquisition, 4*, 5–48.

Tager-Flusberg, H. (1988). On the nature of a language acquisition disorder: The example of autism. In F. Kessel (Ed.), *The development of language and language researchers* (pp. 249–267). Hillsdale, NJ: Lawrence Erlbaum Associates.

Tager-Flusberg, H. (1989a). A psycholinguistic perspective on language development in the autistic child. In G. Dawson (Ed.), *Autism: New directions in diagnosis, nature and treatment* (pp. 92–115). New York: Guilford Press.

Tager-Flusberg, H. (1989b, March). *The development of questions in autistic and Down syndrome children.* Paper presented at the Gatlinburg Conference on Research and Theory in Mental Retardation, Gatlinburg, TN.

Tager-Flusberg, H. (1993). What language reveals about the understanding of mind in children with autism. In S. Baron-Cohen, H. Tager-Flusberg, & D.J. Cohen (Eds.), *Understanding other minds: Perspectives from autism* (pp. 138–157). Oxford, England: Oxford University Press.

Tager-Flusberg, H. (1994). Dissociations in form and function in the acquisition of language by autistic children. In H. Tager-Flusberg (Ed.), *Constraints on language acquisition: Studies of atypical children* (pp. 175–194). Hillsdale, NJ: Lawrence Erlbaum Associates.

Tager-Flusberg, H. (1995a, March). *Language and the acquisition of a theory of mind: Evidence from autism and Williams syndrome.* Paper presented at the Biennial Meeting of the Society for Research in Child Development, Indianapolis, IN.

Tager-Flusberg, H. (1995b). "Once upon a rabbit": Stories narrated by autistic children. *British Journal of Developmental Psychology, 13*, 45–59.

Tager-Flusberg, H. (in press). Language development in atypical children. In M. Barrett (Ed.), *The development of language*, London: University College London Press.

Tager-Flusberg, H., & Anderson, M. (1991). The development of contingent discourse ability in autistic children. *Journal of Child Psychology and Psychiatry, 32*, 1123–1134.

Tager-Flusberg, H., Calkins, S., Nolin, T., Baumberger, T., Anderson, M., & Chadwick-Dias, A. (1990). A longitudinal study of language acquisition in autistic and Down syndrome children. *Journal of Autism and Developmental Disorders, 20*, 1–21.

Tager-Flusberg, H., & Keenan, T. (1987, May). *The acquisition of negation in autistic and Down syndrome children.* Paper presented at the Symposium for Research on Child Language Disorders, Madison, WI.

Tager-Flusberg, H., & Sullivan, K. (1994). Predicting and explaining behavior: A comparison of autistic, mentally retarded and normal children. *Journal of Child Psychology and Psychiatry, 35*, 1059–1075.

Tager-Flusberg, H., & Sullivan, K. (1995). Attributing mental states to story characters: A comparison of narratives produced by autistic and mentally retarded individuals. *Applied Psycholinguistics, 16*, 241–256.

Tager-Flusberg, H., Sullivan, K., Barker, J., & Harris, A. (1994). *Relationships between language and cognition: The case of mental verbs and theory of mind.* Unpublished manuscript, University of Massachusetts, Amherst.

Tomasello, M. (1995). Joint attention as social cognition. In C. Moore & P. Dunham (Eds.), *Joint attention: Its origins and role in development* (pp. 103–130). Hillsdale, NJ: Lawrence Erlbaum Associates.

Wellman, H. (1990). *Children's theories of mind.* Cambridge, MA: MIT Press.

Wetherby, A. (1986). Ontogeny of communication functions in autism. *Journal of Autism and Developmental Disorders, 16*, 295–316.

Wetherby, A., & Prutting, C. (1984). Profiles of communicative and cognitive-social abilities in autistic children. *Journal of Speech and Hearing Research, 27*, 364–377.

Wilkins, W.K., & Wakefield, J. (1995). Brain evolution and neurolinguistic preconditions. *Behavioral and Brain Sciences, 18*, 161–226.

Wing, L., & Gould, J. (1979). Severe impairments of social interaction and associated abnormalities in children: Epidemiology and classification. *Journal of Autism and Developmental Disorders, 9*, 11–30.

# 7

# The Linguistic Profile of SLI

## Implications for Accounts of Language Acquisition

Ruth V. Watkins

Imagine two 5-year-old boys, Mark and Josh, from the same kindergarten class. The boys are similar in many ways. For example, they both enjoy building with blocks and, when asked, report that outdoor play is their favorite time of the school day. When Mark and Josh participated in an investigation of mine, I discovered that they shared additional similarities: Both boys had nonverbal intellectual abilities in the average range, had no difficulties with hearing, and showed no obvious physical or neurological limitations. However, one difference between the two boys was striking. During a play-based conversation, Mark told a complex story about his most recent soccer match and the leg injury a young friend sustained during the game. Mark's sentences were lengthy, nearly adult-like in grammatical complexity, and included rich vocabulary such as "fracture" and "stabilizing pin." In contrast, Josh produced short sentences consisting of simple vocabulary and basic grammatical structures. Several grammatical markers, such as past tense -ed, were missing or inconsistent in Josh's language. Overall, Josh's language sounded like that of a considerably younger child. After talking with both boys during play, I was left with the impression that Mark's language facility allowed him to interact with others with ease, to readily express his ideas and feelings, and to verbally control situations and activities. For Josh, using language seemed effortful and considerably less effective as a tool for interaction.

Preparation of this chapter was supported in part by a grant from the National Institute on Deafness and Other Communication Disorders (R03 DC02218).

A complete assessment revealed that Josh's profile was consistent with a diagnosis of specific language impairment, typically referred to as SLI. In a systematic investigation of kindergarten-age children in the state of Iowa, Tomblin (1993) found that approximately 5% of all youngsters demonstrated difficulties in language expression and/or comprehension as a primary condition. The language difficulties identified by Tomblin were not tied to intellectual impairments (the children Tomblin included showed nonverbal intellectual skills in the average range or above); hearing problems; or physical, neurological, or significant psychosocial limitations. This gap between language and other developmental areas has become the defining feature of SLI; operational variations of it are typically used as research and clinical criteria in the identification of the disability (see Bishop, 1992; Johnston, 1988; Rice, 1991, for comprehensive reviews; for examples of criteria used in SLI identification, see Craig & Evans, 1993; Craig & Washington, 1993; Gillam, Cowan, & Day, 1995; Lahey & Edwards, 1995; Leonard, McGregor, & Allen, 1992; Rice, Wexler, & Cleave, 1995; Watkins, Kelly, Harbers, & Hollis, 1995; Watkins & Rice, 1991; Weismer & Hesketh, 1993).

Since the 1960s, study of the nature and character of SLI has developed into a rich area of scientific inquiry. The impetus for this research has come from two overlapping and interrelated problems. First, clinical concerns have provided strong motivation for the study of SLI; knowledge about plausible sources of the disability, linguistic characteristics associated with it, and the link between language problems and skills in related developmental domains is central to designing and implementing effective intervention approaches. A significant research literature has been generated and framed in a manner that addresses these issues (Camarata, Nelson, & Camarata, 1994; Fey, Long, & Cleave, 1994; Johnston, 1991a; Leonard, 1991; Tomblin, 1991).

The second motivation for inquiry into SLI is theoretical. Scholars from a number of fields have long viewed the language system as a gateway to the capacities and functions of the human mind (Carroll, 1994). Following similar reasoning, many of those who study children with SLI believe that atypical patterns of acquisition can reveal much about the linguistic system and its operation. According to many accounts of language acquisition and human development, the profile of strengths and weaknesses associated with SLI should not exist. For example, the discrepancy between linguistic and cognitive skills demonstrated by children with SLI runs counter to a number of dominant views of the relation between language and thought (Johnston, 1994; Rice & Kemper, 1984). Thus, research on language learning in children with SLI, as well as children with other disabilities, has the potential to provide insights about some of the most central debates on language acquisition (Bates, Dale, & Thal, 1995).

Several related premises underlie the endorsement of this line of work. One such premise is the belief that all children's language, both typical and atypical, must be accounted for by linguistic and developmental theory; that is, any comprehensive theory of language acquisition should encompass the patterns of development exhibited by all learners (Levy, 1994; Roeper & Seymour, 1994). Another premise is that the unique patterns and pathways of language learning associated with particular disabilities can provide insight about the mechanisms and processes of language learning. Here, the logic is that enhanced understanding of how language comes to be can be achieved through exploration of language breakdown (Bates, Bretherton, & Snyder, 1988; Bates & Carnevale, 1993; Bates & Thal, 1991). A final premise is that patterns of individual difference in language acquisition can suggest particular aspects of the linguistic system that are either vulnerable or robust and thus potentially informative for detailed study.

This chapter provides an overview of the nature and character of SLI and highlights some of the theoretical motivations for studying this disability. The chapter begins with an orientation to SLI, including review of the linguistic profile associated with it; the competencies of children with SLI in related developmental domains; and the emerging literature on the long-term nature of SLI. Building on this foundation, key implications of studies of SLI for better understanding the processes and mechanisms of language acquisition are addressed. Three areas in which SLI relates to issues in linguistic theory are presented: 1) dissociations in language development, 2) genetic contributions to language acquisition, and 3) informative approaches to studying the linguistic system. This chapter highlights both the unique aspects of the developmental profile of SLI and the ways in which SLI informs our general knowledge of language acquisition processes.

## OVERVIEW OF SLI

Despite the availability of ample descriptive research on SLI, some of the most fundamental questions about the disability remain difficult to address. For example, when is SLI typically detected? It seems likely that many children with SLI are identified during the preschool period, yet there are limited published reports to confirm this. Research indicates that children with SLI have difficulties with early language milestones, such as word acquisition and initial grammatical skills (Leonard, 1988; Rice, Buhr, & Nemeth, 1990), which are likely to lead to early detection. Furthermore, numerous studies of SLI have involved preschool-age children, and intervention programs have been designed specifically for this age group (Bunce, 1996; Rice & Wilcox, 1995). As demonstrated in several investigations, however, the profile associated with SLI, namely language impairments in conjunction with average or above average nonverbal intellectual skills, can also be identified in older children and even in adults (e.g., Gopnik & Crago, 1991; Tomblin, Freese, & Records, 1992). Different measurement tools are required, but the pattern of SLI can be documented beyond early childhood.

Another fundamental question is whether SLI is a unitary phenomena, that is, whether there is variability in the severity of the disability or in the patterns of strength and weakness displayed by children with SLI. There is evidence of variability on several dimensions. For example, the extent to which language comprehension is compromised appears to vary among children with SLI. Many investigations have used low language comprehension measures as part of the criteria for identifying children with SLI (e.g., Rice et al., 1995; Watkins & Rice, 1991), whereas other studies have not used impairments in comprehension as a criterion skill (e.g., Camarata et al., 1994), and still other investigations have explicitly required average-range comprehension skills (e.g., Whitehurst, Fischel, Arnold, & Lonigan, 1992; children in these studies are often described as specific expressive language impaired/delayed). My investigations suggest that approximately half of the children who show the general SLI profile (i.e., performance below the average range on general language tests and spontaneous sample measures, scores within the average range on nonverbal cognitive indices) will also perform below the average range on standardized measures of vocabulary comprehension, such as the PPVT–R (Peabody Picture Vocabulary Test–Revised) (Dunn & Dunn, 1981); conversely, approximately half will perform within the average range, albeit often below the mean. It may be that comprehension ability actually differentiates children with SLI into distinct populations, but, as yet, comprehension proficiency has not been uniformly controlled in defining and identifying SLI.

Survey of published reports on children with SLI suggests that some diversity in the severity of language disability is also present in children with SLI, at least as evaluated by standardized instruments and language sample measures. For example, individual participant data reported by Camarata et al. (1994) indicated that some children with SLI performed roughly one standard deviation below the mean on expressive language measures, whereas others performed two to three standard deviations below the mean. Participant profiles reported by Rice et al. (1995) suggest similar variability. Also, individual children with SLI differ in the extent to which their language and nonverbal cognitive abilities diverge (e.g., participant profiles reported by Camarata et al., 1994; Rice et al., 1995). Thus, it appears that the disability of SLI can occur across a range of severity. Some caution is warranted when examining discrepancies between individual measures of language proficiency, however; limitations in the precision of various measures may contribute to apparent performance differences.

Another issue is whether SLI involves all language dimensions or yields varied performance across linguistic domains. The following section presents research indicating that the linguistic impairments of children with SLI cluster in certain areas, particularly those involving morphosyntactic and lexical skills. Yet studies have documented both pragmatic and social-interactive difficulties of children with SLI (Fujiki & Brinton, 1994; Windsor, 1995). Although not without dispute, the prevailing view of the pragmatic and social challenges of children with SLI is that they result from more fundamental linguistic difficulties rather than causing them (see Rice, 1993; Windsor, 1995, for discussions).

In summary, throughout this chapter and in much of the existing research literature, SLI is discussed as if it is a unitary disability or a single phenomenon. And certain aspects of the SLI profile are remarkably consistent. In discussing the linguistic characteristics of the disability, however, it is also useful to bear in mind that children with SLI are a heterogeneous group. There is individual variation in both the severity of the disability and the patterns of strength and weakness connected with it.

## Linguistic Profile

Numerous studies have attempted to identify particular challenges associated with SLI, investigating performance on a wide array of specific linguistic skills (Connell & Stone, 1992, 1994; Kelly & Rice, 1994; Oetting & Rice, 1993; Rice et al., 1995; Watkins, 1994; Watkins & Rice, 1994). In these investigations, a research design in which children with SLI are equated to two groups of typically developing peers has been employed (i.e., age- and language-equivalent counterparts). The primary motivation for this design is to differentiate those linguistic competencies that are particularly troublesome for children with SLI, relative to their language-equivalent peers, from those language abilities that are commensurate with either age or general language level. This design is not without problems, and equating participants on general language ability, via mean length of utterance or alternative measures, yields only a gross match (Plante, Swisher, Kiernan, & Restrepo, 1993; Rollins, 1995); nevertheless, use of the design has promoted the overall goal of identifying the central problems constituted by SLI.

From the multiple investigations of SLI, a relatively consistent linguistic profile of the disability is emerging. This profile has been central to the development of theoretical accounts of SLI (Gopnik & Crago, 1991; Leonard, 1989; Rice, 1991; Rice et al., 1995). In turn, the difficulties associated with SLI pertain to views on general processes of language acquisition, as is discussed later in the chapter. Findings in the lexical and morphosyntactic areas are particularly informative and are highlighted in the next section.

***Lexical Skills*** It is well documented that children with SLI do not learn new words as readily or as rapidly as their typically developing counterparts (Leonard, 1988; Rice, 1991). Furthermore, the vocabulary abilities of children with SLI appear to remain depressed throughout the preschool years. Watkins et al. (1995) found that the number of different words used in spontaneous language samples, a measure of lexical diversity or richness, consistently differentiated children with SLI from age-equivalent children with typical language skills. Other investigations have provided details on word-learning processes in the SLI population. For example, Rice et al. (1990) contrasted the aptitude of children with SLI and age- and language-equivalent peers to learn new words through incidental exposure in a video-viewing format (i.e., a Quick Incidental Learning or QUIL paradigm). Children with SLI learned fewer new words in a comprehension format than either comparison group. These findings suggest that children with SLI are less facile than their typically developing counterparts in the process of mapping initial word meanings (see also Rice, 1990).

However, additional investigations suggest that this straightforward characterization of word acquisition difficulties in children with SLI is not complete. Specifically, Dollaghan (1987) did not find differences between children with SLI and matched peers when the word acquisition task involved mapping one novel form in an interactive context. Rice, Oetting, Marquis, Bode, and Pae (1994) discovered that given multiple exposures to novel words (i.e., 10 repetitions), children with SLI made gains in comprehension that were equivalent to those of their same-age counterparts. These outcomes suggest that under optimal learning conditions, where novel words are salient and presented on multiple occasions, children with SLI can perform as well as their typically developing peers.

Other investigations indicate that lexical abilities in children with SLI may also be influenced by grammatical and form-class factors. For example, Watkins, Rice, and Moltz (1993) documented that children with SLI used a less diverse verb vocabulary in spontaneous conversation than did their age- and language-equivalent peers, but used a similar set of high-frequency verb forms. Rice and Bode (1993) found that three preschoolers with SLI relied heavily on a relatively restricted set of general verbs in their language production. Finally, Rice, Cleave, Oetting, and Pae (1993) observed that distinguishing between mass and count nouns in a word-mapping task was difficult for children with SLI (e.g., "a keelwug," "some blick"); children with SLI tended to make errors in associating a novel label with the appropriate novel substance or object. Rice et al. (1994) also found that children with SLI had difficulty retaining newly learned verb forms. Considered together, these studies imply that the profile of lexical difficulties evidenced by children with SLI is not independent of grammatical form-class factors and that aspects of verb learning may be troublesome for children with SLI.

In summary, this survey of selected investigations reveals that lexical difficulties are a component of the SLI profile. Although children with SLI clearly do not map new words with the facility of their typically developing counterparts, their word acquisition profiles can be enhanced given optimal learning conditions.

***Morphological Challenges*** One of the most consistent findings in studies of children with SLI is the substantial difficulty they have in acquiring morphology (Lahey, Liebergott, Chesnick, Menyuk, & Adams, 1992; Leonard, 1989; Leonard, Bortolini, Caselli, McGregor, & Sabbadini, 1992; Rice et al., 1995). The problems that children with SLI have in learning and using grammatical morphology are extensive. Impairments in both morphosyntactic markers, such as regular past tense -ed, and closed-class forms, such as articles and verb particles, have been identified through a range of tasks and activities, including analysis of morpheme use in spontaneous language samples (Hadley & Rice, 1995; Leonard, Bortolini, et al., 1992; Rice & Oetting, 1993; Rice et al., 1995); protocols that elicit production and/or comprehension of target forms (Cleave, 1995; Rice et al., 1995; Watkins, 1994; Watkins & Rice, 1991); tasks that involve training on an invented morphological form in conjunction with probe measures of new learning (Connell & Stone, 1992, 1994; Swisher, Restrepo, Plante, & Lowell, 1995; Swisher & Snow, 1994); and examination of the profile of SLI in languages other than English (e.g., German: Clahsen, 1989; Lindner & Johnston, 1992; Hebrew: Dromi, Leonard, & Shteiman, 1993; Rom & Leonard, 1990; Italian: Leonard, Bortolini, et al., 1992; Swedish: Hansson & Nettelbladt, 1995). Overall, this work suggests that morphological impairments are a central component of the SLI profile.

Although the specific results of these investigations are not entirely uniform, there is a reasonable amount of convergence in findings. For example, many studies of English-speaking children with SLI have identified regular past tense -ed and regular third person -s as particularly troublesome for children with SLI. In contrast, other markers, among them present progressive -ing and regular plural -s, appear less challenging (Leonard, 1994; Rice & Oetting, 1993; Rice et al., 1995).

Despite the overlap in empirical findings, scholars diverge considerably in their accounts of the source of morphological impairments in children with SLI. Two broad orientations have been posited, offering conceptually distinct explanations. First, several accounts cite processing limitations as central to the morphological difficulties of youngsters with SLI. For example, a fundamental processing account is based on the work of Tallal and colleagues, who suggested that the language problems experienced by children with SLI are caused by difficulties in discriminating rapid elements of speech (Tallal et al., 1996; Tallal & Piercy, 1973). In a related and elaborated account, Leonard (1989) proposed that brief, unstressed aspects of the language system are difficult for children with SLI to perceive and process. This difficulty becomes problematic when brief aspects of the language system also carry morphological information and must be recognized, stored in, and retrieved from morphological paradigms (Pinker, 1984, 1989). Another type of processing-based account, offered by Connell and Stone (1992, 1994), is based on the idea that children with SLI have difficulty recognizing patterns and subsequently generating and applying linguistic rules. Connell and Stone (1994) suggested that these problems may also be compounded by difficulties with storage of and access to linguistic knowledge.

In contrast to processing-oriented approaches, other scholars argue for fundamental differences in the underlying grammatical representations of children with SLI. For example, Gopnik and Crago (1991; also Crago & Gopnik, 1994; Gopnik, 1994) proposed that the morphological impairments associated with SLI are accounted for by missing features in the underlying grammar. According to this account, the grammatical mechanisms of individuals with SLI are flawed in that features such as tense, number, and duration are absent from their grammar-making capacity. Rice et al. (1995) also pointed to discrepancies in the underlying grammatical system, but of a more specific nature. Rice et al. (1995) hypothesized that finiteness marking for main verb clauses (i.e., past tense, regular third person, *be* and *do*) is treated as optional by youngsters with SLI for an extended period of time. This extended optional infinitive model seeks to account for a cluster of affected morphemes in the grammars of children with SLI.

These competing theoretical accounts offer an interesting but sometimes perplexing array of explanations for the difficulties that children with SLI display with morphological acquisition. Additional investigation is needed to determine the model(s) that best relates to the constellation of difficulties associated with SLI. Three lines of inquiry may be particularly profitable. First, expanding the range of linguistic phenomena evaluated in children with SLI will be informative. For example, there has been limited consideration of derivational morphology in children with SLI (e.g., acquisition and use of derivations such as -er in teacher, -y in soapy, -ly in quickly, and -able in breakable). Because derivational forms share certain properties of grammatical morphemes but differ in other key ways, evaluating their acquisition can reveal much about the nature of SLI. For example, derivational forms operate through application of rule-based knowledge; however, derivational forms do not serve syntactic functions in the same manner as grammatical morphemes. Second, work by Rice and Wexler (1995; also Rice et al., 1995) suggests that consideration of clusters of affected skills may yield better understanding of the difficulties associated with SLI than a focus on individual morphological forms (e.g., tense marking in English). Finally, cross-linguistic investigations must play a crucial role in identifying universal features of SLI and in differentiating among theoretical accounts (cf. Leonard, 1994; Rice et al., 1995). Based on the configurations of particular languages, predictions can be developed and tested for each competing hypothesis.

In summary, several key points about the linguistic profile of SLI can be made. First, children with SLI display impairments in multiple areas of the linguistic system including the lexicon, but their significant and protracted morphological difficulties are particularly striking. Second, this profile is central to a range of current research applications insofar as it constitutes the phenotype of the disability (i.e., the behavioral profile of SLI), is the source of the majority of theory building about SLI, and has implications for many prevailing views of the language acquisition process. The latter point is addressed later in the chapter.

## Competencies in Related Developmental Areas

A number of investigations have evaluated the abilities of children with SLI in developmental domains that are closely linked to spoken language. Of particular interest are the competencies of children with SLI in interacting with others, learning to read, and cognitive performance. For example, it has been suggested that children with SLI are at risk for difficulties in social interaction and peer relationships (see Fujiki & Brinton, 1994; Rice, 1993; Windsor, 1995, for reviews). Young children with SLI are selected as conversational partners less frequently than peers without disabilities, are more likely to be nominated as disliked by peers in integrated classroom settings, and are perceived as less socially competent by teachers (Gertner, Rice, & Hadley, 1994; Hadley & Rice, 1991; Rice, Hadley, & Alexander, 1993). Furthermore, studies reveal that preschool children with SLI are at risk for reading problems in the school years (Catts, 1993; Catts, Hu, Larrivee, & Swank, 1994; Menyuk et al., 1991). Thus, what appears to begin as a relatively specific difficulty with the acquisition of spoken language subsequently influences broad skill areas. Linguistic challenges have negative consequences for multiple facets of developmental accomplishment.

In terms of intellectual abilities, numerous investigations of the nature and character of SLI have focused on the cognitive domain. Most of these investigations have addressed whether relatively subtle, underlying cognitive weaknesses could contribute to the language-learning problems evidenced by children with SLI (Fazio, 1994; Johnston & Weismer, 1983; Kamhi, 1981; Nelson, Kamhi, & Apel, 1987; Terrell & Schwartz, 1988). Such cognitive difficulties would be subclinical, because average range nonverbal intelligence is a component of virtually all working definitions of the disability (cf. Stark & Tallal, 1981).

At least two general views of the interface between cognitive and language skills for children with SLI have been proposed. The strongest view, often termed the conceptual-representational hypothesis, suggests that limitations in the cognitive mechanisms of children with SLI subsequently constrain their language functioning (i.e., proposed limitations include restricted information-processing capacities, representational skills, and/or reasoning abilities; Johnston, 1988, 1991b, 1994). A somewhat weaker version of this view also has emerged, which emphasizes the interactive nature of the link between language and thought. On this account, subtle cognitive and/or information processing weaknesses slow language learning and, in turn, limited language skills impede cognitive and information-processing capabilities (Johnston, 1994).

Investigations of cognitive skills in children with SLI have used various tasks, including reasoning, representational, and problem-solving exercises. A review of this literature is beyond the scope of this chapter (see Johnston, 1988, 1991b, 1994, for reviews); however, several major points can be summarized.

First, some studies have shown that children with SLI tend to perform below their age-matched peers on representational tasks, yet the cognitive and/or symbolic performance of children with SLI on these tasks often exceeds their general language level, as estimated through the performance of a language-equivalent control group (e.g., Kamhi, 1981). Second, patterns of cognitive strength and weakness are revealed by varied cognitive tasks. For example, Masterson (1993) reported that children with SLI performed as well as their age-matched counterparts on an analysis-synthesis task that required them to select and implement available information in solving a problem. In contrast, children with SLI did not differ from a group of language-equivalent peers on a concept formation problem, which required the generation of a rule-based strategy for problem solving. Other studies have documented similar patterns of strength and weakness for children with SLI on different types of cognitive and problem-solving tasks (Kamhi, Gentry, Mauer, & Gholson, 1990; Nelson et al., 1987; Weismer, 1991).

Overall, there is little question that children with SLI show difficulties with certain cognitive tasks. The more central question, however, is whether these cognitive challenges can convincingly account for the language impairments of children with SLI. What portion of the problems demonstrated by children with SLI merely reflect their partial and/or inefficient use of language as a tool for thinking? The argument that impairments in language competence hinder cognitive performance is as plausible as the opposite position. This problem has been noted by proponents of cognitive accounts of SLI. For example, Johnston (1994) suggested that the inseparability of language and thinking is not problematic for the cognitive perspective, but is the essence of it. From a clinical perspective, this point is no doubt valid. From a theoretical perspective, the problem is unresolved.

Another problem is that specific cognitive difficulties have not been linked to the particular linguistic challenges that constitute SLI, such as morphological impairments. This is a two-sided problem. Research findings indicate that cognitive skills in children with SLI are differentially affected and spared. We also know that certain aspects of the language system are particularly troublesome for children with SLI. However, these observations have not been connected. A persuasive account of cognitive difficulties in children with SLI will be built on linking particular linguistic challenges to identified cognitive weaknesses and, alternatively, associating cognitive and linguistic strengths.

Overall, then, the basic observations are as follows. Children with SLI perform as well as their typically developing peers on standardized measures of nonverbal cognition. Evidence of subtle cognitive differences between children with SLI and their typically developing counterparts is available; however, the data do not rule out the possibility that cognitive challenges are caused by linguistic deficits, nor are the ways delineated in which particular cognitive problems might lead to the linguistic profile of the disability. It will be beneficial if studies in this area work toward delineating the potentially different sources of the linguistic difficulties of children with SLI (i.e., processing or mental resource limitations versus underlying linguistic impairments; see Kail, 1994).

## Continued Language Challenges

Research has established that children with SLI are at risk for reading and academic difficulties in the school years. However, little attention has been directed toward ongoing linguistic differences that older children and adults with histories of SLI might exhibit. Available studies suggest that remnants of early SLI persist into adolescence and even adulthood. Gopnik and Crago (1991; also Crago & Gopnik, 1994; Gopnik, 1994) provided a detailed report on the linguistic skills of individuals from one family with a high concentration of SLI; roughly half of this 32-member family displayed SLI. Affected adults had particular difficulties in using grammatical morphemes to mark tense and number in their language production and could not consistently differentiate grammatical and ungrammatical sentences that involved such constructions. Tomblin et al. (1992) contrasted young adults with histories of SLI with a control population without impairments on a range of receptive and expressive language skills, as well as reading and spelling tasks. Results revealed a fairly consistent pattern in which the individuals with a history of SLI performed more poorly than matched peers. Furthermore, discriminant analyses differentiated with little error the adults with histories of SLI from those with typical language histories.

Close examination of studies suggests that demanding production-based tasks best tap persistent differences between individuals with histories of SLI and same-age peers with typical language acquisition profiles. For example, Tomblin et al. (1992) found that a sentence repetition task contributed much to the differentiation of adults with and without histories of SLI. Using a somewhat different approach, Bishop (1995) evaluated the language skills of two groups of children: one group with ongoing language difficulties and another group with histories of SLI but whose expressive and receptive language difficulties had resolved by age 7–9 years. Although the recovered group performed significantly better than the persistent group on several measures of language skill, findings revealed that the two groups did not differ in their performance on a nonword repetition task. Both groups of children performed lower than typically developing controls on the task. Thus, Bishop (1995) suggested that nonword repetition may serve as a marker of the residual effects of SLI throughout life.

Similar findings have been obtained in follow-up studies of individuals with a history of phonological disability. Lewis and Freebairn (1992) found that school-age children, adolescents, and adults with histories of phonological problems performed more poorly than matched controls on a range of difficult phonological tasks, such as producing multisyllabic words, tongue twisters, and nonsense word repetition. As was the case for language impairments in Bishop's (1995) study, these differences persisted even though phonological and articulatory difficulties in spontaneous speech had resolved.

In summary, these investigations provide important insight on the nature and character of SLI. The disability is not merely slowed development, persistent difficulties and differences are not overcome, and language facility remains out of sync with other aptitudes. For at least some aspects of the language system, the individual with SLI probably never reaches the status of the typical learner. One interesting point is that the tasks that best reveal residual language difficulties share the feature of placing a substantial load on real-time information processing (i.e., repetition of multisyllabic nonwords, sentence repetition). As discussed previously, one line of reasoning is that such information-processing impairments contribute to early language learning difficulties and continue through the adult years (cf. Johnston, 1994; Kail, 1994; Tomblin et al., 1992). Again, however, an equally plausible alternative is that residual, underlying language challenges are best revealed when processing skills and resources are stretched to their limits.

An important question is whether the linguistic challenges of adults with SLI are circumscribed (i.e., restricted to particular aspects of the language system) or whether SLI exerts long-term negative influences on educational achievement, employment, social competence, and general quality-of-life indices. As of 1996, only limited research has addressed these concerns. Records, Tomblin, and Freese (1992) used a self-report questionnaire method to measure quality of life in a group of 29 young adults (21 years of age) with childhood history of SLI and compared these individuals with a same-age control group with no history of language or learning difficulties. The individuals with a history of SLI performed more poorly than controls on a range of language measures at follow-up. Nevertheless, findings revealed no between-group differences in any measure of life quality, including satisfaction with life, family, job, and social situation. The two groups did differ in the amount of education completed (individuals with a history of SLI completed less education than controls) and employment status (more individuals with a history of SLI were employed full-time, relative to controls). An open question is whether differences in educational achievement may influence life satisfaction and/or economic well-being as individuals with histories of SLI age beyond their early 20s. Clearly, it is important that research pursue such concerns.

## THEORETICAL INSIGHTS FROM SLI

From the preceding discussion, it is apparent that children with SLI present a unique profile of weaknesses and strengths. In what ways, then, do these developmental asynchronies inform our general knowledge of language and language development? This section of the chapter considers three areas of insight. First, the issue of modularity of language is addressed, in light of the developmental dissociations evidenced by children with SLI. Second, genetic and biological contributions to language impairment and language acquisition are discussed, with particular attention to findings in behavioral genetics. Third, aspects of language acquisition in children with SLI, which suggest informative approaches for future investigation of both language disorder and language acquisition processes are addressed.

### Developmental Dissociations

Given that particular skill areas appear to dissociate for children with SLI, what does this tell us about how they are constructed in all individuals, both typical and atypical? This question has been the focus of research with many atypical populations. For example, a considerable body of literature on adult aphasia has been devoted to describing and explaining selective impairment and sparing of particular linguistic and cognitive competencies (Bates & Thal, 1991; Caramazza & Berndt, 1978; Grodzinsky, 1986). At issue in much of this work is whether language is a specialized and specific aspect of the human mind or whether generic cognitive mechanisms give rise to linguistic competencies. Often termed modularity, the domain specificity of language is a fundamental feature that differentiates competing linguistic theories and accounts of language acquisition (Bates et al., 1988; Bates et al., 1995; Fodor, 1983, 1985; Levy, 1994; Roeper & Seymour, 1994).

With respect to children with SLI, two developmental dissociations are apparent. The first occurs within the language system. The typical SLI profile involves moderate levels of difficulty with several linguistic domains, such as the lexicon, in conjunction with significant and long-lasting problems with grammatical morphology. Although this asynchrony across language domains is a well-recognized characteristic of SLI, such dissociations apparently do not occur for children following more typical language-learning paths. In a detailed study of individual differences in rate and sequence of language acquisition, Bates et al. (1988) reported on links between lexical and syntactic skills in the transition from first words to grammar. Bates et al. identified discrepancies between comprehension and production during this period but found no evidence of dissociations across linguistic domains. Based on these findings, Bates et al. argued against modular accounts of language. However, data from children with SLI indicate that particular discrepancies within the linguistic system can and do occur, and that they appear relatively early in development and may persist through life. Studies of other atypical populations have also documented dissociations in proficiency across linguistic domains (Curtiss, 1981; Rosenberg & Abbeduto, 1993).

A variety of mechanisms might account for the asynchrony across domains of linguistic competence displayed by children with SLI. Dissociations alone do not reveal discrete processes (see Chapter 4). For example, Leonard's (1989) surface account appeals to impaired general-processing mechanisms, those that deal with the ability to perceive, process, and build paradigms for particular grammatical forms. Although these abilities are critical for learning morphology, they are not necessarily entirely linguistic in nature. In contrast, other accounts of SLI suggest a language-specific deficiency. Gopnik and Crago (1991) proposed a selective deficit in the underlying linguistic features marked by morphology. Rice et al. (1995) suggested an impairment in the underlying linguistic mechanism that marks tense, or finiteness. Thus, evidence exists of developmental discrepancies across language areas for children with SLI. However, the presence of such discrepancies alone does not ensure that underlying language-specific mechanisms are responsible.

The second developmental asynchrony for children with SLI occurs between the domains of language and cognition. Some scholars argue that, under careful scrutiny, gaps between language and cognitive skills disappear. Furthermore, most scholars agree that initial discrepancies are likely to fade over developmental time as limited language skills negatively influence intellectual and problem-solving capabilities. Nevertheless, in the absence of a complete and coherent account of how particular cognitive limitations lead to the specific linguistic profile of SLI, we are left with the fact that children with SLI demonstrate cognitive skills in particular areas that outstrip their linguistic abilities.

Considered alone, this apparent cognitive–language discrepancy may not be particularly informative. Language is a complex achievement that undoubtedly requires complete use of a full set of intellectual resources. Even seemingly trivial cognitive limitations might disrupt linguistic performance (Pinker, 1994). However, the case for dissociation between language and cognitive domains is strengthened by individuals who present a profile opposite that of children with SLI. Available research indicates that there are individuals whose linguistic proficiency markedly exceeds their cognitive competence. For example, Cromer (1976, 1988, 1991) reported on the language and cognitive profiles of several children with severe intellectual impairments; in particular cases, Cromer documented sophisticated use of syntax in the face of significant intellectual delay and lack of functional living skills. Furthermore, available reports suggest that at least some children with Williams syndrome have language capabilities beyond what would be anticipated given their general cognitive level (Bellugi, Bihrle, Neville, Doherty, & Jernigan, 1992; see also Chapter 4). When viewed together, children with SLI and other disabilities support the existence of what has been termed a double-dissociation of language and cognitive capacities (Bates & Thal, 1991; Pinker, 1994).

In summary, the developmental profiles of children with SLI suggest skill discrepancies among the domains of language and between language and cognition. These findings point to a degree of independence both within linguistic abilities and between linguistic and cognitive competencies. We can conclude that the study of children with SLI can inform inquiries as to the domain specificity of language; evidence suggesting developmental asynchrony is sufficient to warrant theoretical consideration and additional investigation; and complex relations should be considered, such as ways in which underlying impairments might unequally influence varied domains, both within language and across language and thought.

Some caveats should also be considered. Although apparent discrepancies are informative, the accumulated evidence is not yet sufficient to differentiate between localized discrepancies and major dissociations. As suggested by Bates and colleagues (Bates et al., 1988), it seems likely that language is neither entirely domain specific nor entirely integrated with other aspects of learning. Whereas some aspects of language proficiency may be specifically linguistic, others may draw on general intellectual and/or processing resources.

## Genetic and Biological Contributions

Since the earliest discussions and studies of language development, a recurring question has been the extent to which acquisition is driven by environmental versus biological contributions. This feature defines and differentiates many theoretical accounts of language development (Bohannon, 1993). Despite the quantity and quality of debate, resolution on the relative contributions of nature and nurture to language learning is incomplete.

Investigations of children with SLI provide some valuable insight on this issue. First, there is little or no empirical support for the view that an impaired language environment leads to difficulties in language learning for children with SLI (Lederberg, 1980; Leonard, 1987). Second, and more important, there is mounting evidence for genetic contributions to SLI. Work in this area has made use of multiple research methodologies, including family report and questionnaire methods (Lahey & Edwards, 1995; Lewis, Ekelman, & Aram, 1989; Tallal, Ross, & Curtiss, 1989; Tomblin, 1989); detailed single-family studies (Gopnik & Crago, 1991); and twin studies (Bishop, North, & Donlan, 1995; Lewis & Freebairn, 1992; Tomblin & Buckwalter, 1994a,b).

Studies of children with SLI and their families are proceeding through a series of steps required to establish the genetic basis of a disorder (cf. Pennington, 1989). The initial step involves documenting the extent to which a particular condition runs in families, also known as familiality. In the case of SLI, multiple studies have demonstrated that SLI occurs at a significantly higher rate in family members of probands (the proband is the affected individual through which the family is identified) than in the general population (Tallal et al., 1989; Tomblin, 1989). For example, Tomblin (1989) found that roughly 23% of proband family members were affected with SLI or a related condition; in contrast, only 3% of the control subjects' family members were identified as affected.

A subsequent step in establishing the genetic basis of a disorder is documenting heritability, the amount of variance in a trait that can be tied to genetic influences. In research on SLI, work on heritability has occurred through twin studies (Bishop et al., 1995; Tomblin & Buckwalter, 1994a). Tomblin and Buckwalter (1994a) reported concordance rates for 71 twin pairs in which one member had been identified as having SLI (concordance rates are measures of the extent to which two individuals have the same trait or disability). Monozygotic twins (MZ twins are identical) had a concordance rate of .79. Dizygotic twins (DZ twins are fraternal) displayed a concordance rate of .56. These findings provide significant support for the heritability and genetic basis of SLI, insofar as MZ twins, who share all genes, displayed relatively high concordance rates for the disorder, rates that were higher than those of the DZ twins, who share 50% of their genes.

The final steps in documenting the genetic basis of a disability involve detailing the mode in which the disorder is transmitted and identifying the location of the gene or genes that influence the condition. In the study of SLI, work in these areas is under way, yet hypotheses regarding plausible modes of transmission and gene locations remain relatively speculative (Crago & Gopnik, 1994; Tomblin & Buckwalter, 1994b).

Overall, the accumulated evidence supports genetic contributions to SLI. These findings generally point to distinct biological underpinnings for language acquisition. Additional work is needed to determine how genetic factors influence neurological structures and/or processes (see Plante, 1991; Plante, Swisher, Vance, & Rapcsack, 1991, for potential neurological influences), as well as which particular aspects of the linguistic system are affected. In this regard, it is essential that future work differentiate the features of SLI that are tied to genetic sources and those that are not (i.e., fully specify the phenotype or behavioral profile of the disorder). Furthermore, although the results of genetic investigations provide evidence of the biological aspects of language, the same genetic mechanisms are not necessarily evoked in typical language-learning processes. For example, if a particular gene or group of genes is ultimately implicated as contributing to SLI, that same genetic material may not direct typical linguistic development. Whereas a single gene or set of genes may interrupt a developmental process, many more may be required for full operation of the process (Pinker, 1994).

In summary, genetics studies represent an important and promising line of inquiry. Investigations of children and families with SLI have revealed much about the biological nature of the disorder, and of language facility in general. These findings do not imply that there is no role for the environment in language acquisition; however, they do suggest that a significant portion of variability in language proficiency is tied to genetic factors.

### Future Studies of Language Acquisition and Disability

In addition to augmenting knowledge of theoretical aspects of language acquisition, investigations of children with SLI have provided insights for scholars in two other ways. First, studies confined to English-speaking children will yield only partial understanding of the disability and of the language-learning patterns associated with it (Leonard, 1994). Expanded cross-linguistic research enables more complete evaluation of whether key characteristics of SLI in English-speaking children are paralleled in children learning other languages (e.g., dissociations between morphological skills and other linguistic abilities, relations between linguistic and cognitive abilities). Full knowledge of the linguistic nature and character of SLI will be gained through detailed, cross-linguistic investigations, a number of which have been completed (Dromi et al., 1993; Hansson & Nettelbladt, 1995; Leonard, Bortolini, et al., 1992; Lindner & Johnston, 1992).

A further insight gained from studies of SLI is the identification of informative linguistic features. The difficulties of children with SLI in the acquisition of grammatical morphology suggest that morphosyntax is a particularly vulnerable and revealing aspect of the language system. Because morphosyntactic abilities appear to pull apart most readily from other aspects of the linguistic system, they may be ideal for disentangling modular versus general components of language and cognitive processing. Inquiries into SLI can capitalize on this by expanding investigations into skill areas closely related to grammatical morphology (e.g., derivational forms) and by using morphological abilities as probes in a range of studies (e.g., evaluations of processing limitations).

Investigations under way in my lab aim to expand knowledge of morphological acquisition in children with SLI by evaluating related skill areas. The primary study involves a comparison of derivational morpheme use by children with SLI and age- and language-equivalent counterparts (Watkins, 1995). In this study, a modified-cloze task was used to elicit nine target derivations (-er, -y, -less, -ful, -ness, -ie, -ish, -able, -ly) in both real word and nonce word contexts. Preliminary results indicate that children with SLI performed more poorly than age-matched peers in using all nine target derivations except -er; however, the children with SLI performed more poorly than language-equivalent peers on only a few derivations. For example, children with SLI used several derivations as well as their language-equivalent counterparts but performed more poorly than their language-matched peers in using -y and -ie. One particularly interesting finding was that all participant groups tended to perform less accurately on nonce items than on real-word items. It is noteworthy that the children with SLI did not have more difficulty than age- and language-equivalent peers with nonce items; several accounts of SLI suggest that a central problem associated with the disability is difficulty in creating and applying generalized linguistic rules (Gopnik & Crago, 1991; Connell & Stone, 1994). Given this view, it would be anticipated that children with SLI would show particular difficulty with nonce forms, forms for which previous vocabulary knowledge could not assist performance. The data from this study did not support this prediction.

A secondary study involves longitudinal monitoring of derivational morpheme acquisition in a subgroup of the participants with SLI from the larger investigation. Longitudinal tracking reveals that the acquisition of derivations proceeds slowly for children with SLI, with levels of accuracy remaining below age-equivalent peers for sustained periods of time.

On the basis of preliminary data, these studies indicate that the difficulties of children with SLI extend beyond inflectional morphology into the area of derivational morphology, but perhaps not to the same degree. The problems evidenced by the children with SLI in learning and using derivations did not appear equal across forms. Furthermore, the finding that children with SLI did not find nonce forms any more difficult than did their typical counterparts runs counter to predictions of rule-learning accounts of SLI. Thus, like grammatical morphology, derivational morphology is an informative aspect of the linguistic system. Investigations of derivational morpheme acquisition in children with SLI can assist in discerning the relative merits and weaknesses of available accounts of SLI, thereby expanding knowledge of the disability.

## CONCLUSION

This chapter reflects a commitment to the belief that children with SLI and the pathways of language acquisition that these children follow can and must assist in the formulation and evaluation of theoretical perspectives on language learning. SLI presents a particularly intriguing language-learning puzzle. Striking linguistic challenges and unevenness in the language profile itself, in the face of at least generally typical cognitive abilities, suggest some level of independence in particular language functions and structures. Furthermore, work in the area of behavioral genetics provides solid foundation for biological contributions to language acquisition and disruption.

Many scholars pursue the study of SLI in search of guidance with intervention programming and related clinical concerns. This is vital work with direct application. However, it is also valuable to consider the unique route of linguistic development followed by children with SLI; although not commonplace, the pathways of their language-acquisition journey are pertinent to our understanding of linguistic development and may ultimately contribute much toward the advancement of both clinical and theoretical science. Returning to the two children introduced at the beginning of the chapter, by contrasting the rate, patterns, and ultimate language proficiency of Mark and Josh, we gain insight into the mechanisms of language learning and performance.

## REFERENCES


Bates, E., Bretherton, I., & Snyder, L. (1988). *From first words to grammar: Individual differences and dissociable mechanisms.* Cambridge, England: Cambridge University Press.

Bates, E., & Carnevale, G. (1993). New directions in research on language development. *Developmental Review, 13,* 436–470.

Bates, E., Dale, P., & Thal, D. (1995). Individual differences and their implications for theories of language development. In P. Fletcher & B. MacWhinney (Eds.), *Handbook of child language* (pp. 96–151). Oxford, England: Blackwell.

Bates, E., & Thal, D. (1991). Associations and dissociations in child language development. In J. Miller (Ed.), *Research in child language disorders: A decade of progress* (pp. 147–168). Austin, TX: PRO-ED.

Bellugi, U., Bihrle, A., Neville, H., Doherty, S., & Jernigan, T. (1992). Language, cognition, and brain organization in a neurodevelopmental disorder. In M. Gunnar & C. Nelson (Eds.), *Developmental behavioral neuroscience: Minnesota symposia on child psychology.* Hillsdale, NJ: Lawrence Erlbaum Associates.

Bishop, D.V.M. (1992). The underlying nature of specific language impairment. *Journal of Child Psychology and Psychiatry and Allied Health Disciplines, 33*(1), 3–66.

Bishop, D.V.M. (1995, June). *Nonword repetition as a phenotypic marker for inherited language impairment.* Paper presented at the Symposium on Research in Child Language Disorders, Madison, WI.

Bishop, D.V.M., North, T., & Donlan, C. (1995). Genetic basis of specific language impairment: Evidence from a twin study. *Developmental Medicine and Child Neurology, 37,* 56–71.

Bohannon, J.N. (1993). Theoretical approaches to language acquisition. In J.B. Gleason (Ed.), *The development of language* (3rd ed., pp. 239–298). New York: Merrill/Macmillan.

Bunce, B.H. (1996). *Building a language-focused curriculum for the preschool classroom: Vol. II. A planning guide.* Baltimore: Paul H. Brookes Publishing Co.

Camarata, S., Nelson, K.E., & Camarata, M. (1994). Comparison of conversational recasting and imitative procedures for training grammatical structures in children with specific language impairment. *Journal of Speech and Hearing Research, 37,* 1414–1423.

Caramazza, A., & Berndt, R. (1978). Semantic and syntactic processes in aphasia: A review of the literature. *Psychological Bulletin, 85,* 898–918.

Carroll, D. (1994). *Psychology of language* (2nd ed.). Pacific Grove, CA: Brooks/Cole.

Catts, H.W. (1993). The relationship between speech-language impairments and reading disabilities. *Journal of Speech and Hearing Research, 36,* 948–958.

Catts, H.W., Hu, C.F., Larrivee, L., & Swank, L. (1994). Early identification of reading disabilities in children with speech-language impairments. In R.V. Watkins & M.L. Rice (Eds.), *Communication and language intervention series: Vol. 4. Specific language impairments in children* (pp. 145–160). Baltimore: Paul H. Brookes Publishing Co.

Clahsen, H. (1989). The grammatical characterization of developmental aphasia. *Linguistics, 27,* 897–920.

Clark, E.V., & Hecht, B.F. (1982). Learning to coin agent and instrument nouns. *Cognition, 12,* 1–14.

Cleave, P.L. (1995, June). *The acquisition of the morpheme be in children with specific language impairment.* Paper presented at the Symposium on Research in Child Language Disorders, Madison, WI.

Connell, P.J., & Stone, C.A. (1992). Morpheme learning of children with specific language impairment under controlled instructional conditions. *Journal of Speech and Hearing Research, 35*, 844–852.

Connell, P.J., & Stone, C.A. (1994). The conceptual basis for morpheme learning problems in children with specific language impairment. *Journal of Speech and Hearing Research, 37*, 389–398.

Crago, M.B., & Gopnik, M. (1994). From families to phenotypes: Theoretical and clinical implications of research into the genetic basis of specific language impairment. In R.V. Watkins & M.L. Rice (Eds.), *Communication and language intervention series: Vol. 4. Specific language impairments in children* (pp. 35–51). Baltimore: Paul H. Brookes Publishing Co.

Craig, H., & Evans, J.L. (1993). Pragmatics and SLI: Within-group variations in discourse behaviors. *Journal of Speech and Hearing Research, 36*, 777–789.

Craig, H., & Washington, J. (1993). Access behaviors of children with specific language impairment. *Journal of Speech and Hearing Research, 36*, 322–337.

Cromer, R. (1976). The cognitive hypothesis of language acquisition and its implications for child language deficiency. In D.M. Morehead & A.E. Morehead (Eds.), *Normal and deficient child language* (pp. 283–333). Baltimore: University Park Press.

Cromer, R. (1988). The cognition hypothesis revisited. In F.S. Kessel (Ed.), *The development of language and language researchers* (pp. 223–248). Hillsdale, NJ: Lawrence Erlbaum Associates.

Cromer, R. (1991). *Language and thought in normal and handicapped children.* Cambridge, England: Blackwell.

Curtiss, S. (1981). Dissociations between language and cognition: Cases and implications. *Journal of Autism and Developmental Disorders, 11*, 15–30.

Dollaghan, C. (1987). Fast mapping in normal and language-impaired children. *Journal of Speech and Hearing Disorders, 52*, 218–222.

Dromi, E., Leonard, L.B., & Shteiman, M. (1993). The grammatical morphology of Hebrew-speaking children with specific language impairment: Some competing hypotheses. *Journal of Speech and Hearing Research, 36*, 760–771.

Dunn, L.M., & Dunn, L.M. (1981). *Peabody Picture Vocabulary Test–Revised.* Circle Pines, MN: American Guidance Service.

Fazio, B. (1994). The counting abilities of children with specific language impairment: A comparison of oral and gestural tasks. *Journal of Speech and Hearing Research, 37*, 358–368.

Fey, M.E., Long, S.H., & Cleave, P.L. (1994). Reconsideration of IQ criteria in the definition of specific language impairment. In R.V. Watkins & M.L. Rice (Eds.), *Communication and language intervention series: Vol. 4. Specific language impairments in children* (pp. 161–178). Baltimore: Paul H. Brookes Publishing Co.

Fodor, J. (1983). *The modularity of mind.* Cambridge, MA: MIT Press.

Fodor, J. (1985). Precis of the modularity of mind. *Behavioral and Brain Sciences, 8*, 1–42.

Fujiki, M., & Brinton, B. (1994). Social competence and language impairment in children. In R.V. Watkins & M.L. Rice (Eds.), *Communication and language intervention series: Vol. 4. Specific language impairments in children* (pp. 123–143). Baltimore: Paul H. Brookes Publishing Co.

Gertner, B., Rice, M.L., & Hadley, P.A. (1994). Influence of communicative competence on peer performance in a preschool classroom. *Journal of Speech and Hearing Research, 37*, 913–923.

Gillam, R.B., Cowan, N., & Day, L.S. (1995). Sequential memory in children with and without language impairment. *Journal of Speech and Hearing Research, 38*, 393–402.

Gopnik, M.L. (1994). Theoretical implications of inherited dysphasia. In Y. Levy (Ed.), *Other languages, other children: Issues in the theory of language acquisition* (pp. 331–358). Hillsdale, NJ: Lawrence Erlbaum Associates.

Gopnik, M., & Crago, M. (1991). Familial aggregation of a developmental language disorder. *Cognition, 39*, 1–50.

Grodzinsky, Y. (1986). Language deficits and the theory of syntax. *Brain and Language, 27*, 135–159.

Hadley, P.A., & Rice, M.L. (1991). Conversational responsiveness of speech- and language-impaired preschoolers. *Journal of Speech and Hearing Research, 34*, 1308–1317.

Hadley, P.A., & Rice, M.L. (1995, June). *The use of finiteness markers among children with SLI: A longitudinal perspective*. Paper presented at the Symposium on Research in Child Language Disorders, Madison, WI.

Hansson, K., & Nettelbladt, U. (1995). Grammatical characteristics of Swedish children with SLI. *Journal of Speech and Hearing Research, 38*, 589–598.

Johnston, J.R. (1988). Specific language disorders in the child. In N. Lass, L. McReynolds, J. Northern, & D. Yoder (Eds.), *Handbook of speech-language pathology and audiology* (pp. 685–715). Toronto, Ontario, Canada: B.C. Decker.

Johnston, J.R. (1991a). The continuing relevance of cause. *Language, Speech, and Hearing Services in Schools, 22*, 75–79.

Johnston, J.R. (1991b). Questions about cognition in children with specific language impairment. In J.F. Miller (Ed.), *Research on child language disorders: A decade of progress* (pp. 299–308). Austin, TX: PRO-ED.

Johnston, J.R. (1994). Cognitive abilities of children with language impairment. In R.V. Watkins & M.L. Rice (Eds.), *Communication and language intervention series: Vol. 4. Specific language impairments in children* (pp. 107–121). Baltimore: Paul H. Brookes Publishing Co.

Johnston, J.R., & Weismer, S. (1983). Mental rotation abilities in language-disordered children. *Journal of Speech and Hearing Research, 26*, 397–403.

Kail, R. (1994). A method of studying the generalized slowing hypothesis in children with specific language impairment. *Journal of Speech and Hearing Research, 37*, 418–421.

Kamhi, A. (1981). Nonlinguistic symbolic and conceptual abilities of language-impaired and normally developing children. *Journal of Speech and Hearing Research, 24*, 446–453.

Kamhi, A., Gentry, B., Mauer, D., & Gholson, B. (1990). Analogical learning and transfer in language-impaired children. *Journal of Speech and Hearing Disorders, 55*, 140–148.

Kelly, D.J., & Rice, M.L. (1994). Preferences for verb interpretation in children with specific language impairment. *Journal of Speech and Hearing Research, 37*, 182–192.

Lahey, M., & Edwards, J. (1995). Specific language impairment: Preliminary investigation of factors associated with family history and with pattern of language performance. *Journal of Speech and Hearing Research, 38*, 643–657.

Lahey, M., Liebergott, J., Chesnick, M., Menyuk, P., & Adams, J. (1992). Variability in children's use of grammatical morphemes. *Applied Psycholinguistics, 13*, 373–398.

Lederberg, A. (1980). The language environment of children with language delays. *Journal of Pediatric Psychology, 5*, 141–159.

Leonard, L.B. (1987). Is specific language impairment a useful construct? In S. Rosenberg (Ed.), *Advances in applied psycholinguistics: Disorders of first language development* (Vol. 1, pp. 1–39). New York: Cambridge University Press.

Leonard, L.B. (1988). Lexical development and processing in specific language impairment. In R.L. Schiefelbusch & L.L. Lloyd (Eds.), *Language perspectives: Acquisition, retardation, and intervention* (2nd ed., pp. 69–87). Austin, TX: PRO-ED.

Leonard, L.B. (1989). Language learnability and specific language impairment in children. *Applied Psycholinguistics, 10*, 179–202.

Leonard, L.B. (1991). Specific language impairment as a clinical category. *Language, Speech, and Hearing Services in Schools, 22*, 66–68.

Leonard, L.B. (1994). Some problems facing accounts of morphological deficits in children with specific language impairments. In R.V. Watkins & M.L. Rice (Eds.), *Communication and language intervention series: Vol. 4. Specific language impairments in children* (pp. 91–105). Baltimore: Paul H. Brookes Publishing Co.

Leonard, L.B., Bortolini, U., Caselli, M.C., McGregor, K.K., & Sabbadini, L. (1992). Morphological deficits in children with specific language impairment: The status of features in the underlying grammar. *Language Acquisition, 2*, 151–179.

Leonard, L.B., McGregor, K.K., & Allen, G. (1992). Grammatical morphology and speech perception in children with specific language impairment. *Journal of Speech and Language Research, 35*, 1076–1085.

Lewis, B.A., Ekelman, B.L., & Aram, D.M. (1989). A familial study of severe phonological disorders. *Journal of Speech and Hearing Research, 32*, 713–724.

Lewis, B., & Freebairn, L. (1992). Residual effects of preschool phonology in grade school, adolescence, and adulthood. *Journal of Speech and Hearing Research, 35*, 819–831.

Levy, Y. (1994). Concluding chapter: Modularity reconsidered. In Y. Levy (Ed.), *Other languages, other children: Issues in the theory of language acquisition* (pp. 383–400). Hillsdale, NJ: Lawrence Erlbaum Associates.

Lindner, K., & Johnston, J.R. (1992). Grammatical morphology in language-impaired children acquiring English or German as their first language: A functional perspective. *Applied Psycholinguistics, 13*, 115–129.

Masterson, J.J. (1993). The performance of children with language-learning disabilities on two types of cognitive tasks. *Journal of Speech and Hearing Research, 36*, 1026–1036.

Menyuk, P., Chesnick, M., Liebergott, J., Korngold, B., D'Agostino, R., & Belanger, A. (1991). Predicting reading problems in at-risk children. *Journal of Speech and Hearing Research, 34*, 893–903.

Nelson, L., Kamhi, A., & Apel, K. (1987). Cognitive strengths and weaknesses in language-impaired children: One more look. *Journal of Speech and Hearing Disorders, 52*, 36–43.

Oetting, J.B., & Rice, M.L. (1993). Plural acquisition in children with specific language impairment. *Journal of Speech and Hearing Research, 36*, 1236–1249.

Pennington, B.F. (1989). Using genetics to understand dyslexia. *Annals of Dyslexia, 39*, 81–93.

Pinker, S. (1984). *Language learnability and language development*. Cambridge, MA: Harvard University Press.

Pinker, S. (1989). *Learnability and cognition: The acquisition of argument structure*. Cambridge, MA: MIT Press.

Pinker, S. (1994). *The language instinct: How the mind creates language*. New York: William Morrow.

Plante, E. (1991). MRI findings in the parents and siblings of specifically language-impaired boys. *Brain and Language, 41*, 67–80.

Plante, E., Swisher, L., Kiernan, B., & Restrepo, M.A. (1993). Language matches: Illuminating or confounding? *Journal of Speech and Hearing Research, 36*, 772–776.
Plante, E., Swisher, L., Vance, R., & Rapcsack, S. (1991). MRI findings in boys with specific language impairment. *Brain and Language, 41*, 52–66.
Records, N.L., Tomblin, J.B., & Freese, P.R. (1992). The quality of life of young adults with histories of specific language impairment. *American Journal of Speech-Language Pathology, 1*(2), 44–53.
Rice, M.L. (1990). Preschoolers' QUIL: Quick incidental learning of words. In G. Conti-Ramsden & C. Snow (Eds.), *Children's language* (Vol. 7, pp. 171–195). Hillsdale, NJ: Lawrence Erlbaum Associates.
Rice, M.L. (1991). Children with specific language impairment: Toward a model of teachability. In N. Krasnegor, D.M. Rumbaugh, R.L. Schiefelbusch, & M. Studdert-Kennedy (Eds.), *Biological and behavioral determinants of language development* (pp. 447–480). Hillsdale, NJ: Lawrence Erlbaum Associates.
Rice, M.L. (1993). "Don't talk to him; he's weird": A social consequences account of language and social interactions. In A.P. Kaiser & D.B. Gray (Eds.), *Communication and language intervention series: Vol. 2. Enhancing children's communication: Research foundations for intervention* (pp. 139–158). Baltimore: Paul H. Brookes Publishing Co.
Rice, M.L., & Bode, J.V. (1993). Gaps in the verb lexicons of children with specific language impairment. *First Language, 13*, 113–131.
Rice, M.L., Buhr, J.C., & Nemeth, M. (1990). Fast mapping word learning abilities of language-delayed preschoolers. *Journal of Speech and Hearing Research, 55*, 33–42.
Rice, M.L., Cleave, P.L., Oetting, J.B., & Pae, S. (1993, November). *SLI children's use of syntactic cues in lexical acquisition.* Paper presented at the American Speech-Language-Hearing Association Convention, Anaheim, CA.
Rice, M.L., Hadley, P.A., & Alexander, A. (1993). Social biases toward children with speech and language impairments: A correlative causal model of language limitations. *Applied Psycholinguistics, 14*, 443–471.
Rice, M.L., & Kemper, S. (1984). *Child language and cognition.* Baltimore: University Park Press.
Rice, M.L., & Oetting, J.B. (1993). Morphological deficits of children with SLI: Evaluation of number marking and agreement. *Journal of Speech and Hearing Research, 34*, 1249–1257.
Rice, M.L., Oetting, J.B., Marquis, J., Bode, J., & Pae, S. (1994). Frequency of input effects on word comprehension of children with specific language impairment. *Journal of Speech and Hearing Research, 37*, 106–122.
Rice, M.L., & Wexler, K. (1995, June). *TNS as a clinical marker of specific language impairment.* Paper presented at the Symposium on Research in Child Language Disorders, Madison, WI.
Rice, M.L., Wexler, K., & Cleave, P. (1995). Specific language impairment as a period of extended optional infinitive. *Journal of Speech and Hearing Research, 38*, 850–863.
Rice, M.L., & Wilcox, K. (1995). *Building a language-focused curriculum for the preschool classroom: Vol. 1. A foundation for lifelong communication.* Baltimore: Paul H. Brookes Publishing Co.
Roeper, T., & Seymour, H.N. (1994). The place of linguistic theory in the theory of language acquisition and language impairment. In Y. Levy (Ed.), *Other languages, other children: Issues in the theory of language acquisition* (pp. 305–330). Hillsdale, NJ: Lawrence Erlbaum Associates.
Rollins, P.R. (1995, June). *MLU as a matching variable: Understanding its limitations.*

Paper presented at the Symposium on Research in Child Language Disorders, Madison, WI.

Rom, A., & Leonard, L. (1990). Interpreting deficits in grammatical morphology in specifically language-impaired children: Preliminary evidence from Hebrew. *Clinical Linguistics and Phonetics*, *4*, 93–105.

Rosenberg, S., & Abbeduto, L. (1993). *Language and communication in mental retardation*. Hillsdale, NJ: Lawrence Erlbaum Associates.

Stark, R.E., & Tallal, P. (1981). Selection of children with specific language deficits. *Journal of Speech and Hearing Disorders*, *46*, 114–122.

Swisher, L., Restrepo, M.A., Plante, E., & Lowell, S. (1995). Effect of implicit and explicit "rule" presentation on bound-morpheme generalization in specific language impairment. *Journal of Speech and Hearing Research*, *38*, 168–173.

Swisher, L., & Snow, D. (1994). Learning and generalization components of morphological acquisition by children with specific language impairment: Is there a functional relation? *Journal of Speech and Hearing Research*, *37*, 1406–1413.

Tallal, P., Miller, S.L., Bedi, G., Byma, G., Wang, X., Nagarajan, S.S., Schreiner, C., Jenkins, W., & Merzenich, M.M. (1996). Language comprehension in language-learning impaired children with acoustically modified speech. *Science*, *271*, 81–84.

Tallal, P., & Piercy, M. (1973). Deficits of nonverbal auditory perception in children with development aphasia. *Nature*, *241*, 468–469.

Tallal, P., Ross, P., & Curtiss, S. (1989). Familial aggregation in specific language impairment. *Journal of Speech and Hearing Research*, *54*, 167–173.

Terrell, B., & Schwartz, R. (1988). Object transformations in the play of language-impaired children. *Journal of Speech and Hearing Disorders*, *53*, 459–466.

Tomblin, J.B. (1989). Familial concentration of developmental language impairment. *Journal of Speech and Hearing Development*, *54*, 287–295.

Tomblin, J.B. (1991). Examining the cause of specific language impairment. *Language, Speech, and Hearing Services in Schools*, *22*, 69–74.

Tomblin, J.B. (1993, November). *The genetic epidemiology of specific language impairment*. Paper presented at the Merrill Advanced Studies Institute, Toward a Genetics of Language, University of Kansas, Lawrence.

Tomblin, J.B., & Buckwalter, P. (1994a, June). *Preliminary results of a twin study of SLI*. Paper presented at the Symposium on Research in Child Language Disorders, University of Wisconsin, Madison.

Tomblin, J.B., & Buckwalter, P.R. (1994b). Studies of genetics of specific language impairment. In R.V. Watkins & M.L. Rice (Eds.), *Communication and language intervention series: Vol. 4. Specific language impairments in children* (pp. 17–34). Baltimore: Paul H. Brookes Publishing Co.

Tomblin, J.B., Freese, P., & Records, N. (1992). Diagnosing specific language impairment in adults for the purpose of pedigree analysis. *Journal of Speech and Hearing Research*, *35*, 832–843.

Watkins, R.V. (1994). Grammatical challenges for children with specific language impairments. In R.V. Watkins & M.L. Rice (Eds.), *Communication and language intervention series: Vol. 4. Specific language impairments in children* (pp. 53–68). Baltimore: Paul H. Brookes Publishing Co.

Watkins, R.V. (1995, December). *Production of derivational morphemes by children and adults*. Paper presented at the American Speech-Language-Hearing Association Convention, Orlando, FL.

Watkins, R.V., Kelly, D.J., Harbers, H.M., & Hollis, W. (1995). Measuring children's lexical diversity: Differentiating typical and atypical language learners. *Journal of Speech and Hearing Research*, *38*, 1349–1355.

Watkins, R.V., & Rice, M.L. (1991). Verb particle and preposition acquisition in language-impaired preschoolers. *Journal of Speech and Hearing Research, 34*, 1130–1141.

Watkins, R.V., & Rice, M.L. (Eds.). (1994). *Communication and language intervention series: Vol. 4. Specific language impairments in children*. Baltimore: Paul H. Brookes Publishing Co.

Watkins, R.V., Rice, M.L., & Moltz, C. (1993). Verb use by language-impaired and normally developing children. *First Language, 13*, 133–143.

Weismer, S. (1991). Hypothesis testing abilities of language-impaired children. *Journal of Speech and Hearing Research, 34*, 1329–1339.

Weismer, S., & Hesketh, L. (1993). The influence of prosodic and gestural cues on novel word acquisition by children with specific language impairment. *Journal of Speech and Hearing Research, 36*, 1013–1025.

Whitehurst, G.J., Fischel, J.E., Arnold, D.S., & Lonigan, C.J. (1992). Evaluating outcomes with children with expressive language delay. In S.F. Warren & J. Reichle (Eds.), *Communication and language intervention series: Vol. 1. Causes and effects in communication and language intervention* (pp. 277–313). Baltimore: Paul H. Brookes Publishing Co.

Windsor, J. (1994). Children's comprehension and production of derivational suffixes. *Journal of Speech and Hearing Research, 37*, 408–417.

Windsor, J. (1995). Language impairment and social competence. In M.E. Fey, J. Windsor, & S.F. Warren (Eds.), *Communication and language intervention series: Vol. 5. Language intervention: Preschool through the elementary years* (pp. 213–238). Baltimore: Paul H. Brookes Publishing Co.

# 8

# Comprehension and Language Acquisition

## Evidence from Youth with Severe Cognitive Disabilities

Rose A. Sevcik and Mary Ann Romski

By the time Benjamin, a typically developing child, utters his first words at age 15 months, he can identify by name many objects, familiar people, and some body parts and can carry out simple commands (e.g., "Bring Mommy her shoes"). This early ability to comprehend words is a component of early language acquisition that is often taken for granted by researchers in child language acquisition (Adamson, 1996). Even though the onset of early word comprehension precedes word production by a considerable period, when young typically developing children begin to speak, traditionally the majority of research attention has been placed on their language productions rather than on their skill at comprehending language (Benedict, 1979; Hirsh-Pasek & Golinkoff, 1991; Huttenlocher, 1974). Thus, the role and function that early language comprehension plays in language development are somewhat obscured.

This chapter is an expanded version of papers presented as part of a symposium entitled "Language Learning Research and Mental Retardation: Contributions to Developmental Research" at the 26th Gatlinburg Conference on Research in Mental Retardation and Developmental Disabilities, March 1993, and a symposium entitled "Early Language Acquisition: Basic Research with Children with Developmental Disabilities" at the biennial meeting of the Society for Research in Child Development, March 1993, New Orleans, Louisiana.

The preparation of this chapter was funded by NICHD Grant No. 06016, the Department of Communication, College of Arts and Sciences, and a Research Enhancement Grant from Georgia State University.

This chapter explores the role of early comprehension in language development. Extending the theme of this book, we employ data from youth who encounter serious difficulty learning to speak—youth with severe cognitive disabilities—to examine early comprehension. The first section of this chapter provides a brief synopsis of the literature on the early word comprehension skills of young typical language learners. The second section presents findings from two related but distinct studies about symbol acquisition and use by youth with severe cognitive disabilities who did not learn to speak. These studies emphasize the relationship between the youths' spoken language comprehension skills and their subsequent abilities to use symbols for communication in an alternate mode. The extant spoken language comprehension skills some of these youth brought to the task permitted them to rapidly enter into the world of productive language when an alternate mode was provided. Their performance is contrasted with that of youth who did not bring such comprehension skills to the augmented language-learning task. The final section revisits the function spoken word comprehension skills play in early language development and outlines the contributions derived from research with children and youth with severe cognitive disabilities.

## EARLY WORD COMPREHENSION

Young children first hear language during rich social-communicative interactions that include reoccurring familiar situations or events (Bruner, 1983; Nelson, 1985). Before children actually produce words, the social and environmental interactional contexts converge with the available linguistic information to produce understandings (Huttenlocher, 1974). By the time typical children are 12–15 months of age, they understand, on average, about 50 words (Benedict, 1979; Snyder, Bates, & Bretherton, 1981). As they move through their second year of life, they quickly begin to understand relational commands, such as "Give Daddy a kiss," and can carry them out.

What does comprehension provide the young language learner? First, it focuses the child's attention on word forms and their referents in the environment. Second, it permits the caregiver to create new learning opportunities by capitalizing on well-established routines (Oviatt, 1985).

The limited literature on early word comprehension has focused on describing the emergence of word comprehension (e.g., Benedict, 1979; Huttenlocher, 1974) and examining experimentally the contextual influences on its development (Oviatt, 1980; Resnick & Goldfield, 1992). The findings from both of these methodologies provide evidence that early word comprehension precedes early word production. Young typically developing children, however, quickly move on to word production, and comprehension of words becomes a given. Because word production skills emerge so quickly in typical children, they may mask and overshadow the continuing role speech comprehension plays in early language development. After a young typically developing child starts talking, it is difficult, if not impossible, to independently examine speech comprehension skills without considering the impact of word production skills on the findings. What is still missing is a precise identification and analysis of the skills that must operate in concert to comprehend a word. This chapter considers some skills (e.g., representational abilities) that appear to underlie early word comprehension.

## CHILDREN AND YOUTH WITH SEVERE COGNITIVE DISABILITIES

In sharp contrast to young typical children, children and youth with severe cognitive disabilities encounter serious difficulty acquiring their first productive spoken words (Romski & Sevcik, 1996). Children and youth with severe cognitive disabilities, by definition, have significant intellectual impairments as evidenced by extremely low scores on intelligence tests (Snell, 1993). Far from presenting a homogeneous profile, children and youth with severe cognitive disabilities typically exhibit a range of accompanying disabilities that may include, though are not limited to, cerebral palsy, sensory impairments, seizure disorders, other medical conditions, or maladaptive behaviors (Guess & Horner, 1978; Snell, 1993). They require extensive ongoing support in major life activities, especially communication, to participate in their communities (Luckasson et al., 1993). Some children and youth with severe cognitive disabilities acquire oral communication skills, albeit slowly and often incompletely, and exhibit varying degrees of impairment in the comprehension and production of the semantics, syntax, pragmatics, and/or phonology of language (see Rosenberg & Abbeduto, 1993, for a review). The majority of these individuals, however, fail to develop functional spoken communication skills, sometimes even if they have had considerable speech and language instruction directed toward that goal. We are interested in youth with such profiles because they have not developed word production skills even though they have been exposed to spoken language since birth. First, for children and youth with severe disabilities who do not speak, exploring the foundation on which initial language and communication production skills can be built is a critical task for their subsequent success as communicators. Second, given their lack of productive language skills, findings about their language learning can also provide a unique window into the role early word comprehension plays in overall language development.

## STUDIES OF AUGMENTED LANGUAGE DEVELOPMENT

In this section, we discuss two studies about augmented language development by youth with severe disabilities using the System for Augmenting Language (SAL) (Romski & Sevcik, 1996). The first study examined patterns of language achievement when youth with severe disabilities who did not talk were provided with the SAL. After the use of the SAL was well established, the second study was undertaken to manipulate experimentally the learning of novel words by these same youth.

## Participants

The participants in these two studies were male school-age youth with severe disabilities. Thirteen male youth participated in the first study (mean CA=12 years, 3 months; mean nonverbal MA=3 years, 6 months) and 12 of the 13 youth participated in the second study (mean CA=17 years, 5 months; mean nonverbal MA=3 years, 8 months). Each participant had moderate or severe cognitive disabilities and severe spoken language impairments, resided at home, and attended a special education program at his local public school. They all demonstrated intentional communication abilities (e.g., gestures, vocalizations) but no more than 10 intelligible word approximations at the onset of the first study. Table 1 provides a general description of the participants at the onset of Study 1. When Study 2 was begun, the participants had 5 years of experience with the SAL and had working symbol vocabularies that ranged from 23 to 104 symbols (mean=66).

## System for Augmenting Language

Because the participants in these two studies had no functional expressive communication system in place before the initiation of the first study, they had to

Table 1. Participants' description at the onset of Study 1

| P | CA (years:months) | Medical etiology | Level of retardation[a] | PPVT–R[b] (years:months) | Leiter[c] (years:months) |
|---|---|---|---|---|---|
| BB | 13:5 | Cerebral palsy | Severe | <1:6[d] | 3:0 |
| FG | 20:1 | Cerebral palsy | Severe | <1:6[d] | <2:0[d] |
| GJ | 6:2 | Unknown | Severe | <1:6[d] | <2:0[d] |
| KH | 10:8 | Unknown | Severe | <1:6[d] | <2:0[d] |
| DC | 8:9 | Unknown | Moderate | 4:7 | 5:1 |
| DE | 11:11 | Down syndrome | Severe | 2:7 | 4:0 |
| EC | 16:7 | Autism | Severe | 3:1 | 5:0 |
| JA | 13:3 | Unknown | Moderate | 2:3 | 7:0 |
| JL | 20:5 | Unknown | Severe | <1:6[d] | <2:0[d] |
| KW | 13:2 | Down syndrome | Severe | <1:6[d] | 4:2 |
| MH | 7:3 | Autism | Moderate | <1:6[d] | 5:0 |
| TE | 11:9 | Cerebral palsy | Severe | <1:6[d] | 3:3 |
| TF | 6:11 | Reye syndrome | Severe | <1:6[d] | <2:0[d] |

P=participant.

[a]Level of retardation, as defined by Grossman (1983), was assigned as a result of psychological evaluations conducted by certified school psychologists before the onset of the study. These evaluations took into account both IQ, as measured by the Stanford-Binet Intelligence Scale (Terman & Merrill, 1960), and adaptive behavior, as measured by the AAMD Adaptive Behavior Scale (Lambert, Windmiller, Cole, & Figueroa, 1975). Moderate and severe mental retardation were defined as IQs of 50–70 and 20–40, respectively (Grossman, 1983).

[b]PPVT–R=the Peabody Picture Vocabulary Test–Revised (Dunn & Dunn, 1981).

[c]Leiter=the Arthur Adaptation of the Leiter International Performance Scale (Arthur, 1952).

[d]No basal was achieved and the participant's age-equivalent score was estimated as being below the lowest age-equivalent score available on the test.

learn language through instruction in an alternate modality. To provide such experience, we created an instructional approach, called SAL, using visual-graphic symbols coupled with speech-output communication devices to teach the participants to communicate symbolically. The SAL consists of five integrated components designed to supplement the youth's natural, albeit severely limited, language abilities with a symbol-embossed computerized keyboard that produced synthesized speech. Table 2 lists the five components of the SAL.

***Speech-Output Communication Device*** The first component of the SAL was a speech-output communication device. This component permitted the participant to communicate by touching a visual-graphic symbol on a computer-based display. The computerized device produced a synthetic spoken word that corresponded to the symbol that was touched. Because the participants were unable to read, spell, or write and could not access the computer keyboard in a conventional manner, the use of such a device permitted a translation between the visual symbol and the spoken, albeit synthetic, word. It facilitated use of the SAL in a variety of environments, including initially home or school and later a range of community settings.

For the first study, we employed a Words + Portable Voice II (Words +, Inc., 1985) augmentative communication device consisting of a specially modified Epson HX-20 Notebook computer and an adapted Votrax Personal Speech System. A touch-sensitive Unicorn Expanded Keyboard was used to access the Words + system. To optimize portability in the home and school settings, the entire system was transported on a modified luggage cart. We later employed a WOLF (Adamlab, 1988). This device functioned like the Words + system but was considerably smaller and significantly reduced in weight. The participants readily transferred their symbol use skills from the Words + system to the WOLF (Romski & Sevcik, 1996). The WOLF was employed in Study 2.

***Symbol Vocabulary*** The second component consisted of the symbol vocabulary. Lexigrams (Rumbaugh, 1977), arbitrary visual-graphic symbols,

Table 2. Five components of the System for Augmenting Language

- Electric computer-based speech-output communication devices are available for use in natural communicative environments.
- Appropriate, initially limited, symbol vocabularies with the printed English word above each symbol are placed on the devices.
- Participants are encouraged, though not required, to use the device during loosely structured naturalistic communicative exchanges.
- Communicative partners are taught to use the device to augment their speech input to the participants with symbol input.
- Ongoing resource and feedback mechanisms are provided to support the participants and their partners in their communication efforts.

From Romski, M.A., & Sevcik, R.A. (1996). *Breaking the speech barrier: Language development through augmented means*, p. 54. Baltimore: Paul H. Brookes Publishing Co.; reprinted by permission.

were chosen because they ensured that none of the participants was familiar with the symbols and that there was an arbitrary relationship between the symbol and its meaning. The symbols were placed on the display panel with the corresponding English word or phrase placed above each symbol to facilitate interpretation by unfamiliar partners. A lexigram was activated by touching it on the display and resulted in the production of a synthesized equivalent of the spoken word for that symbol. Vocabulary was individually chosen for each participant by his parents and teacher in conjunction with the investigators. Initial vocabulary included referential (e.g., baseball, Coca Cola, Walkman) and social-regulative words (e.g., I want, please, more). Vocabulary was expanded during Study 1 and updated and increased as needed thereafter.

***Naturalistic Teaching Strategies*** The third component of the SAL was the naturalistic teaching strategy. Communicative use of the device was not taught in the traditional sense. The use of the device was integrated into each youth's ongoing daily activities. Partners were asked to use the device as part of their own spoken communications to the participant. The participant was always encouraged, but never required, to use the device whenever communicative opportunities arose. The use of this approach permitted each individual to feel comfortable with the device and to facilitate its use in communicative exchanges as they occurred in everyday activities.

***Role of Communicative Partners*** The fourth component was the role played by communicative partners (i.e., parents, teachers). They were taught to use the device to augment their speech input to the participants with symbol input (e.g., "MORE MILK PLEASE"; "Let's ride BIKES") where the words were spoken and symbols touched in sequence. The parents and teachers themselves participated in a series of instructional sessions in which the communicative use of the SAL was emphasized. Included was an orientation to the operation of the computer-linked device and to its use as a communicative tool through videotaped examples and role playing.

***Resource and Feedback Mechanism*** The fifth and final component of the SAL was the provision of an ongoing resource and feedback mechanism to support the youth and their partners' use of the SAL. This component consisted of obtaining regular and systematic feedback by using a questionnaire (QUEST) with the participant's primary partner about the participant's use of the device. It permitted the investigators to monitor communicative use and deal with any challenges (e.g., computer breakdown) that arose.

## Study 1: Patterns of Vocabulary Achievement

Study 1 addresses vocabulary achievement during the first 2 years of the longitudinal study. During Year 1, participants took part in daily communicative interactions with adult partners at home or school employing the SAL. During Year 2, use of the SAL was expanded to include home and school for all participants. The immersion and use of the SAL within the participants' daily lives produced notable acquisition and use of symbols during communicative exchanges (Romski & Sevcik, 1996; Romski, Sevcik, Robinson, & Bakeman, 1994; Romski, Sevcik, & Wilkinson, 1994). By the end of the study's first year, however, there was considerable variability evident in the quantity of different symbols each participant employed in comprehension and production. Although slightly less than half of the vocabulary was comprehended and produced (43%), a visual inspection of the data indicated that the participants fell into one of two nonoverlapping categories based on the proportion of vocabulary they did not understand or produce. Nine of the 13 participants comprehended and produced the majority of their referential vocabularies. The remaining four participants were more likely to comprehend a symbol than to produce it. Their performance also included a much larger proportion of vocabulary that they neither comprehended nor produced (.43 versus .12).

This variability suggested that, based on their vocabulary performance, there might be at least two distinct groups of participants. Because we had studied the participants' performances in a variety of domains across the 2-year period, we were able to examine how individual participants performed across domains and if there were any similarities or differences that emerged (Romski & Sevcik, 1996).

We selected the following seven domains from the longitudinal study in which to examine performance: 1) communicates with adults (Romski, Sevcik, Robinson, & Bakeman, 1994); 2) communicates with peers (Romski, Sevcik, & Wilkinson, 1994); 3) produces symbol combinations (Wilkinson, Romski, & Sevcik, 1994); 4) maintains vocabulary from Year 1 to Year 2 (Romski & Sevcik, 1996); 5) has a vocabulary greater than 35 symbols at 2 years (Romski & Sevcik, 1996); 6) improves speech intelligibility (Romski, Sevcik, Robinson, & Wilkinson, 1990); and 7) recognizes printed English words (Sevcik, Romski, & Robinson, 1991). A dichotomous coding scheme (yes or no) was employed; each participant's documented achievement was then coded in every domain based on his performance within the domain. Table 3 presents the results of this coding for each participant in each domain.

A review of the individual performance patterns in Table 3 suggests that the two distinct patterns evidenced in vocabulary performance were maintained across other domains as well (Romski & Sevcik, 1992). Nine (DC, DE, EC, JA, JL, KW, MH, TE, and TF) participants demonstrated achievement in at least five of the seven domains. DC, JA, MH, and TE evidenced skill in every domain while DE, EC, JL, KW, and TF achieved skill in at least five of the seven domains. They encountered difficulty with only a few domains: maintaining their vocabularies across years (DE, JL, TF), generating symbol combinations (EC, TF, KW), increasing speech intelligibility (DE, JL, EC), or recognizing printed English words (KW).

The achievements of BB, KH, FG, and GJ were much more modest. All four of them communicated with adults. By the end of Year 2, BB showed

Table 3. Patterns of achievement

| Domain | Participants | | | | | | | | | | | | |
|---|---|---|---|---|---|---|---|---|---|---|---|---|---|
| | Beginning achievers (Comprehended vocabulary) | | | | Advanced achievers (Comprehended and produced vocabulary) | | | | | | | | |
| | BB | KH | FG | GJ | DC | TF | EC | DE | JL | JA | KW | MH | TE |
| Communicates with adults | Y | Y | Y | Y | Y | Y | Y | Y | Y | Y | Y | Y | Y |
| Communicates with peers | N | N | N | N | Y | Y | Y | Y | Y | Y | Y | Y | Y |
| Produces symbol combinations | N | Y | N | N | Y | N | N | Y | Y | Y | N | Y | Y |
| Maintains vocabulary from YR1 to YR2 | N | N | N | N | Y | N | Y | N | N | Y | Y | Y | Y |
| Two-year vocabulary>35 symbols | N | N | N | N | Y | Y | Y | Y | Y | Y | Y | Y | Y |
| Speech intelligibility improves | N | N | N | N | Y | Y | N | N | N | Y | Y | Y | Y |
| Recognizes printed English words | Y | N | N | N | Y | Y | Y* | Y | Y | Y* | N | Y* | Y |

Adapted from Table 7.1 of Romski, M. A., & Sevcik, R. A. (1996). *Breaking the speech barrier: Language development through augmented means* (p. 140). Baltimore: Paul H. Brookes Publishing Co.; reprinted by permission.

Y=yes, N=no, *=recognized printed English words at the onset of the study.

some minimal recognition of printed English words and KH produced a few ordered symbol combinations.

These nine participants evidenced what we described as an advanced achievement pattern, composed of the rather swift acquisition of symbols followed by the emergence of symbol combinations and other symbolic skills (e.g., printed word recognition). We described this pattern as advanced because it permitted the participants to use basic skills as a firm foundation to progress from and develop skills in other related domains. The four remaining participants (BB, FG, GJ, KH) evidenced a second distinct pattern that we referred to as a beginning achievement pattern. This pattern consisted of the slow acquisition of a small set (less than 35) of single visual-graphic symbols in comprehension and production. We labeled this pattern "beginning" because it suggested that the participants had developed a set of basic skills from which they could build additional communication skills. Although they had not, as yet, generalized their skills to other domains, two of them were showing signs of new skill development.

***Factors Contributing to Achievement Patterns*** It appears that these differences in initial SAL learning resulted in distinct achievement patterns across the 2 years of the study. What factors may have contributed to these distinct achievement patterns? Although all participants were matched on productive language skills at the outset of the study—all participants had fewer than 10 intelligible spoken words—a number of related factors varied across participants at the beginning of the study and may have contributed to their distinct achievement patterns.

First, the initial SAL instructional group (home or school) in which the participants were placed did not appear to contribute to the differences beccause the four beginning achievers were equally distributed across both instructional groups. Second, the participants' level of intellectual functioning was probably not a determining factor in achievement. Participants evidencing severe cognitive disabilities were represented in both achievement patterns. All the beginning achievers had a diagnosis of severe mental retardation while the advanced achievers had mixed diagnoses (moderate and severe, see Table 1).

Third, it may be a combination of factors related to speech comprehension that contribute to these two patterns of achievement. The participants' performance on the battery of formal and informal cognitive and language measures, administered before their participation in the study, may help to uncover those factors that distinguish the two patterns of achievement. These measures included standardized instruments (i.e., The Leiter International Performance Scale [Arthur, 1952]) as well as informal assessments of matching/sorting (for objects/colors) skills and representational matching (identity and nonidentity) skills. No specific cognitive skills, however, differentiated the four beginning participants from the other participants, although GJ's matching/sorting skills fell below those of all the other participants. A description of the participants' representational abilities clearly indicated that FG's and GJ's ability to grasp representational relations fell consistently below the remaining participants. The four participants with a beginning pattern did not obtain a basal score on the Peabody Picture Vocabulary Test–Revised (Dunn & Dunn, 1981) and had fairly low vocabulary scores on the Assessing Children's Language Comprehension (Foster, Giddan, & Stark, 1983). In addition, while all participants understood, in a very general sense, that spoken words represented real-world items, the four beginning achievers had not established specific word–referent relationships when single-word comprehension was systematically assessed through nonstandardized means.

In general, this review suggests that matching/sorting and representational skills distinguished two of the beginning achievers (FG, GJ) from the other participants. Restricted formal and informal speech comprehension skills also was a common characteristic of the four beginning achievers. These findings, though certainly preliminary given the small sample size, suggest that multiple factors related to speech comprehension influenced these two achievement patterns. Two additional investigations provide support for these findings. Romski, Sevcik, and Pate (1988) studied older adolescents and young adults with severe cognitive disabilities who had been explicitly taught symbol production skills. They described distinct symbol acquisition and generalization patterns that were linked to the participants' extant speech comprehension skills. Franklin, Mirenda, and Phillips (1996) reported that learners with severe cognitive disabilities who comprehended spoken words were better able to perform on visual matching tasks than learners who did not comprehend spoken words.

With the SAL approach, the participant is not overtly taught relationships between symbols and their referents. Instead, the participant must extend already extant learning abilities to acquire new relationships that involve the learning of the rule that "symbols refer." If the relationship between a spoken word and its referent was established during a participant's previous life experience, and subsequently the SAL is provided, existing receptive and cognitive skills may serve as a foundation on which the participant could build a relationship between the visual symbols he is acquiring and already established understandings of spoken words. Perhaps, however, the beginning achiever's difficulties may be even more basic than an individual's ability to use speech comprehension skills as a foundation for augmented language learning. It may be that he has not established the underlying ability to establish equivalence relationships (McIlvane, Dube, Green, & Serna, 1993). The advanced achievers would use the generalized rule that each symbol represents a real-world referent to pair the symbol with the spoken synthetic word that is produced when the symbol is activated. The beginning achievers, evidencing little or no speech comprehension, had a less stable foundation of word understanding with which to link visual symbols to their referents. Thus, they began the acquisition process by establishing the relationship between a visual symbol and its referent, relying on cues in the communicative environment to extract visual symbol meaning. Given the small number of symbols learned and the lack of generalization to other domains, the beginning achievers may have been using a different, less sophisticated learning strategy than the advanced achievers. Different types of learning provide one view of what factors might distinguish beginning and advanced symbol achievers.

Overall, these findings suggest that there appear to be skills, such as the establishment of equivalence relations, that underlie the ability to comprehend speech in children and youth with severe cognitive disabilities. Such skills have been alluded to in the child language literature on typically developing children (e.g., Oviatt, 1985). Perhaps children and youth with cognitive disabilities afford us a unique opportunity to delineate some of these specific parameters that form the cognitive substrate for early word comprehension. The variability of such skills in children and youth with severe cognitive disabilities underscores the impact of spoken language comprehension skills on subsequent language learning.

### Study 2: Learning Novel Symbols

Once the participants' communication skills were in place, we wanted to understand further the differences between the two achievement patterns. We undertook an experimental study (Study 2) to assess the participants' ability to learn the meanings of new symbols for novel objects (Romski, Sevcik, Robinson, Mervis, & Bertrand, 1996). Child language researchers have argued that lexical acquisition proceeds rapidly in typically developing children because the child has a set of operating principles that guides the learning of words (e.g., Golinkoff, Mervis, & Hirsh-Pasek, 1994; Mervis & Bertrand, 1993, 1994). One of the more advanced principles that directs the child's learning is called the novel name–nameless category (N3C) principle. This principle states that when a child hears a novel word in the presence of an unknown object, he or she will immediately map the novel name onto the novel entity. Therefore, the N3C principle enables the young typically developing child to map the meanings of new words at a rapid rate and with very little exposure to the new words. The behavioral demonstration of the N3C principle is known as fast mapping. We were interested in determining if and how the participants used this principle to learn symbol meanings.

As previously mentioned, all participants, with the exception of one advanced achiever (TF), participated in Study 2. Using an adaptation of the procedure described by Mervis and Bertrand (1994), we assessed the participants' abilities to learn novel symbols when they were first given exposure to them. Participants were presented with sets of four known objects and their corresponding words symbols and one unknown object and its corresponding novel word symbol and were asked to select the novel word symbol. To ensure that none of the participants could have had experience with these novel words + symbols before the study, we gave the unknown words + symbols nonsense names, such as "gegot" and "wiztor." All known objects were individualized for each participant and were part of the participant's assessed symbol comprehension vocabulary. The experimental protocol consisted of four conditions: 1) exposure to new symbols, 2) immediate comprehension and production assessment, 3) 1-day delayed comprehension and production assessments, and 4) 15-day extended delayed comprehension and production assessments.

After one exposure to these novel words + symbols, seven of the eight advanced achievers (DC, DE, EC, JA, KW, MH, TE) were able to choose the novel object that represented the nonsense word + symbol. The remaining advanced achiever (JL) and the four beginning achievers (BB, KH, FG, GJ) were unable to do so.

We then conducted three assessments of the participants' knowledge: 1) assessment immediately following the participants' initial experience, 2) assessment 1 day after the original exposure, and 3) assessment 15 days after the original exposure. During these three assessments, we measured both comprehension and production of the nonsense words + symbols.

The seven advanced achievers retained comprehension of more than half of the novel words + symbols for delays of more than 2 weeks with no intervening experience. They also generalized their comprehension knowledge to production of the novel symbols. The eighth advanced achiever (JL) and the beginning achievers did not retain any word + symbol knowledge in comprehension or production. An examination of JL's errors during the fast-mapping comprehension assessment task, however, indicated that his errors were different from those of the beginning achievers. Although 63% of his errors consisted of choosing the distractor novel object that was added to the stimulus set for the assessment, there was no pattern to the errors of the beginning achievers. This error analysis suggested that JL understood a portion of the strategy (novelty) but had not completely worked out the entire principle.

With one exception, then, the advanced achievers were able to rapidly map, retain, and generalize the names of novel words + symbols even though they had little exposure and no intervening naturalistic communicative experience with the novel words + symbols. These findings suggest that the use of the N3C principle may provide one post hoc explanation of how the advanced achievers learned to use symbols during exposure to them. Furthermore, these findings support our previously articulated interpretation for how our advanced achievers learned symbols. They employed extant comprehension skills and used them to expand their vocabularies into production when provided with the opportunity to use the SAL.

## REEXAMINING THE ROLE OF SPEECH COMPREHENSION

Together these studies suggest that the paths taken by these youth to learn and use symbols illustrate the important role speech comprehension can play in initial language learning when spoken language production is not a viable output option. We believe that these findings highlight how speech comprehension for words can function in the initial language acquisition process. The ability to comprehend spoken words permits the children to bootstrap their way into the world of productive language in an alternate mode. When children do not have such a foundation, their productive language learning is slow and constrained, even in an alternative mode. Our understanding of one of the intricacies of very initial language development, the critical role speech comprehension skills play in facilitating early language acquisition, is strengthened by a precise examination of the visual symbol acquisition of children and youth with such severe language impairments (Romski & Sevcik, 1996). Studying children and youth with severe cognitive disabilities who do not speak reveals information about the underlying cognitive skills that unfold as early word comprehension.

Like the process observed when typical children develop their first words, comprehension permits the child to observe and to actively engage in the communicative process before actually taking on the role of speaker (e.g., Huttenlocher, 1974). In her 1973 monograph, Nelson proposed that typical children who, early in the language development process, produced little speech may have been relying on an internal processing of the language they heard to advance their underlying linguistic competence. Conclusions from children and youth with cognitive disabilities provide additional empirical evidence that supports Nelson's hypothesis.

Data from children and youth with cognitive disabilities are supported by findings from another distinct group learning language through an alternative means—nonhuman primates. Research with bonobos, also known as pygmy chimpanzees (*Pan paniscus*), suggests that they too used speech comprehension skills as a path for acquiring the productive use of arbitrary visual-graphic symbols or lexigrams (Savage-Rumbaugh, 1991; Savage-Rumbaugh, Sevcik, Brakke, Rumbaugh, & Greenfield, 1990; Sevcik, 1989; Sevcik & Savage-Rumbaugh, 1994). For example, Mulika, an infant ape, comprehended symbols that she never productively used (Sevcik, 1989; Sevcik & Savage-Rumbaugh, 1994). The symbol acquisition sequence that the young apes appeared to have followed was comprehension of spoken words, comprehension of symbols, and symbol production. Receptive skills served as the foundation for productive symbol communication for these apes, as well.

## CONCLUSION

Research from individuals using an alternative pathway to productive language acquisition strengthens the modest findings about early comprehension from the typical development literature and broadens our perspective on the language development process in general. Speech comprehension provides an essential foundation upon which individuals can build productive language competence. It can develop even when an individual does not learn to speak and can be a link across modalities (e.g., auditory to visual) when speech is not a viable productive mode. We have now shifted our focus to toddlers with developmental disabilities who are at significant risk for not developing spoken language. Adopting a longitudinal outlook, we are both characterizing and facilitating the language and communication development of these children in an effort to understand the skills and abilities that subserve the development of language and its comprehension. Research with atypical populations offers promising avenues for investigation of these previously elusive capacities.

## REFERENCES

Adamlab. (1988). *WOLF manual.* Wayne, MI: Author.

Adamson, L.B. (1996). *Communication development during infancy.* Boulder, CO: Westview.

Arthur, G. (1952). *The Arthur Adaptation of the Leiter International Performance Scale.* Chicago: C.H. Steolting.

Benedict, H. (1979). Early lexical development: Comprehension and production. *Journal of Child Language, 6,* 183–200.

Bruner, J. (1983). *Child's talk: Learning to use language.* New York: Norton.

Dunn, L.M., & Dunn, L.M. (1981). *Peabody Picture Vocabulary Test–Revised.* Circle Pines, MN: American Guidance Service.

Foster, C.R., Giddan, J.J., & Stark, J. (1983). *Assessment of Children's Language Comprehension–1983 Edition.* Palo Alto, CA: Consulting Psychologists Press.

Franklin, K., Mirenda, P., & Phillips, G. (1996). Comparison of five symbol assessment protocols with nondisabled preschoolers and learners with severe intellectual disabilities. *Augmentative and Alternative Communication, 12,* 63–77.

Golinkoff, R.M., Mervis, C.B., & Hirsh-Pasek, K. (1994). Early object labels: The case for lexical principles. *Journal of Child Language, 21,* 125–155.

Grossman, H. (1983). *Classification in mental retardation.* Washington, DC: American Association on Mental Retardation.

Guess, D., & Horner, R. (1978). The severely and profoundly handicapped. In E.L. Meyen (Ed.), *Exceptional children and youth: An introduction* (pp. 218–268). Denver: Love Publishing.

Hirsh-Pasek, K., & Golinkoff, R. (1991). Language comprehension: A new look at some old themes. In N. Krasnegor, D. Rumbaugh, R. Schiefelbusch, & M. Studdert-Kennedy (Eds.), *Biological and behavioral determinants of language development* (pp. 301–320). Hillsdale, NJ: Lawrence Erlbaum Associates.

Huttenlocher, J. (1974). The origins of language comprehension. In R.L. Solso (Ed.), *Theories of cognitive psychology* (pp. 331–368). Hillsdale, NJ: Lawrence Erlbaum Associates.

Lambert, N.M., Windmiller, M., Cole, L., & Figueroa, R.A. (1975). Standardization of a public school version of the AAMD Adaptive Behavior Scale. *Mental Retardation, 13,* 3–7.

Luckasson, R., Coulter, D.L., Polloway, E.A., Reiss, S., Schalock. R.L., Snell, M.E., Spitalnik, D.M., & Stark, J.A. (1993). *Mental retardation: Definition, classification, and systems of supports* (9th ed.). Washington, DC: American Association on Mental Retardation.

McIlvane, W.J., Dube, W.V., Green, G., & Serna, R.W. (1993). Programming conceptual and communication skill development: A methodological stimulus-class analysis. In A.P. Kaiser & D.B. Gray (Eds.), *Communication and language intervention series: Vol. 2. Enhancing children's communication: Research foundations for intervention* (pp. 243–286). Baltimore: Paul H. Brookes Publishing Co.

Mervis, C.B., & Bertrand, J. (1993). Acquisition of early object labels: The role of operating principles and input. In A.P. Kaiser & D.B. Gray (Eds.), *Communication and language intervention series: Vol. 2. Enhancing children's communication: Research foundations for intervention* (pp. 287–316). Baltimore: Paul H. Brookes Publishing Co.

Mervis, C.B., & Bertrand, J. (1994). Acquisition of the novel name-nameless category (N3C) principle. *Child Development, 63*, 1646–1662.

Nelson, K. (1973). Structure and strategy in learning to talk. *Monographs of the Society for Research in Child Development*, 38 (1–2, Serial No. 139).

Nelson, K. (1985). *Making sense: The acquisition of shared meaning*. New York: Academic Press.

Oviatt, S.L. (1980). The emerging ability to comprehend language: An experimental approach. *Child Development, 51*, 97–106.

Oviatt, S.L. (1985). Tracing developmental change in language comprehension ability before twelve months of age. *Papers and Reports on Child Language Development, 24*, 87–94.

Resnick, J.S., & Goldfield, B.A. (1992). Rapid change in lexical development in comprehension and production. *Developmental Psychology, 28*, 406–413.

Romski, M.A., & Sevcik, R.A. (1992). Developing augmented language in children with severe mental retardation. In S.F. Warren & J. Reichle (Eds.), *Communication and language intervention series: Vol. 1. Causes and effects in communication and language intervention* (pp. 113–130). Baltimore: Paul H. Brookes Publishing Co.

Romski, M.A., & Sevcik, R.A. (1996). *Breaking the speech barrier: Language development through augmented means*. Baltimore: Paul H. Brookes Publishing Co.

Romski, M.A., Sevcik, R.A., & Pate, J.L. (1988). The establishment of symbolic communication in persons with severe retardation. *Journal of Speech and Hearing Disorders, 53*, 94–107.

Romski, M.A., Sevcik, R.A., Robinson, B.F., & Bakeman, R. (1994). Adult-directed communications of youth with mental retardation using the System for Augmenting Language. *Journal of Speech and Hearing Research, 37*, 617–628.

Romski, M.A., Sevcik, R.A., Robinson, B.F., Mervis, C.B., & Bertrand, J. (1996). Mapping the meanings of novel visual symbols by youth with moderate or severe mental retardation. *American Journal on Mental Retardation, 100*, 391–402.

Romski, M.A., Sevcik, R.A., Robinson, B.F., & Wilkinson, K.M. (1990, November). *Intelligibility and form changes in the vocalizations of augmented language learners.* Paper presented at the annual meeting of the American Speech-Language-Hearing Association, Seattle, WA.

Romski, M.A., Sevcik, R.A., & Wilkinson, K.M. (1994). Peer-directed communicative interactions of augmented language learners with mental retardation. *American Journal on Mental Retardation, 98*, 527–538.

Rosenberg, S., & Abbeduto, L. (1993). *Language and communication in mental retardation: Development, processes, and intervention*. Hillsdale, NJ: Lawrence Erlbaum Associates.

Rumbaugh, D.M. (Ed.). (1977). *Language learning by a chimpanzee: The LANA Project*. New York: Academic Press.

Savage-Rumbaugh, E.S. (1991). Language learning in the bonobo: How and why they learn. In N. Krasnegor, D.M. Rumbaugh, R.L. Schiefelbusch, & M. Studdert-

Kennedy (Eds.), *Biological and behavioral determinants of language development* (pp. 209–233). Hillsdale, NJ: Lawrence Erlbaum Associates.

Savage-Rumbaugh, E.S., Sevcik, R.A., Brakke, K.E., Rumbaugh, D.M., & Greenfield, P.M. (1990). Symbols: Their communicative use, comprehension, and combination by bonobos (*Pan paniscus*). In C. Rovee-Collier & L.P. Lipsitt (Eds.), *Advances in infancy research* (Vol. 6, pp. 221–278). Norwood, NJ: Ablex.

Sevcik, R.A. (1989). *A comprehensive analysis of graphic symbol acquisition and use: Evidence from an infant bonobo (Pan paniscus).* Unpublished doctoral dissertation, Georgia State University, Atlanta.

Sevcik, R.A., Romski, M.A., & Robinson, B.F. (1991, November). *Printed English word recognition by nonspeaking children with mental retardation.* Poster presented at the annual convention of the American Speech-Language-Hearing Association, Atlanta, GA.

Sevcik, R.A., & Savage-Rumbaugh, E.S. (1994). Language comprehension and use by great apes. *Language and Communication, 14,* 37–58.

Snell, M. (1993). *Instruction of students with severe disabilities.* Columbus, OH: Charles E. Merrill.

Snyder, L., Bates, E., & Bretherton, I. (1981). Content and context in early lexical development. *Journal of Child Language, 8,* 565–582.

Terman, L.M., & Merrill, M.A. (1960). *Stanford-Binet Intelligence Scale.* Newton, MA: Houghton Mifflin.

Wilkinson, K.M., Romski, M.A., & Sevcik, R.A. (1994). Emergence of visual-graphic symbol combinations by youth with moderate or severe mental retardation. *Journal of Speech and Hearing Research, 37,* 883–895.

Words +, Inc. (1985). *Words + Portable Voice II User's Manual.* Sunnyvale, CA: Author.

9

# Different Modes, Different Models

## Communication and Language of Young Deaf Children and Their Mothers

Patricia Elizabeth Spencer and Amy R. Lederberg

Since the 1970s, the general public's attitudes and information about deafness have undergone significant change: Sign interpretations of the national anthem appear on television as we watch major sporting events, political candidates are routinely accompanied by sign interpreters, and actors "speak" their lines with their hands. It has become clear even to those who do not study linguistics that language can be learned and messages transmitted without access to the spoken word.

Since Stokoe and his colleagues (Stokoe, 1960; Stokoe, Casterline, & Croneberg, 1965) demonstrated that the complexity, abstractness, and systematicity of spoken language are also characteristic of ASL (American Sign Lan-

Spencer's projects were funded by Grant Nos. MCJ-110563 (Maternal and Child Health Research Program, U.S. Department of Health and Human Services) and HO23C10077 (Office of Special Education and Rehabilitation Services, U.S. Department of Education). Additional support was provided by the Center for Studies in Education and Human Development, Gallaudet University. Data reported here were collected by a team of researchers including Kathryn P. Meadow-Orlans, Donald F. Moores, Robert H. MacTurk, and Lynne S. Koester. Gratitude is expressed to Robyn Waxman, Barbara Gleicher, Linda Stamper, Natalie Grindstaff, Arlene B. Kelly, Patricia Albee, Lynne Siegal, Karen Soloman, Michael Tierney, Laine Podell, and Silvio Menzano for their assistance with literature reviews, data collection, data coding, preparation of communication transcripts, and helpful discussions about "what it all means."

Lederberg's research was partially supported by grants from the Office of Special Education Programs and the March of Dimes Foundation. She wishes to thank Vicki S. Everhart, Caryl Mobley, Lisa B. Mongoven, Martha Kenny-Marks, Angie Love, Margaret Yebra, and Amy Prezbindowski for their aid in data collection and coding.

guage), those who study language development have increasingly sought insights into basic language processes through comparisons of sign and spoken language (e.g., Bellugi & Fischer, 1972; Meier & Newport, 1990; Orlansky & Bonvillian, 1985; Petitto, 1988). Studies of the language development of children who are deaf allow investigation of two questions of interest in the field of language acquisition: 1) What characteristics of language development are universal to the extent that they are consistent even when language is expressed in different modalities? 2) What aspects of communication and language are resilient and will appear even when children are deprived of normal levels of linguistic input (regardless of the modality used)? These two questions can be addressed by reference to two different subgroups of children who are deaf: those with deaf parents and those with hearing parents. The language-learning experiences of these two groups of children differ both from each other and from those of hearing children acquiring spoken language.

Approximately 1 of every 1,000 American children is born deaf (National Institutes of Health, 1993). Of those, approximately 10% have deaf parents and learn a sign language (usually ASL) as their first language. Just as hearing children do, deaf children with deaf parents acquire language through naturally occurring interactions. Thus, this group of deaf children can provide information useful for differentiating modality-specific from more general amodal acquisition patterns and processes.

Deaf children with hearing parents, comprising more than 90% of deaf children, face a language-learning situation different from that of both hearing children with hearing parents and deaf children with deaf parents. This group can provide unique information about the course of language development by children who are relatively deprived of linguistic input. Limited access to a language model is, of course, the case when hearing parents decide to rely exclusively on spoken language with deaf children. It is unfortunately also usually the case even when hearing parents decide to supplement their spoken language with a signing system. As new learners of the system, hearing parents are frequently unable to provide the kind of expert tutelage typical of parents using a language in which they are fluent. Thus, the language input typically available to deaf children with hearing parents generally fails to match the richness or consistency of models provided for hearing children by their hearing parents or for deaf children by signing, deaf parents.

We know that, as a group, deaf children with hearing parents display significant language deficits by school age, having limited vocabularies as well as difficulties with English syntactic structures (Meadow, 1980; Moores, 1987; Rodda & Grove, 1987). Investigation of these children's prelinguistic and early language development can illuminate the pervasiveness of effects of lack of typical rates of exposure to language, perhaps identifying communicative components that are relatively resistant to differences in language experience.

This chapter reviews information available about language acquisition patterns of deaf infants and young children to address effects of modality and consistency of language experience on the acquisition of language. We first focus on selected aspects of mothers' communication and language directed to infants to better explicate similarities and differences in the communicative experiences of the two groups of deaf infants and those of hearing infants. Then, we visit a cornerstone of language acquisition, the ability to establish joint attention during interactions with parents. Subsequently, deaf children's progress through the stage of intentional prelinguistic communication is reviewed. The emergence of early one-word/one-sign productions and trends in acquisition of vocabulary are then addressed. Finally, information about the transition to multiword/multisign expressions is provided.

Information presented in this chapter has been obtained from a number of reports available from language researchers focusing on signed and spoken language development of deaf children. In addition, we draw from our own work in this area. Spencer has completed longitudinal investigations of communication and language development of deaf infants with deaf and with hearing parents at 9, 12, and 18 months of age. This chapter reviews some previously published findings from those investigations (Spencer, 1993a,b; Spencer & Waxman, 1995; Waxman & Spencer, in press). In addition, some new analyses are reported. Each group (deaf infants with hearing parents [dH], deaf infants with deaf parents [dD], and hearing infants with hearing parents [hH]) included 19–20 infant–mother dyads. Lederberg conducted a similar investigation of deaf children with hearing parents at 22 months and 3 years of age (Lederberg & Everhart, 1996). This study included 20 dyads of deaf infants and hearing mothers and 20 dyads in which both infant and mother were hearing. The participants in both of these studies were advantaged in that they and their families had potential benefits of relatively early identification of hearing loss (before 9 months in Spencer's studies and at an average of 10 months in Lederberg's study). The mothers who participated had relatively high levels of education (all had graduated from high school) and had been provided information about deafness and communication methods by the family-focused early intervention programs in which they were participating.

## THE MODEL: MATCHING INPUT TO ATTENTION AND COMMUNICATION ABILITIES

### Hearing Mothers/Hearing Infants

Hearing mothers' communications to young infants differ in a number of ways from those addressed to older children or adults. Modifications occurring in interactions with infants include use of exaggerated facial expressions, increased tactile contact, increased production of gesture, and a characteristic set of changes in prosodic aspects of speech (Papoušek, Papoušek, & Bornstein, 1985). Speech to infants is characterized by strong rhythmicity, frequent repetition, high pitch, and exaggerated intonation patterns. All of these modifications appear suited to attracting and maintaining infants' attention to communicative input (Cooper & Aslin, 1990; Fernald, 1985).

As hearing infants near 1 year of age and give evidence of receptive and emerging expressive language skills, mothers' language becomes characterized by short, well-formed utterances that tend to highlight relations between the language and the objects or events in the immediate environment to which it refers (Murray, Johnson, & Peters, 1990; Sherrod, Friedman, Crawley, Drake, & Devieux, 1977; Snow, 1972, 1977). These simplifications in mothers' language support acquisition of vocabulary as well as development of receptive and expressive syntax (Cross, 1977).

Based on studies of hearing infants and their hearing parents, Papoušek and Papoušek (1987) proposed that modifications in maternal communication behaviors are "intuitive" and are a naturally occurring process which is prompted by interaction with an infant. Will "intuitions" lead deaf mothers, whose language is expressed through the gestural mode and whose infants depend on vision for receptive language, to make modifications parallel to those of hearing mothers? To the degree that the processes of modification are generalizable and amodal rather than modality specific, we would expect to see modifications made by deaf mothers, albeit in a different form from those of hearing mothers. However, it is not clear, even if modifications can be made across modalities, whether mothers who are hearing and whose own language experiences are primarily auditory-oral can generate and employ modifications appropriate for their deaf infants' visual needs.

### Deaf Mothers Who Sign

A number of reports confirm that deaf mothers modify communications with their infants and toddlers in ways analogous to the modifications of hearing "motherese," thus indicating that the modification process is not limited to auditory-oral communication channels. The modifications employed by signing deaf mothers appear to be especially responsive to their infants' visual attention. For example, both American (Erting, Prezioso, & Hynes, 1990/1994) and Japanese (Musataka, 1992) deaf mothers produce signs that are larger, slower, and have more exaggerated movements and rhythmic repetitions when communicating with infants than with adults. These "dance-like" sign productions serve to attract the infants' visual attention and provide a longer time for processing. As Musataka commented, these prosodic modifications in signing evoke "more robust responses" from deaf infants than does adult-like signing (p. 459).

Another modification in communications addressed by deaf mothers to deaf infants serves to make signed messages available to infants even when they do not look up from their play to see them. This modification occurs when deaf mothers move their hands to sign on or near an object toward which the infant is already looking. (This change in the location at which a sign is produced differs considerably from the usual practice of producing signs within the space directly in front of the signer's head and chest area.) Modification is also indicated when deaf mothers sit and wait for their infants to look at them before beginning to sign. This latter tendency explains in part the lower rate of language produced by deaf than by hearing mothers during interactions with their infants (Harris, Clibbens, Chasin, & Tibbits, 1989; Spencer, Bodner-Johnson, & Gutfreund, 1992). Modifications such as these, which accommodate immature patterns of infant attention, decrease as infants mature. Thus, there is less frequent displacement of signs and more frequent signed utterances by deaf mothers of 18-month-olds compared with 12- and 9-month-old deaf infants in Spencer's study (Waxman & Spencer, in press).

Similar to hearing mothers, deaf mothers also produce communicative behaviors designed to direct their infants' attention to objects of interest (e.g., tapping on an object or shaking it in front of the child). But unlike hearing mothers, deaf mothers quite frequently tap on their infants' shoulders or wave a hand in front of their faces to redirect the infants' attention back to mother herself. These signals are cultural conventions used even with older children and adults in the deaf community. However, they are used more frequently and persistently with infants.

As do hearing mothers, deaf mothers simplify language to deaf infants when evidence of understanding and emerging expression appears. Simplification is found in the content of mothers' language that generally relates to objects and events that are clearly evident in the current setting. Syntactic simplifications are also common. Most maternal utterances to 12-month-old deaf infants in Spencer's study were short and composed of a single sign (although perhaps with many rhythmic repetitions of the sign), a sign plus a point, or two or three signs. Like hearing mothers, deaf mothers' utterances again became longer when their infants began to produce utterances of more than one or two semantic units—a linguistic development demonstrated at 18 months of age by the more advanced dD (deaf infants/deaf mothers) infants in Spencer's study.

Another type of syntactic simplification evident in the deaf mothers' language is that of "breaking apart" and expressing morphemes linearly instead of in the simultaneous, layered fashion typical of many signs in adult-directed ASL. For example, WALK-QUICKLY can be differentiated from WALK-SLOWLY by the manner in which the verb is produced; no additional sign is required. When conversing with an infant, however, deaf mothers tend to produce a separate sign for the "manner" information.

Kantor (1982) observed an example of another kind of syntactic simplification when a deaf mother signed "SHE (is) WATCH(ing) YOU" to her young child. If signed to an adult, the sign for WATCH would have been started from the direction of the location of the agent (SHE)—in this case, the woman who was behind the video camera—and moved in the direction of the patient (YOU), with no separate handshape made to indicate either agent or patient. The mother made two modifications for her daughter. First, she indicated the agent (SHE) by pointing directly toward the person indicated. Then, she began the sign for WATCH in front of her own face (in its citation or most basic form) before directing it toward the patient (YOU). Spencer has observed similar syntactic modifications in which the agent is clearly marked by a separate sign when it is not linguistically necessary and other modifications in which adverbs and adjectives are signed separately instead of being incorporated into the verb or noun signs.

One example observed on Spencer's videotapes included a number of the modifications typical in deaf mothers' infant-directed expressions: Reaching around to sign between her daughter and the doll toward which she was looking, the mother signed, YOU-YOU-YOU FEED-DOLL FEED-DOLL FEED-DOLL. As above, the agent of the action was indicated by a direct point to the little girl. (With an adult, directional production of FEED-DOLL would have been grammatically sufficient to indicate both agent and patient.) In addition, the mother actually touched her daughter when signing YOU (adding a tactile component), and the sign repetitions increased the time during which the child could perceive the message. The utterance was signed slowly, signs were made larger than usual, and there was a rhythmic quality to the timing of the repetitions.

Thus, although the exact form of modifications made by deaf mothers and by hearing mothers differs, the modifications appear to represent similar underlying processes. Language to young infants emphasizes features that appear to match infant attention preferences (rhythmicity, repetition, increased emphasis), suggesting underlying infant amodal sensitivities that can be accommodated across modalities. Language to older infants appears to be modified to present a simplified, clear, more learnable model of the adult language.

Differences due to the modalities through which communications proceed are also found; for example, deaf mothers employ a set of attention-accommodating and redirecting strategies not commonly used by hearing mothers of hearing infants. It is of particular interest to determine whether these modifications that seem suited to communication in visual-gestural modalities are spontaneously generated by hearing mothers of deaf infants.

## Hearing Mothers of Deaf Children

There have been numerous reports of a relative lack of reciprocity and mutual responsiveness in dyads of hearing mothers and young deaf children (e.g., Meadow, Greenburg, Erting, & Carmichael, 1987; Wedell-Monnig & Lumley, 1980; White & White, 1984). These findings raise the possibility that hearing mothers are relatively unsuccessful in modifying their communications to suit deaf infants' attention and perceptual needs. However, analyses of the communicative behaviors of this group are complicated by some hearing parents deciding to use signing systems with their infants with others specifically rejecting gesturally based language. Furthermore, the families' decisions concerning communication mode often change over time. For example, only one quarter of the mothers in Lederberg's study used some sign language with their children at 22 months of age, but three quarters of the mothers were learning signs by the time the children were 3 years old. In Spencer's study, a number of families changed from oral programs to signing programs over the course of a year, while others moved from signing programs to programs using various oral language approaches.

***Spoken Language*** Whether or not hearing mothers use sign, speech accounts for the bulk of their linguistic-level communications to deaf infants and children. Hearing mothers in Spencer's study (about half of whom participated in educational programs emphasizing the use of signs) produced spoken utterances to their deaf children at the same rate as that of hearing mothers to hearing children (i.e., about 15 spoken utterances per minute). Lederberg similarly found no differences in the number of spoken utterances produced by hearing mothers to deaf and hearing 22-month-olds. However, by the time the children reached 3 years of age, the pattern was changing: Mothers spoke less often to deaf children than to hearing children. This difference may reflect growing differences in the children's language abilities.

No studies of which we are aware have specifically addressed the existence of prosodic modifications in speech by hearing mothers to deaf infants and toddlers. However, both authors have informally noted a relative lack of prosodic modifications in the speech of a number of the hearing mothers of deaf infants and toddlers in our studies. For example, several of the hearing mothers in our studies lowered the volume of their voices, essentially whispering to their deaf infants and toddlers. It is possible that prosodic modifications typical of maternal speech to hearing infants are less consistent when hearing mothers know their infants are deaf.

In contrast, several researchers have reported modifications in syntactic complexity of language spoken to deaf infants and children by their hearing mothers. For example, Spencer (1993a) noted that these mothers make syntactic simplifications (including shortening of utterances) typically made for hearing infants and toddlers. Cross (1977), as well as Wedell-Monnig and Lumley (1980), reported that such syntactic modifications continue to be made for deaf preschool children whose language level is delayed. Lederberg (1984) noted that even hearing women who are not mothers of deaf children and who have no experience with deafness simplify their language during interactions with deaf children.

Thus, at least some modifications common in speech to hearing infants occur with deaf infants and toddlers. When considering the potential impact of speech addressed to deaf children, however, it is important to consider Harris's

(1992) cogent distinction between language "input" (the amount of language produced by the mothers) and language "uptake" (the amount received by the child). Spoken language input and uptake may be at best marginally associated for deaf children. Regardless of the presence or absence of modifications in mothers' speech, the model of spoken language accessible to deaf children will not match that available to hearing children at similar language levels.

***Gestural Communication*** Hearing mothers observed in both of our studies showed inconsistent patterns of accommodation to deaf infants' and toddlers' visual needs. A lack of accommodation is indicated in that many of the mothers who were participating in signing programs failed to produce more than a few signs during the play sessions we observed. Furthermore, the sign language of hearing mothers we have observed lacks the rhythmic, exaggerated "prosodic" character of that of deaf mothers.

Hearing mothers' attention-directing behaviors also differ from those of deaf mothers. Although hearing mothers use the tapping signal more often to redirect the attention of deaf than of hearing infants, the frequency of usage falls far below that of deaf mothers. Hearing mothers observed by Waxman and Spencer (in press) seemed to work to establish a joint focus of attention with deaf infants primarily by directing attention to objects, a strategy they employed more often than either deaf mothers or hearing mothers of hearing infants.

However, there is some evidence of positive accommodation by hearing mothers. For example, although the mothers of 12- and 18-month-old deaf infants failed to increase their rate of production of conventional gestures over that typical in interactions with hearing infants, Lederberg found such an increase occurring by 22 months and continuing through 3 years. In addition, a few of the mothers in Spencer's study actually matched the mean rate of deaf mothers' production of signed utterances (5–6 per minute) and modified the location of a proportion of their signs and gestures (placing them within the infant's existing attention focus) similar to that shown by deaf mothers.

Syntactic modifications have been observed in hearing mothers' signed utterances, which (like those of deaf mothers) tend to be short and contain few signs. In this respect, hearing mothers' sign language appears to be adapted for the attention patterns of language-learning toddlers. However, the hearing mothers' productions often fail to meet the "well-formed" characteristic of language appropriately adapted for infants and toddlers. Because hearing mothers have rarely been taught ASL, most of them use signing systems artificially created to mimic the semantic and syntactic structures of the spoken language (English in most parts of the United States) that the signs are expected to accompany. In these signing systems, morphemes are combined linearly, new "signs" for grammatical morphemes (e.g., indicating tense, number, negation) have been created, and spoken word order is followed. Although hearing mothers have been noted to maintain English word order in their production of base or content signs, there are numerous reports that hearing signers tend to omit the grammatical morphemes and to frequently misarticulate signs (e.g., Spencer, 1993b; Swisher, 1984). Thus, the model of sign language available to deaf infants with hearing parents is less consistent and less grammatical than the ASL model presented to infants of deaf parents and also fails to match the grammaticality of spoken language available to hearing infants.

### Intuitions, Modifications, and Perceptual Processes

The existence of intuitive parenting behaviors, which results in parents directing toward infants the kinds of behaviors that best match their processing abilities, is supported by cross-modality (and cross-cultural) observations of communication modifications made by deaf mothers that seem suited to their deaf infants' perceptual and attention needs. Furthermore, similarity in the underlying characteristics of modifications in deaf mothers' signs and hearing mothers' speech (emphasizing rhythm, changes in intensity, and repetitiveness) suggests that infants are most sensitive to and most likely to attend to communicative stimuli with these characteristics, regardless of the modality through which they are expressed.

Despite exposure to information about deafness, hearing mothers evidence some limitations in their abilities to accommodate deaf infants' perceptual needs. Some sensitivity to the infants' visual needs is shown in modifications in attention-directing and gestural communication behaviors; however, hearing mothers often fail to spontaneously produce other useful communicative strategies. Characteristics of hearing mothers' signs suggest that ability to represent presumably amodal characteristics such as increased rhythmicity and prosody is limited when they must be expressed in a modality different from the one in which the speaker is most experienced, or perhaps in a language system with which the mother is not fluent. These limits to the ability to respond intuitively to young children whose sensory processing differs from that of the adult indicate that ability to modify communications to young language learners is intimately tied to adults' own communicative experience. As a result, deaf children with hearing parents are frequently provided communicative input that not only fails to meet their sensory processing needs but that, even when presented in visual form, fails to match the quality of that provided to deaf children by their signing deaf parents.

## CHILDREN'S COMMUNICATIVE DEVELOPMENT

### Infants' Engagement in Joint Attention Episodes

Episodes in which hearing mothers and hearing infants are engaged with the same object provide particularly potent opportunities for the acquisition of vocabulary when mothers provide language about the object of interest (Smith, Adamson, & Bakeman, 1988; Tomasello, 1988). Such episodes become increasingly frequent during the first 2 years of life. Bakeman and Adamson (1984) found that episodes of mother–infant joint attention focus are plentiful by 12 months of age, but the joint focus is frequently due to mothers joining in with their infants' previously established focus. Episodes in which infants actively coordinate glances between objects and their communication partners are relatively rare until 12 months of age but increase rapidly thereafter.

Because deaf infants are unable to auditorily process their mothers' spoken language, it is unlikely that much linguistic benefit accrues from episodes of joint attention unless they are characterized by the infants' coordinating visual attention to mother (thus visually receiving information from her hands and face) and to object. Despite their increased need for flexible person–object attention, the possibility has been raised that deaf children may have difficulty developing such higher-level visual attention skills. For example, Wood (1989) reported that preschool deaf children in oral language programs commonly showed delays in coordinating attention between people and objects. Wood implicated the children's inability to process auditory information and integrate it with visual information in the delays he observed. Similarly, Quittner, Smith, Osberger, Mitchell, and Katz (1994) reported that deaf school-age children (in both sign and oral programs) performed less well than hearing children on selective attention tasks. However, the deaf children's attention skills improved after cochlear implants increased their access to auditory stimuli. In contrast, Harris et al. (1989) found no negative impact on early attention skills from lack of auditory input. They reported that deaf children with deaf parents show patterns of "switching attention" reliably at about the same age as hearing children.

To further investigate effects of audition on attention development, Spencer and Waxman (1995) studied the patterns of visual attention demonstrated by infants in three groups (deaf infants with deaf mothers, deaf infants with hearing mothers, hearing infants with hearing mothers) who were observed at three ages (9, 12, and 18 months). Infant attention was coded using a system developed by Bakeman and Adamson (1984) in which qualitatively different attention patterns are represented by a set of six mutually exclusive "states." The two states of most relevance to this discussion are those of supported joint and coordinated joint attention. The former includes episodes of mutual infant–mother attention to the same object when the infant remains focused on the object, although being influenced by the mother's actions with it. The latter state includes episodes in which infants actively alternate their gaze between mother and object.

The patterns of performance of the three groups indicate that deafness does not necessarily cause delays in development of attention during infancy. No significant differences were found between the three groups in time in the supported joint attention state. Nor did time in this state change significantly within the age range observed. In contrast, time in coordinated joint attention increased significantly for all groups between 9 and 18 months of age. As Figure 1 shows, only deaf infants with deaf mothers had any measurable time in this state at 9 months. This group continued to have the greatest mean time at 12 and 18 months, and their overall time in the coordinated joint state significantly exceeded that of the deaf infants with hearing mothers.

Hearing infants did not differ significantly from either deaf group. This suggests fairly strong maturation influences on development of attention during infancy. This suggestion is supported by Lederberg's observations that her deaf (with hearing parents) and hearing subjects at 22 and 36 months did not differ significantly in visual "vigilance" or attention to communications. However, given a dependence on vision for reception of communication and language, even small differences in attention skills may have significant developmental consequences.

The difference in performance between the two groups of deaf infants observed by Spencer and Waxman (1995) suggests that interactive experiences significantly affect attention development when auditory information is not available. The role of experience on attention development of deaf infants was further investigated by comparing time in supported and coordinated joint attention for the two groups of deaf infants with three composite measures of the mothers' attention strategies discussed previously. The first measure, direct-to-self, included the tactile and visual signals of tapping on the infant, waving in the infant's visual field, and hitting on the floor. A second measure, direct-to-object, included moving objects and demonstrating activities with objects as well as tapping on objects. A third measure was the frequency of signing or gesturing by the mothers, activities that were assumed to be salient prompts for visual attention.

Direct-to-self, produced most often by the deaf mothers, was found to be significantly associated with their infants' time in coordinated joint attention. For the deaf infants with hearing mothers, who generally produced few direct-

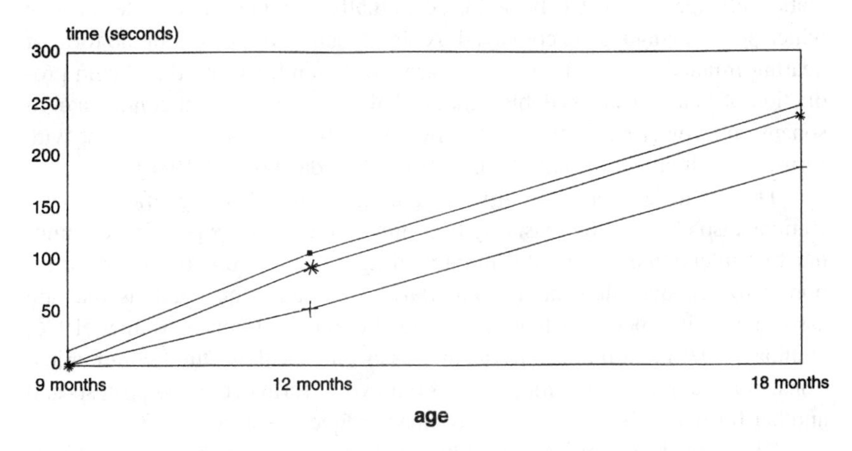


Figure 1. Time in coordinated joint attention during 10 minutes of dyadic play (dD = deaf infants/deaf mothers; dH = deaf infants/hearing mothers; hH = hearing infants/hearing mothers; • = group dD; * = group hH; + = group dH).

to-self behaviors, time in coordinated joint attention was associated significantly with the mothers' frequency of production of signs and/or gestures, a behavior for which there was considerable variance. Direct-to-object behaviors, which were produced most often by hearing mothers of deaf infants, were not associated systematically with infants' coordinated attention; instead, this category of attention strategy was associated with time in the supported joint attention state for both deaf groups.

Preliminary analyses comparing time in coordinated joint attention and language development of a portion of the deaf and hearing children participating in Spencer's study (13 dD, 15hD, 15hH) suggested different relations between attention and language across the groups. Language skills at 18 months for the deaf infants with deaf parents were significantly correlated with their 12-month ($r$=.65, $p$<.01) and 18-month ($r$=.59, $p$<.05) times in coordinated joint attention. Hearing infants' 18-month language skills were also correlated significantly with 12-month ($r$=.42, $p$=.06) and 18-month ($r$=60, $p$<.05) coordinated attention. In contrast, the association between 18-month language skills and time in coordinated joint attention at 12 ($r$=.32) and 18 months ($r$=.22), although positive, failed to approach significance for deaf infants with hearing parents. Because these children were less likely than those in the other two groups to receive language input during coordinated joint episodes (given that their mothers were less likely to sign than deaf mothers), it appears that the importance of such episodes for language development is due to their serving as sources of readily "uptaken" language rather than their being simply an index of general development.

## Prelinguistic Intentional Communication

***Vocal Communication.*** Soon after birth, infants produce nonvegetative and nonreflexive vocalizations. Over time, both the form and function of vocalization change, and vocal behaviors eventually become the vehicle through which spoken language is conveyed. A significant development in the form of hearing infants' vocalizations occurs around 7 months, when they begin production of "canonical" syllables, that is, babbled syllables that contain a consonant and vowel element with timing and thus articulation consistent with forms in adult language (e.g., "ba," "bee," "da-da") (Oller, 1980).

During the last part of the first year, the function of hearing infants' vocalizations also changes, increasingly becoming a means for expressing communicative intentions. By about 9 months of age, hearing infants have been reported to produce idiosyncratic but fairly consistent vocalizations that are associated with specific situations (Dore, Franklin, Miller, & Ramer, 1976; Halliday, 1975) and that are frequently associated with gestural communications. For example, a child may use a certain vocal form to express protests and another fairly consistent form to accompany request gestures.

There has been considerable interest in the vocalizations of deaf infants because of the natural experiment they provide regarding whether changes in phonetic or phonological form (at least through the prelinguistic stage) are prompted by general physiological maturation or result from infants' auditory experience. Although Lenneberg, Rebelsky, and Nichols (1965) and Mavilya (1969) are often quoted as having found no differences in the prelinguistic vocalizations of deaf and hearing infants, Oller, Eilers, Bull, and Carney (1985) pointed out that neither Lenneberg et al. nor Mavilya distinguished between precanonical and canonical babbling as described above. Oller's own investigations of deaf and hearing infants' prelinguistic vocalizations have shown a significant delay for deaf infants in the onset of canonical-level babbling.

Yoshinaga-Itano and Stredler-Brown (1992) as well as Spencer (1993a) presented data on vocalizations of fairly large samples of deaf infants that are consistent with those of Oller and colleagues (Oller & Eilers, 1988; Oller et al., 1985). For example, Spencer (1993a) found that despite early identification of hearing loss and early use of amplification, deaf subjects with hearing parents lagged significantly behind hearing peers in production of vocalizations containing canonical syllables at 12 months. Although the deaf children continued to lag at 18 months, their production of canonical syllables significantly increased over the 6 months, providing more evidence for Oller's thesis that the quantity of listening experience affects the form of children's vocal productions and indicating that these children's ability to profit from auditory experience (provided in some degree to most of the children by their hearing aids) had not yet diminished significantly. Such continued growth is important, especially in light of the suggestion by Oller and Eilers (1994) that canonical babbling may be a necessary precursor of productive use of spoken language. In this regard, Spencer (1993a) found that the frequency of deaf and hearing infants' canonical babbling at 12 months was positively associated with their rate of spoken language production at 18 months, although the strength of association was somewhat weaker for deaf than hearing infants.

Less research emphasis has been placed on the communicative function of vocalizations for deaf infants. Given less ability to monitor their own vocal productions, will deaf infants and young children continue to produce them in communicative situations? Spencer (1993a) found that deaf infants with hearing parents produced vocalizations judged to represent communicative intent no less frequently than hearing infants at 12 and 18 months. The amplification (hearing aids) used by the deaf infants allowed most of them awareness of their own as well as others' vocalizations. Furthermore, their hearing parents responded frequently to vocalizations.

The infants' vocal performance was consistent with the performance of Lederberg's sample of slightly older deaf children with hearing parents. The children she observed at approximately 22 and 36 months of age vocalized at frequencies similar to those of hearing children of the same age (although more of the hearing children's vocal productions were actual spoken words). Lederberg's deaf subjects used vocalizations more often than gestures or signs for expressive communication.

In contrast, a preliminary analysis of communication behaviors of Spencer's sample of deaf infants with deaf parents who were not using hearing aids and whose parents were not apt to reinforce infant vocalizations indicates that those infants relatively rarely produced vocalizations marked for communicative intent (as indicated by looking at their mothers or by accompanying the vocalization with a gestural communication) during toy-play interactions at 12 and 18 months. Comparisons of this group with the deaf children with hearing parents suggests that by 12 months of age, the rate of vocalization, phonological form of vocalizations, and use of vocalizations for intentional communication are dependent on experience rather than physiological or cognitive maturation.

***Gestural Communication*** Despite the frequency of vocalizations, meaningful prelinguistic communication is accomplished most often even by hearing infants through manual gestures such as showing and giving objects, reaching, pointing, and referential gestures (e.g., sniffing the air to mean smell, raising arms high to signify "so big"). Gestures begin to be used for intentional communication by most hearing infants before or around 1 year of age (about the same age at which intentional vocal communications emerge). Infants' intentional use of gestures is potentiated by a convergence of the acquisition of means–ends relations (in both social and cognitive domains) with the development of a general symbolic function (Piaget, 1952; Werner & Kaplan, 1963).

Research on hearing infants' communicative development (Fenson et al., 1994) indicates that use of gestures for intentional communication is closely associated with the level of receptive, but not expressive, language skills. This suggests that expressive gesture use is motivated at least in part by the relative acceleration of receptive over expressive language skills common around 1 year of age, that is, infants use gestures to express meanings they understand but for which they cannot yet express a formal linguistic symbol. (See Thal & Tobias, 1992, for data from hearing children with language delays that support this proposition.) If gestural communication is motivated by greater receptive than expressive language, might deaf infants who have hearing parents (and who are likely to have receptive as well as expressive delays at this age) be less likely to use expressive gestural communication than their typically developing peers?

This was not the case for the deaf infants with hearing parents observed by Spencer. Those infants, like the hearing infants and deaf infants with deaf parents in the study, produced approximately one intentionally communicative gesture per minute during the 12-month toy-play session. Although use of expressive gestures may reflect cognitive skills in advance of expressive linguistic skills, it does not seem to require relatively advanced formal receptive linguistic abilities.

It is possible that the similar rates of gestural expression by the three groups of infants observed by Spencer reflected the similar rates documented for their mothers. Other studies have provided suggestions of an association between frequency of gestures modeled and children's rate of gesture production. Accredolo and Goodwyn (1990) reported that hearing infants and toddlers increased the rate and variety of gestures produced when their parents artificially increased their own rate. Oral deaf mothers observed by de Villiers, Bibeau, Ramos, and Gatty (1993) accompanied their speech with an unusually high frequency of gestures, and their deaf toddlers also displayed high rates of gesture production. Lederberg and Everhart (1996) also found increased rates of gesture use by both hearing mothers and their deaf children (at 22 and 36 months) compared with dyads of hearing mothers and hearing children. These reports suggest that increased use of gestures by mothers is accompanied by increased use by their children.

However, mothers do not appear to spontaneously increase the frequency of gestures with younger deaf infants, with whom most communication focuses on the immediately perceptual environment (Spencer, 1993b). Instead, gestures are more likely to be used communicatively with somewhat older children, when mothers have reason to believe that children's cognitive abilities and communicative needs outstrip their language-processing abilities (Lederberg & Everhart, 1996). In turn, deaf children with language delays who have access to gestural but not formal language communication models may use gestures for their own expressive communications, even elaborating systems beyond the simple single gestures used by their mothers as Goldin-Meadow and her colleagues (Goldin-Meadow & Feldman, 1977; Goldin-Meadow & Morford, 1985) have reported. However, given adequate formal language models (whether in speech or in sign), infants' use of gesture for intentional communication is soon supplanted by acquisition and use of their parents' language.

## EMERGENCE OF WORDS AND SIGNS

### Acquisition of Vocabulary

Hearing children are generally reported to produce their first expressive words between 10 and 13 months of age (Bates, O'Connell, & Shore, 1987). They then gradually add to their lexicon until approximately 50 words are acquired (usually around 17 or 18 months of age), after which vocabulary size increases exponentially for most children (Bates, Bretherton, & Snyder, 1988; Bloom & Capatides, 1987; Goldfield & Reznick, 1990).

There are reports that the rate of hearing children's vocabulary growth is related to the frequency of language input they receive, but this association remains somewhat controversial. Vocabulary growth has also been reported to be related to gender, at least through 18 months (Huttenlocher, Haight, Bryk, Seltzer, & Lyons, 1991), and to contingency and semantic force of parents' language (Akhtar, Dunham, & Dunham, 1991). Furthermore, associations between parental language frequency and children's vocabulary development fade as development proceeds (Hart, 1991).

Because deaf children with deaf or with hearing parents generally receive less language input than hearing children (i.e., deaf mothers sign fewer utterances than hearing mothers speak and language "uptake" is generally decreased for deaf children with hearing parents), Harris (1992) suggested that the rate of vocabulary acquisition would be slower for deaf than for hearing children. Moreover, because deaf children with hearing parents generally have access to very low rates of language input, they may provide information about threshold levels required to support initial acquisition and subsequent vocabulary development.

### Deaf Children with Deaf Parents

***Initial Production of Signs*** There has been considerable debate about the age at which infants with signing deaf parents begin to sign expressively and thus demonstrate initial vocabulary acquisition. However, counter to Harris's (1992) suggestion, this debate has not centered on whether these infants "trail" hearing children; it has centered on whether deaf infants with deaf parents begin to sign significantly *earlier* than hearing children begin talking.

Since the 1970s, there have been reports that infants (both hearing and deaf) with signing deaf parents begin to sign as early as 5–9 months of age, significantly earlier than hearing infants first use spoken words (Bonvillian, Orlansky, Novack, & Folven, 1983; Maestas y Moores, 1980; McIntire, 1977; Orlansky & Bonvillian, 1985; Prinz & Prinz, 1979). These reports suggested that formal signing can occur before or concurrently with the first use of gestures for intentional communication. Orlansky and Bonvillian (1985) suggested that early signing indicates that cognitive capacity for formal language is available before its typical emergence in hearing infants around 12 months. They posited that spoken language is in effect "delayed" while it awaits maturation of oral articulators, and that the earlier maturation of manual articulators allows linguistic expression more representative of cognitive capabilities.

Petitto (1988) as well as Caselli and Volterra (1990/1994) disagreed strongly with the conclusions of Bonvillian et al. (1983), reporting that first signs of deaf children with deaf parents occur at about 12 months of age, similar to the age at which hearing children commonly express their first spoken words. Meier and Newport (1990), in a review of available reports of age of onset of expressive signing, concluded that the first context-bound signs may occur at an earlier age than hearing children's first words, but that any advantage for signs completely disappears before the stage at which utterances of more than one sign or word are produced.

Part of the confusion about the so-called "gestural advantage" in language development has undoubtedly resulted from different definitions of "sign" being used across studies. For example, it is not clear whether some early reports (see Bonvillian, Orlansky, & Folven, 1990/1994) differentiated between signs used only in routines or imitative contexts and those used at a referential level. Petitto (1988) argued strongly that many of the signs reported to occur early are gestures produced by both deaf and hearing infants that have been misinterpreted as signs. Petitto and Marentette (1991) have also reported a phenomenon referred to as manual babbling that has been observed in deaf infants at approximately the same age as hearing infants' canonical vocal babbling, and at the same age as some of the reports of early occurring signs. It is possible that such babbling (which involves the noncommunicative production of handshapes that will be used later in signs) may in some cases have been overinterpreted by parents as being meaningful signs. In fact, Bonvillian et al. (1990/1994) revisited their data and, using a definition of sign restricted to those that were clearly referential, found first signs occurred on average at 12.6 months of age.

Spencer analyzed sign production of the deaf infants of deaf parents in her study using a definition of sign based on that developed by Huttenlocher et al. (1991) to identify hearing infants' spoken words. Infant signs included those manual productions that correctly represented at least two of the three parameters of the presumed sign's articulation (or phonology), had an apparent meaning that was supported by context, and were not immediate imitations of parents' productions. (This definition allows for some "misarticulations," which are characteristic of early signs as well as of early spoken words.) Using this definition, no infant was observed to sign expressively during the 9-month session. Furthermore, the number of hearing infants and deaf infants with deaf parents who produced formal words or signs at 12 and 18 months was almost identical (with a slight advantage for the hearing infants). In addition, the vocabulary sizes reported at 18 months for the two groups of children by their mothers were similar.

Interpretation of findings from Spencer's study must be tentative due to the length of time between observations and the relatively brief time periods in which dyads were observed. However, the preponderance of evidence available fails to reliably support significantly earlier onset of signing compared with spoken language. Even if signs are not produced earlier than spoken words on average, however, it is clear that there is *no delay* in initial sign production by deaf infants with deaf parents. This is the case despite the fact that the quantity of language modeled by their mothers is less than that typically provided to hearing infants.

***Rate of Vocabulary Growth*** Just as data are inconclusive about the age of onset of expressive signing, so too is there disagreement about the rate of subsequent acquisition of signs. Bonvillian et al. (1990/1994) suggested that subsequent acquisition occurs more rapidly than for hearing children's acquisition of spoken words. Provine, Reilly, and Anderson (1993), who are collecting data to create norms for an ASL version of the Communicative Development

Inventory (CDI), however, have reported cross-sectional findings that sign vocabulary size during the second year of life for deaf children with deaf parents falls within the range typically found for hearing children's spoken vocabulary. This range is, of course, quite broad.

Although more data are needed, those available show no negative effects on sign vocabulary growth from the generally low rate of deaf mothers' utterance production. It is tempting to conclude that rate of language acquisition by deaf children with deaf parents is not related to the amount of input. However, Spencer found a within-group association, with language levels of 18-month-old deaf infants with deaf parents (based on the number of different signs demonstrated as well as the length of signed utterance) being significantly positively correlated with their mothers' frequency of signed utterances at both 12- and 18-month sessions. Although these findings are only correlational, they raise the possibility that the quantity of language input is related to language growth for these children as well as for hearing children, but that less sign than speech input is necessary to support lexical acquisition.

Why might this be true? There are at least two potential explanations. The first may be that for some as yet unexplained reason, language seen is more readily remembered and retrieved than language heard. (For example, the generally slower production of signs may allow more processing and storage time than does spoken language.) A second explanation is based on the high degree of visual contingency in signs produced by deaf mothers. That is, deaf mothers almost invariably produce signs where they can be seen (and sometimes felt) by their children. There is a generally high probability, therefore, that the deaf mothers' signing is uptaken by their children. In contrast, although hearing mothers speak more frequently to their hearing infants, it is not always evident how much of that language is actually processed by children who are engaged in object exploration or other kinds of play. This may be the reason semantic contingency of mothers' utterances on hearing children's existing focus of attention is so strongly associated with child language growth (e.g., Tomasello, 1988). Such contingency may increase the probability of the children actually processing the spoken language and relating it to their current attention focus.

### Deaf Children with Hearing Parents

***Initial Signs and Words*** Wide variations in the age of diagnosis of hearing loss and subsequent language-learning experiences of this group of children have made obtaining anything approximating "normative" information difficult. In addition, interpretation of some information available about this group is complicated by the inclusion of infants with disabilities unrelated to their hearing loss (e.g., Yoshinaga-Itano & Stredler-Brown, 1992). Spencer's group of deaf subjects with hearing parents represents a cohort that benefited from early diagnosis and intervention as well as being free (to the extent possible to evaluate during infancy) of cognitive, motor, and social disabilities. This group's rate of acquisition of first words may, therefore, be particularly illuminating.

The mothers in this group, approximately half of whom were participating in programs using signing systems, did not direct large amounts of signing to their children. However, half of the children in the group produced single-sign or single spoken-word utterances by 18 months (Spencer, 1993a,b). Several of the children in oral programming were reported to have an expressive vocabulary (recognized at least by their mothers) of 10 or more spoken words by 18 months of age. They were matched or exceeded by infants whose mothers had signed as few as .5 utterances per minute in the 12-month session. These infants were reported to produce their first sign between 13 and 15 months of age and had expressive vocabularies of 10–50 signs at 18 months.

Taken as a group, the deaf children with hearing parents in this study trailed both hearing children and deaf children with deaf parents in mean vocabulary size, and fully half of the group had no formal language at 18 months. The more successful portion of the group shows that initial vocabulary development can be supported by far less language input than might be expected from observations of hearing children. However, the less successful portion, as well as most of the preschool deaf children observed by Lederberg and Everhart (1996), shows that there are input limits below which acquisition of language is severely delayed.

***Rate of Vocabulary Growth*** Effects of the generally low rate of language input available to the deaf infants with hearing parents in Spencer's study are especially evident in their rate of vocabulary development subsequent to initial use of signs or spoken words. Follow-up data available for 11 of the deaf children with hearing parents and an equal number of hearing children at 24 and 30 months of age present a sobering assessment of the deaf children's progress. Parental reports (using the CDI: Toddler, modified when appropriate for use of signs instead of spoken words) indicated that the deaf children's rate of vocabulary development (in sign and/or in speech) increasingly deviated with age from that of hearing children. Thirty-month expressive vocabularies of the deaf children in oral programming ranged from 16 to 328 words. The range for signing children was 97–232 signs (but note that the two signing children with the largest reported vocabularies at 18 months did not have a 30-month CDI). In comparison, CDIs for the hearing subjects indicated a range of 465–661 expressive words at 30 months. All but four of the hearing children had expressive vocabularies at 24 months that exceeded the largest reported for a deaf child with hearing parents at 30 months.

Data from Lederberg's subjects also show increasing deviation between the language skills of deaf children with hearing parents and their hearing peers during the preschool years. It should be noted, however, that such a deviation is not inevitable. Notoya, Suzuki, and Furukawa (1994) reported that two Japanese deaf children whose hearing parents consistently exposed them to sign, vocal language, and print from an early age developed vocabularies (considering all lexical units regardless of modality) within the typical range for Japanese hearing children at least through 48 months of age.

## TRANSITION TO SYNTAX

It should not be thought that onset of expressive spoken language signals the end of hearing children's dependence on gestures that have previously been critical for communication. Indeed, gestures (albeit modified when they accompany speech) remain an important companion of spoken language throughout adulthood (McNeill, 1993). Furthermore, it appears that pointing gestures fill an important role in hearing children's transition from single-word to multiword utterances. Multiword utterances are preceded by hearing children's simultaneous production of a point with a single spoken word (Goldin-Meadow & Morford, 1985; Iverson, Volterra, Pizzuto, & Capirci, 1994). In the earliest such productions, the pointing gesture and the word are redundant (i.e., the word labels the object toward which the point is directed). Somewhat later, however, the point and the spoken word can represent different functions in a single utterance. In this case, the point and word supplement each other in that they provide nonredundant information, with the word indicating a nonlabel characteristic of the object or event toward which the point is directed. Nonredundant point–word combinations appear immediately before the first spoken multiword productions, apparently signaling a cognitive readiness for the expression of relations between symbolic elements.

Hearing children generally produce their first true multiword utterances several months after the onset of the acceleration in vocabulary growth. Although different styles have been noted among hearing children, it is most common for their first productive multiword utterances to consist of two words and, for the most part, to be "telegraphic," with grammatical morphemes omitted. By 3 years of age, however, most hearing children learning English produce varied and relatively complex English syntactic structures.

### Deaf Children with Deaf Parents

Deaf children who are acquiring sign language also combine points with their one-sign utterances (Kantor, 1982; Newport & Meier, 1985). In this case, the production of the point and sign usually occur in sequence, with the point coming either before or after the sign. A review of the 12- and 18-month signed utterances of deaf infants with deaf parents in Spencer's study showed that, like those of hearing children, both point and sign in the deaf children's earlier occurring productions have the same referent: Children point to an object and sign its name. By 18 months, utterances in which the point and sign were nonredundant (that is, they represent several different aspects of the referent) were common, and two-sign utterances were produced by several of the children.

The similarity in these structures produced by children who are acquiring spoken language and those who are acquiring sign language is striking, especially considering that pointing serves a strictly linguistic function as sign language development proceeds.

An additional syntactic similarity between children learning spoken English and those learning ASL is seen in the morphological simplicity of their productions. Early multisign productions tend to be bereft of grammatical morphemes, with sign order generally used to mark grammatical or semantic roles (Kantor, 1982). Before acquiring the inflectional system of ASL (which has been noted to emerge at about 3 years of age), the signed utterances of deaf children are structured much like hearing children's early spoken utterances.

On a related issue, Newport and Ashbrook (1977) as well as Kantor (1982) reported that the developmental sequence in which semantic relations are expressed in multisign utterances is the same as that reported for hearing children's spoken productions. Thus, modality of language seems to have little impact on the structure of the earliest word or sign combinations, even though the structure of signed language and spoken English are different in later stages.

### Deaf Children with Hearing Parents

The few available data suggest that these children, like the other deaf and hearing children, also progress through an initial stage in which points are combined with a single sign or word, followed by production of utterances with multiple signs or spoken words (Day [Spencer], 1986). However, these developments are almost always significantly delayed.

Grammatical morphemes tend to be omitted from the early multiword and multisign utterances of deaf children with hearing parents just as they are from those of hearing children or deaf children with deaf parents. However, it is not clear that the same process is occurring across the three groups. Deaf children with hearing parents are provided language models that are usually neither ASL nor complete models of English, and hearing signers tend to omit the grammatical signs created for the artificial English-based signing systems. In addition, such grammatical morphemes are unstressed in vocal productions and are therefore among the linguistic elements least available auditorily, making them essentially disappear for a child with a significant hearing loss. Thus, the grammatical model presented to deaf children of hearing parents tends to preserve English word order but lack markings of tense, number, and other information carried by grammatical morphemes.

Not surprisingly, given deficiencies in the language model they are provided and their typically late onset of expressive language, deaf children with hearing parents show continued slow growth in syntactic abilities. Although some students in programs using signing systems acquire relatively good understanding of major types of English sentence structures, Schick and Moeller (1992) reported that their use of English grammatical morphemes remains problematic even through adolescence.

## SUMMARY

In this chapter, we aimed to identify aspects of language acquisition that were universal, or amodal, and aspects that were resilient in the face of deprivation of a complete and fluent language model, by reviewing and comparing data on the language acquisition of deaf and hearing children. We posited that amodal characteristics would be demonstrated in similarities found between the acquisition process of deaf children with signing deaf parents and the process of hearing children exposed to a spoken language model. Resilience would be demonstrated for characteristics that were shared between the communication and language behaviors of hearing children and deaf children with hearing parents, most of whom have access only to a language model lacking both consistency and completeness.

The difference in language modality did not prevent deaf mothers from accomplishing communicative modifications that, like those of hearing mothers of hearing infants, are tuned to their infants' attention needs and proclivities. The major difference between language of deaf and hearing mothers was the decreased frequency of utterances produced by deaf mothers. This difference appears to be a positive adaptation to visual communication with an infant whose attention skills are still developing, but it results in deaf infants with deaf parents being presented with a lesser quantity of language than hearing children.

Despite this quantitative difference, the course of prelinguistic and early linguistic development of deaf infants with deaf parents shows a strong pattern of convergence with that of hearing infants. Episodes in which infants actively coordinate visual attention to mother and to an object occur at least as early for deaf infants of deaf parents as for hearing infants and are strongly associated with language development in both groups of infants. The development and use of gestures for intentional prelinguistic communication also appears to progress similarly for the two groups. Although there is some evidence that initial expressive signs occur earlier than hearing infants' spoken words, that evidence is clouded by definitional problems and small sample sizes and is countered by other reports indicating a similar age of onset for signs and speech. Sign vocabulary size appears to fall within the normal range compared with spoken word vocabularies of hearing children during the second year of life, but the scarcity of data leaves this an open issue in need of further research. Finally, there are striking similarities in the syntax of early sign and spoken word combinations. Both deaf and hearing infants produce combinations of pointing with single signs or words, followed by combinations of more than one unmodulated lexical unit. Neither early structures nor the range of semantic relations expressed in those structures appears to be sensitive to modality differences.

The similarities in early development of deaf infants with deaf parents and hearing infants with hearing parents have two implications. First, even if sign acquisition occurs at the same and not an earlier age than spoken language, deaf infants appear to require less sign input to perform at a given level expressively compared with the spoken language model typically available to hearing infants. This suggests that although there may be no "gestural advantage" in the sense of onset of expressive language, there may be an advantage in the amount of input required to acquire knowledge of signs compared with speech. Second, modality-specific influences on linguistic structures are not clearly apparent until almost 3 years of age; thus, more general amodal processes characterize early development. This suggests a developmental discontinuity, or at least an increased sensitivity to language experience, as the processes of initial prelinguistic and early one-sign (or word) communication give way to those involved in the rapid expansion of syntactic abilities that occurs after initial vocabulary is established.

Such a discontinuity is also indicated by observations that the course of acquisition of prelinguistic communication is more resilient, thus more robust, than that of formal language in the face of deficiencies in the available language model. Although deaf infants with hearing parents trailed their deaf peers with deaf parents in time in coordinated joint attention (suggesting that their later development may be hampered by a lack of optimal visual attention skills), their patterns of visual attention did not differ significantly from those of their hearing peers through 18 months of age. Deaf infants with hearing mothers also acquired and used gestures for prelinguistic intentional communication at the same age and at a similar rate as hearing infants. Thus, prelinguistic use of gestures does not appear to be strongly influenced by the infants' receptive language skills or the amount or fluency of their mothers' linguistic expressions and attention-directing behaviors. Even the onset of expressive language, that is, the production of the first signs or spoken words, appears to be somewhat resilient under adverse conditions. Given uptake of far less language than is available to hearing infants, some deaf infants with hearing parents acquire first signs or words near the beginning to middle of the second year of life. Of course, there are limits to this ability. If almost no uptake is possible, no formal language will develop.

The pattern of language development of this group of children suggests that, in addition to sensitivity at the syntactic level to differences in input, lexical acquisition beyond initial signs or words is also more sensitive, and less resilient, than acquisition of the first few items. Even those deaf infants of hearing parents who demonstrated their first expressive signs within the age range typical for hearing infants' first spoken words fell progressively behind their hearing peers in vocabulary growth.

Few of the deaf children with hearing parents in our studies had begun to combine signs or words at the termination of the studies. In general, data on the process of acquisition of syntactic patterns are especially scarce for younger children in this population. However, data available from older children suggest that formal syntax is highly sensitive to variations in input. This at least appears to be true for that aspect of English syntax involving use of grammatical morphemes combined linearly with base words.

It is important to note here that similarities in the process of communication and language acquisition of deaf and hearing infants and young children are only apparent when modality of expression is ignored. Use of the vocal mode for expression at both prelinguistic and linguistic levels is especially sensitive to variations in ability to process auditory stimuli. Although use of vocalizations for prelinguistic communication develops when hearing aids or other amplification devices allow some processing of sound, deaf infants with little to no awareness of sound and no environmental support for vocal communication vocalize infrequently. Acquisition of phonological characteristics of spoken language is even more sensitive to variations in auditory processing abilities.

## CONCLUSION

Children who are born deaf or lose their hearing early in infancy provide a unique perspective on processes of language acquisition and development. Because more than half of these children have no disabilities beyond the inability to process auditory information, they possess normal neurological and cognitive potential for communication and language. Studies of this portion of the population of deaf children, therefore, allow us a naturally occurring window through which to observe effects of experiential differences on the developing communication and language systems. The findings reviewed in this chapter reveal many similarities in early communication and language acquisition despite experiential differences in modality, quantity, and even quality of language available for uptake in deaf infants and toddlers compared with hearing infants and toddlers. Effects of modality in the earliest stages of language acquisition appear to be limited to a possibility that acquisition of sign vocabulary requires less input than spoken language. Effects of relative deprivation of language input, although not strongly evident during the first year of life and in early prelingual communication, become more pervasive as children move beyond the age at which prelingual communication is developmentally appropriate. Characteristics of the available language model have increasingly differential effects during the toddler and preschool years, with ASL-signing deaf children and English-speaking hearing children incorporating progressively more of the syntactic conventions of their specific languages. In addition, deaf children who are provided minimally accessible language models fall farther behind the other two groups of children with age, sometimes turning to increased use of gestures to provide themselves with a means of communication.

## REFERENCES

Accredolo, L., & Goodwyn, S. (1990). Sign language in babies: The significance of symbolic gesturing for understanding language development. In R. Vasta (Ed.), *Annals of child development* (pp. 1–42). London: Jessica Kingsley Publishers.

Akhtar, N., Dunham, F., & Dunham, P. (1991). Directive interactions and early vocabulary development: The role of joint attention focus. *Journal of Child Language, 18*, 41–49.

Bakeman, R., & Adamson, L. (1984). Coordinating attention to people and objects in mother–infant and peer–infant interaction. *Child Development, 55*, 1278–1289.

Bates, E., Bretherton, I., & Snyder, L. (1988). *From first words to grammar: Individual differences and dissociable mechanisms.* Cambridge, England: Cambridge University Press.

Bates, E., O'Connell, B., & Shore, C. (1987). Language and communication in infancy. In J. Osofsky (Ed.), *Handbook of infant development* (pp. 149–230). New York: John Wiley & Sons.

Bellugi, U., & Fischer, S. (1972). A comparison of sign language and spoken language. *Cognition, 1*, 173–200.

Bloom, L., & Capatides, J. (1987). Expression of affect and the emergence of language. *Child Development, 58*, 1513–1522.

Bonvillian, J., Orlansky, M., & Folven, R. (1990/1994). Early sign language acquisition: Implications for theories of language acquisition. In V. Volterra & C. Erting (Eds.), *From gesture to language in hearing and deaf children* (pp. 219–232). Berlin: Springer-Verlag (1990); Washington, DC: Gallaudet University Press (1994).

Bonvillian, J., Orlansky, M., Novack, L., & Folven, R. (1983). Early sign language acquisition and cognitive development. In D. Rogers & J. Sloboda (Eds.), *The acquisition of symbolic skills* (pp. 207–214). New York: Plenum.

Caselli, M., & Volterra, V. (1990/1994). From communication to language in deaf and hearing children. In V. Volterra & C. Erting (Eds.), *From gesture to language in hearing and deaf children* (pp. 263–278). Berlin: Springer-Verlag (1990); Washington, DC: Gallaudet University Press (1994).

Cooper, R., & Aslin, R. (1990). Preference for infant-directed speech in the first month after birth. *Child Development, 61*, 1584–1595.

Cross, T. (1977). Mothers' speech adjustments: The contribution of selected child listener variables. In C. Snow & C. Ferguson (Eds.), *Talking to children: Language input and acquisition* (pp. 151–188). New York: Cambridge University Press.

Day (Spencer), P. (1986). Deaf children's expression of communicative intentions. *Journal of Communication Disorders, 19*, 367–386.

deVilliers, J., Bibeau, L., Ramos, E., & Gatty, J. (1993). Gestural communication in oral deaf mother–child pairs: Language with a helping hand? *Applied Psycholinguistics, 14*, 319–347.

Dore, J., Franklin, M., Miller, R., & Ramer, A. (1976). Transitional phenomena in early language acquisition. *Journal of Child Language, 3*, 13–28.

Erting, C., Prezioso, C., & Hynes, M. (1990/1994). The interactional context of deaf mother–infant interaction. In V. Volterra & C. Erting (Eds.), *From gesture to lan-*

*guage in hearing and deaf children* (pp. 97–106). Berlin: Springer-Verlag (1990); Washington, DC: Gallaudet University Press (1994).

Fenson, L., Dale, P., Reznick, J., Bates, E., Thal, D., & Pethick, S. (1994). Variability in early communicative development. *Monographs of the Society for Research in Child Development, 595*, Serial No. 242).

Fernald, A. (1985). Four-month-old infants prefer to listen to motherese. *Infant Behavior and Development, 8*, 181–195.

Goldfield, B., & Reznick, J. (1990). Early lexical acquisition: Rate, content, and the vocabulary spurt. *Journal of Child Language, 17*, 171–183.

Goldin-Meadow, S., & Feldman, H. (1977). The development of language-like communication without a model. *Science, 197*, 401–403.

Goldin-Meadow, S., & Morford, M. (1985). Gesture in early child language: Studies of deaf and hearing children. *Merrill-Palmer Quarterly, 31*, 145–176.

Halliday, M. (1975). *Learning how to mean.* London: Arnold.

Harris, M. (1992). *Language experience and early language development: From input to uptake.* Hillsdale, NJ: Lawrence Erlbaum Associates.

Harris, M., Clibbens, J., Chasin, J., & Tibbits, R. (1989). The social context of early sign language development. *First Language, 9*, 81–97.

Hart, B. (1991). Input frequency and children's first words. *First Language, 11*, 289–300.

Huttenlocher, J., Haight, W., Bryk, A., Seltzer, M., & Lyons, T. (1991). Early vocabulary growth: Relation to input and gender. *Developmental Psychology, 27*, 236–248.

Iverson, J., Volterra, V., Pizzuto, E., & Capirci, O. (1994, June). *The role of communicative gesture in the transition to the two-word stage.* Poster presented at International Conference of Infant Development, Paris, France.

Kantor, R. (1982). Communicative interaction: Mother modification and child acquisition of American Sign Language. *Sign Language Studies, 36*, 233–282.

Lederberg, A. (1984). Interaction between deaf preschoolers and unfamiliar hearing adults. *Child Development, 55*, 598–606.

Lederberg, A., & Everhart, V. (1996). *Communicative interactions between deaf toddlers and their hearing mothers.* Manuscript submitted for review.

Lenneberg, E., Rebelsky, F., & Nichols, I. (1965). The vocalization of infants born to deaf and to hearing parents. *Human Development, 8*, 23–37.

Maestas y Moores, J. (1980). Early linguistic environment: Interactions of deaf parents with their infants. *Sign Language Studies, 26*, 1–13.

Mavilya, M. (1969). *Spontaneous vocalization and babbling in hearing impaired infants.* Unpublished doctoral dissertation, Teachers College, Columbia University, New York.

McIntire, M. (1977). The acquisition of American Sign Language hand configurations. *Sign Language Studies, 16*, 247–266.

McNeill, D. (1993). The circle from gesture to sign. In M. Marschark & D. Clark (Eds.), *Psychological perspectives on deafness* (pp. 153–184). Hillsdale, NJ: Lawrence Erlbaum Associates.

Meadow, K. (1980). *Deafness and child development.* Berkeley: University of California Press.

Meadow, K., Greenberg, M., Erting, C., & Carmichael, H. (1987). Interactions of deaf mothers and deaf preschool children: Comparisons with three other groups of deaf and hearing dyads. *American Annals of the Deaf, 126*, 454–468.

Meier, R., & Newport, E. (1990). Out of the hands of babes: On a possible sign advantage in language acquisition. *Language, 66*, 1–23.

Moores, D. (1987). *Educating the deaf: Psychology, principles and practices.* Boston: Houghton Mifflin.

Murray, A., Johnson, J., & Peters, J. (1990). Fine-tuning of utterance length to preverbal infants: Effects on later language development. *Journal of Child Language, 17*, 511–525.

Musataka, N. (1992). Motherese in a signed language. *Infant Behavior and Development, 15*, 453–460.

National Institutes of Health. (1993). Early identification of hearing impairment in infants and young children. *NIH Consensus Statement, 11*(1).

Newport, E., & Ashbrook, E. (1977). The emergence of semantic relations in American Sign Language. *Papers and Reports on Child Language Development, 13*, 16–21.

Newport, E., & Meier, R. (1985). The acquisition of American Sign Language. In D. Slobin (Ed.), *The cross-linguistic study of language acquisition: Vol. 1. The data* (pp. 881–938). Hillsdale, NJ: Lawrence Erlbaum Associates.

Notoya, M., Suzuki, S., & Furukawa, M. (1994). Effects of early manual instruction on the oral-language development of two deaf children. *American Annals of the Deaf, 139*, 348–351.

Oller, D. (1980). The emergence of the sounds of speech in infancy. In G. Yeni-Komshian, J. Kavanagh, & C. Ferguson (Eds.), *Child phonology: Vol. 1. Production* (pp. 93–112). New York: Academic Press.

Oller, D., & Eilers, R. (1988). The role of audition in infant babbling. *Child Development, 59*, 441–449.

Oller, D., & Eilers, R. (1994). Infant vocalizations and the early diagnosis of severe hearing impairment. *Journal of Pediatrics, 124*, 199–203.

Oller, D., Eilers, R., Bull, D., & Carney, A. (1985). Prespeech vocalizations of a deaf infant: A comparison with normal metaphonological development. *Journal of Speech and Hearing Research, 28*, 47–63.

Orlansky, M., & Bonvillian, M. (1985). Sign language acquisition: Language development in children of deaf parents and implications for other populations. *Merrill-Palmer Quarterly, 31*, 127–143.

Papoušek, H., & Papoušek, M. (1987). Intuitive parenting: A dialectic counterpart to the infant's precocity in integrative capacities. In J. Osofsky (Ed.), *Handbook of infant development* (2nd ed., pp. 669–720). New York: John Wiley & Sons.

Papoušek, H., Papoušek, M., & Bornstein, M. (1985). The naturalistic vocal environment of young infants: On the significance of homogeneity and variability in parental speech. In T. Field & N. Fox (Eds.), *Social perception in infants.* Norwood, NJ: Ablex.

Petitto, L. (1988). "Language" in the prelingusitic child. In F. Kessel (Ed.), *The development of language and language researchers* (pp. 187–221). Hillsdale, NJ: Lawrence Erlbaum Associates.

Petitto, L., & Marentette, P. (1991). Babbling in the manual mode: Evidence for the ontogeny of language. *Science, 25*, 1493–1496.

Piaget, J. (1952). *The origins of intelligence in infants.* New York: Norton.

Prinz, P., & Prinz, E. (1979). Simultaneous acquisition of ASL and spoken English. *Sign Language Studies, 25*, 283–296.

Provine, K., Reilly, J., & Anderson, D. (1993, November). *Language development of deaf children: The CDI for ASL.* Poster presented at the American Speech-Language-Hearing Association Annual Convention, Anaheim, CA.

Quittner, A., Smith, L., Osberger, M., Mitchell, T., & Katz, D. (1994). The impact of audition on the development of visual attention. *Psychological Science, 5*, 347–353.

Rodda, M., & Grove, C. (1987). *Language, cognition, and deafness.* Hillsdale, NJ: Lawrence Erlbaum Associates.

Schick, B., & Moeller, M. (1992). What is learnable in manually coded English? *Applied Psycholinguistics, 13*, 313–340.

Sherrod, K., Friedman, S., Crawley, S., Drake, D., & Devieux, J. (1977). Maternal language to prelinguistic infants: Syntactic aspects. *Child Development, 48*, 1662–1665.

Smith, C., Adamson, L., & Bakeman, R. (1988). Interactional predictors of early language. *First Language, 8*, 143–156.

Snow, C. (1972). Mothers' speech to children learning language. *Child Development, 43*, 549–566.

Snow, C. (1977). Development of conversation between mothers and babies. *Journal of Child Language, 4*, 1–22.

Spencer, P. (1993a). Communication behaviors of infants with hearing loss and their hearing mothers. *Journal of Speech and Hearing Research, 36*, 311–321.

Spencer, P. (1993b). The expressive communication of hearing mothers and deaf infants. *American Annals of the Deaf, 138*, 275–283.

Spencer, P., Bodner-Johnson, B., & Gutfreund, M. (1992). Interacting with infants with a hearing loss: What can we learn from mothers who are deaf? *Journal of Early Intervention, 16*, 64–78.

Spencer, P., & Waxman, R. (1995). Joint attention and maternal attention strategies: 9, 12, 18 months. In *Maternal responsiveness and child competency in deaf and hearing children.* Final Report, Grant HO23C10077. Washington, DC: U.S. Department of Education, Office of Special Education and Rehabilitation Services.

Stokoe, W. (1960). Sign language structure: An outline of the visual communication system of the American deaf. *Studies in Linguistics, Occasional Papers No. 8*. Buffalo, NY: University of Buffalo, Department of Anthropology and Linguistics.

Stokoe, W., Casterline, D., & Croneberg, C. (1965). *A dictionary of American Sign Language on linguistic principles.* Washington, DC: Gallaudet University Press.

Swisher, M. (1984). Signed input of hearing mothers to deaf children. *Language Learning, 34*, 69–85.

Thal, D., & Tobias, S. (1992). Communicative gestures in children with delayed onset of oral expressive vocabulary. *Journal of Speech and Hearing Research, 35*, 1281–1289.

Tomasello, M. (1988). The role of joint attentional processes in early language development. *Language Sciences, 10*, 69–88.

Waxman, R., & Spencer, P. (in press). What mothers do to support infant visual attention: Sensitivities to age and hearing status. *Journal of Deaf Studies and Deaf Education.*

Wedell-Monnig, J., & Lumley, J. (1980). Child deafness and mother–child interaction. *Child Development, 51*, 766–774.

Werner, H., & Kaplan, B. (1963). *Symbol formation.* New York: John Wiley & Sons.

White, S., & White, R. (1984). The deaf imperative: Characteristics of maternal input to hearing-impaired children. *Topics in Language Disorders, 4*, 38–49.

Wood, D. (1989). Social interaction as tutoring. In M. Bornstein & J. Bruner (Eds.), *Interaction in human development* (pp. 59–80). Hillsdale, NJ: Lawrence Erlbaum Associates.

Yoshinaga-Itano, C., & Stredler-Brown, A. (1992). Learning to communicate: Babies with hearing impairments make their needs known. *Volta Review, 94*, 107–129.

# III

# DEVELOPMENT IN ATYPICAL CONTEXTS

# 10

# Language Processes in Context

## Language Learning in Children Reared in Poverty

Grover J. Whitehurst

Since the 1970s, most theory within developmental psycholinguistics has focused on processes thought to be general to all cultures and driven by an inherited, language-specific set of neurological mechanisms. Thus, Brown and Hernstein (1975, p. 479) said about language acquisition, "One irresistibly has the impression of a biological process developing in just the same way in the entire human species," and Pinker (1984, p. 29) maintained that language acquisition is such a robust process that "there is virtually no way to prevent it from happening short of raising a child in a barrel."

Following this lead, researchers with an interest in language development in typically developing children have generally observed small numbers of children, have largely ignored individual differences, and have not used the statistical or research design tools that are employed extensively in other areas of social and behavioral science to study complex phenomena (see Bates, Bretherton, Beeghly-Smith, & McNew, 1982). After all, if the important processes in language development are universal and the final product of the language ac-

This work was supported by grants to the author from the Pew Charitable Trusts (91-01249-000) and the U.S. Administration for Children and Families (90CD095701 & 90CD096201). Research by the author in child care settings reported herein was supported by a grant from a private foundation that prefers not to be identified publicly. Views expressed are the author's and have not been cleared by the grantors. The author is deeply appreciative of the cooperation of the administration, staff, and families of Long Island Head Start and the Children's Community Head Start. This chapter has been improved by comments on a draft made by Dorothy Bishop, Jim Stevenson, Christopher Lonigan, and the editors of this book, for which the author is appreciative.

quisition process is essentially the same across all typically developing children, 1 subject can be as edifying as 1,000 subjects.

Research on children with language and communication impairments has occupied an awkward position with respect to the mainstream of work on language acquisition. For that segment of the community of researchers whose focal concern has been therapy and intervention, the literature on typical development has occasionally proven useful in conceptualizing instructional sequences. For example, a clinical researcher working with children with severe language delays might structure instructional goals around the stages in the development of early grammatical forms laid out by Brown (1973) and Ruder and Smith (1984). However, clinicians and researchers attempting to develop interventions have had little reason to seek guidance on designing treatments from a literature that has largely downplayed the role of social and environmental processes. For that reason, interventions have typically been drawn from the literature on social learning or have been created from amalgams of clinical experience, prior intervention research, and disconnected hints from disparate programs of research and theory (Whitehurst et al., 1991).

Correspondingly, researchers and theorists in the mainstream of work on typical language development have had little interest in the nature or efficacy of interventions for children with language impairments, reasoning that special teaching evironments are necessary for these children because their language acquisition device is not typical.

A second component of research on language impairments has had closer links to the mainstream of research on language development. This is research that describes and characterizes specific language impairments (e.g., Bishop, 1992; Watkins & Rice, 1994; Whitehurst & Fischel, 1994). This research appeals to theorists who view typical language development as a function of an innate language acquisition device because it helps to identify the outlines of that device and perhaps some of its mechanisms. For example, if there are individuals who function cognitively at much lower levels than they function linguistically (Bellugi, Marks, Bihrle, & Sabo, 1988), one might think of the language acquisition device as a relatively independent neurological module (Fodor, 1983) as opposed to a set of general information-processing mechanisms that support language acquisition (MacWhinney, 1993). As another example, if children with language impairments can be shown to have a specific impairment in language processing such as phonological memory (Gathercole & Braddeley, 1990), then a part of the structure of the language acquisition device begins to be visible. Thus, research on syndromes of language impairment has served a function for theories of typical language development much like research on brain injury has served for theories of normal neurological functions: to map the limits and functions of the underlying mechanisms.

This chapter focuses on a population of children who fall between these research traditions described and cannot continue to be neglected by theorists who aim to develop general theories of language acquisition. Children reared in poverty are an important challenge to our understanding of language acquisition. As a group, their profile of language skills is typically closer to that of children with mild mental retardation than to that of middle-class children. Yet for the vast majority of children reared in poverty, language differences are clearly attributable to environmental circumstances rather than biological impairments. Language quotients below 80 during the preschool years for children who are biologically intact are problematic for Pinker's (1984) position that there is no way to stop language acquisition from occurring short of raising a child in a barrel. As the evidence in this chapter and elsewhere indicates, conditions far less severe than being raised in a barrel can adversely affect the rate and form of development in many areas of language.

This chapter documents some of the language characteristics of children reared in poverty, describes some of the social–cultural conditions that affect those characteristics, and points out the implications of these findings for theories of language acquisition and for future research on language development. Although this chapter focuses on social effects on language acquisition, I do not present this material in opposition to theory and research suggesting that language development is driven by innately acquired, language-specific mechanisms. My work with a different population of children with language delays has led me toward a substantially congenital account of the etiology of that population's problem (Whitehurst & Fischel, 1994). Neither does this work stand in opposition to environmental effects on language that are nonsocial, such as brain injury, maternal substance abuse, or poor nutrition. A full account of typical language development will have to be interactionist, combining language-specific cognitive mechanisms (e.g., Fodor, 1983), with non–language-specific cognitive mechanisms (e.g., MacWhinney, 1993), with social–cultural mechanisms (e.g., Bloom, 1993; Whitehurst & DeBaryshe, 1989), and with nonsocial environmental and biological mechanisms (e.g., Malakoff, Mayes, & Schottenfeld, 1994). I believe that language theorists who pay attention to the language characteristics of children reared in poverty will have to expand their models to include more social–cultural processes.

## DEFICITS VERSUS DIFFERENCES

Data on levels of language skill in children from low-income backgrounds run into the differences versus deficits debate. A history of this debate since the 1970s might begin with the work of the British sociologist Bernstein (1971), though a wider history would include philosophers such as Durkheim, anthropologists such as Sapir and Whorf, and psychologists such as Vygotsky. Bernstein's research led him to distinguish between uses of language that are restricted or context bound and uses of language that are more elaborated and less dependent on context. For example, the same scene might be described as "It went through and broke it," or "The boy kicked the football and it went through the window of the school and broke it." Understanding the former utterance depends on the listener's having considerable implicit knowledge about its context, perhaps even observing the event along with the speaker of the message. The meaning of the latter utterance, in contrast, is much more explicit. It can be understood by someone at a distance based on the words alone. It is relatively context free and universalistic compared with the former utterance.

Bernstein's (1971) research indicated that working-class children in England were more likely than middle-class children to produce restricted code and less likely to produce elaborated code. Correspondingly, mothers of working-class children were less likely than mothers of middle-class children to use elaborated code in socializing their children. Bernstein (1971) went to considerable lengths to distance himself from a frequent interpretation of his work, that it meant that working-class children were linguistically deficient: "This does not mean that working-class mothers are non-verbal, only that they differ from the middle-class mothers in the *contexts* which evoke universalistic meaning. They are *not* linguistically deprived, neither are their children" (p. 196).

Despite these disclaimers, Bernstein's work created controversy. In his own summary of critical responses to his work, Bernstein (1971) wrote the following:

> The concept of restricted code was said to impose a humiliating uniformity upon the diversity and imaginative potential of cultural forms. At the level of the classroom, the same concept was said to have lowered the expectations teachers held of their children, whereas the concept of elaborated code legitimized the teacher's own middle-class conception of appropriate communication. (p. 19)

While Bernstein attempted to distance himself from the deficit interpretation, Hunt, a scholar whose work on intelligence and experience was an intellectual force behind early intervention initiatives such as Head Start, published a series of studies with his colleagues that supported the deficit model. In separate investigations involving concepts of color, position, shape, and number, 4-year-olds from low-income families attending Head Start were compared with children from middle-class backgrounds attending nursery school (Hunt, Kirk, & Lieberman, 1975; Hunt, Kirk, & Volkmar, 1975; Kirk, Hunt, & Lieberman, 1975; Kirk, Hunt, & Volkmar, 1975). The procedure of each study was first to test children on perceptual discrimination of a concept, for example, by asking the child to "find the one that is different" in an array of differently colored blocks. Subsequently children were tested on their linguistic knowledge of the same concept, for example, by being asked to "point to the red block" or by being asked "what color is this" as each block was presented. The rationale for the two different test conditions, one perceptual and one semantic, was to demonstrate that the test conditions themselves, with their possible middle-class bias, did not prevent children from low-income backgrounds from demonstrating competence.

Findings were similar across each of the concept categories. On the perceptual tasks, Head Start children performed roughly equivalent to the middle-class nursery school sample. However, on the semantic tasks, performance by the children from low-income families was dramatically lower than that of children from middle-class backgrounds. For example, only approximately 24% of Head Start children could point to all six test colors when they were named by the examiner, compared with 89% of nursery school children. The researchers summarized their findings by writing:

> The finding of a deficiency in semantic mastery for such an elementary abstraction as color is highly dissonant with the contention that children of poverty . . . are without cognitive or linguistic deficit, and that they fail in school only because they use a dialect differing from standard English. The finding supports the contention that children of poverty do have a cognitive and linguistic deficit which may, and probably does, derive from the rearing conditions in their homes during the preschool years. (Kirk, Hunt, & Lieberman, 1975, p. 299)

Scholarly support for the differences model of the language of children reared in poverty has come largely from linguists and anthropologists. The linguist Labov (1972), focusing on phonology and grammar, pointed out that Black English, a group of similar dialects spoken by many low-income African Americans, is as rule governed and logical as Standard American English, the dialect used in the media and by most middle-class Americans. Thus, the typical dropping of the verb *to be* in the vernacular of Black English (e.g., "She the first one," "He fast") is logically and informationally identical to the contractions used in Standard English in the same contexts (e.g., "She's the first one," "He's fast").

The anthropologist Heath (1983, 1989), emphasizing the social, pragmatic functions of language, documented the rich oral tradition of African Americans in the form of rhymes, stories, music, sermons, and joking. This cultural tradition places a premium on children's development of group-oriented forms of language that allow adaptation within frequently shifting contexts of extended families, community institutions, and the streets. "Adults expect children *to show* what they know rather than *to tell* what they know" (Heath, 1989, p. 369). Viewed through this lens, testing children on discrete formal language elements such as vocabulary or grammar or metalinguistic awareness is inherently biased against African American children from low-income families because these children's culture emphasizes the social functions of language. The distinction being made implicitly by Heath is among the social, functional, cooperative, or illocutionary functions of language versus the truth, structural, reality, or locutionary functions of language, as has been discussed in detail by authors such as Austin (1962); Clark and Clark (1977); Olson and Hildyard (1981); and Searle (1969).

Notice the relationship between Bernstein's (1971) conclusion that working-class children and their parents are more likely to use restricted linguistic code and Heath's (1989) conclusion that low-socioeconomic status African Americans are more likely to emphasize the social over the formal functions of language. Although these scholars have been seen as on the opposite side of the differences versus deficits debate, both appear to be describing the same phenomenon: People from poverty backgrounds are less likely to use language in which meaning adheres to the spoken or written word itself and more likely to use language that is adjusted to and depends on a particular social context for meaning.

## A Synthesis: Differences and Different Types of Deficits

This chapter distinguishes between comparative differences and subsets of comparative differences that entail either competitive or absolute disadvantages. In a *comparative difference*, one person or group of people can be demonstrated to have less of some measurable characteristic than another person or group of people (e.g., less body hair, fewer vocabulary words, less height). Comparative differences are always relative to some comparison group and in the meaning ascribed here are entirely descriptive; that is, they do not entail value judgments. Thus, we may describe a person or group of people as having less body hair or less melanin or less money than another person or group of people, and at the level of comparative differences, we need to be concerned only with the empirical accuracy of the description.

A subset of comparative differences is *competitive deficits*. These are differences among people to which consequences are attached because of social and cultural realities that can vary across settings. For example, the grammar and phonology of Black English may place people who use it at a competitive disadvantage in U.S. schools and workplaces because of cultural preferences, even though there is no inherent logical advantage of Standard English over Black English in terms of the information it can carry, and even though one can imagine a culture in which the tables would be turned. The empirical operation for demonstrating a competitive deficit is first to demonstrate a quantitative difference and then to demonstrate that people with that difference are more likely to encounter barriers to achievement within particular cultural settings which they engage.

A subset of comparative differences, *absolute deficits* place individuals at a competitive disadvantage for reasons that are relatively independent of changing cultural settings. Examples are impaired sense organs, intellectual functioning at mentally retarded levels, severe social skills deficits, and perhaps, as Hunt and colleagues argued, linguistic inabilities that prevent people from describing or comprehending descriptions of such basic aspects of their environment as shape, color, position, or number (e.g., Hunt, Kirk, & Volmar, 1975). The measurement requirement for demonstrating an absolute deficit is evidence that people with that deficit are differentially likely to encounter barriers to achievement within most or all of the cultural settings which they engage.

Concepts such as cultural settings and achievement are abstract, admit of no precise definition, and vary over time and setting. They can, however, be operationalized in ways that are more or less useful for a particular task. I would imagine, for example, that without putting the reader through the actual exercise, few would doubt that I could operationalize terms so as to reliably and usefully categorize people with schizophrenia as having a comparative difference that is also an absolute deficit, and people with tone deafness as having a comparative difference that becomes a competitive deficit only if they try to achieve musically.

Most proponents of the traditional differences perspective on the development of children from poverty or minority backgrounds argue that the language dimensions on which children are said to be deficient exist only at the level of comparative differences but are turned by society into competitive deficits and often interpreted by the mainstream culture as absolute deficits. That is, the mainstream culture turns the use of Black English into a competitive deficit by basing instruction in the schools on Standard English and treats Black English as an absolute deficit by attributing less intelligence and motivation to people who use it. The political imperative from the differences perspective is to create a more pluralistic society in which purely comparative differences are not turned into competitive deficits.

However, we cannot dismiss the previously described possibility raised by Hunt, Kirk, and Lieberman (1975) that aspects of the language development of children in poverty fall into the category of absolute deficits. Consider this description by Heath (1989), who is perhaps the most prominent current proponent of the differences view, of her research on the interactions between a mother and her preschool children. The mother is said to be prototypical of many poor urban African American mothers who live in small apartments or public housing, isolated from supportive family or community:

> One mother agreed to tape-record her interactions with her children over a two-year period and to write notes about her activities with them. . . . Within approximately 500 hours of tape and over 1,000 lines of notes, she initiated talk to . . . her three preschool children (other than to give them a brief directive or query their actions or intentions) in only 18 instances. (pp. 369–370)

As a working hypothesis, we must be willing to consider the possibility that rearing conditions in which three preschool children receive only 18 linguistically informative utterances over a 2-year period can produce absolute deficits in language skills of the sort that would compromise functioning in virtually any culture or subculture. At the same time, we must be careful not to interpret competitive deficits as absolute deficits without clear supporting evidence.

In general, the whole issue of how much language input, in what form, and at what time is necessary for language development in what area and for what ultimate outcome requires more research attention. We have evidence, for example, that typical hearing children raised by deaf mothers develop normal oral language and can combine imitation of the stress patterns of "deaf speech" with standard phonological characteristics (Schiff-Myers, 1988). However, in this work the frequency of typical language input from sources other than the mother is not controlled, nor are the effects of signed language input as a substitute for aural stimulation, nor are the effects of the mothers' responsiveness to their children's efforts to communicate. We also have reports of so-called wild children who have been described as developing sophisticated language abilities later in life despite very limited early language exposure (Curtiss, 1977; Rymer, 1994). However, the actual conditions of early rearing are uncertain in these cases, and to the extent that typical language functions eventually develop, the issue becomes one of critical periods, not of the role of language input itself. In addition to these problems of interpretation, the very limited literature on the role of input available to children has not included ultimate language outcomes or different components of language. For instance, finding that the phonological development of 2-year-old children of deaf mothers is similar to that of children of hearing mothers is different from proposing that children who received limited language input and limited responsiveness to their own language productions over extended periods of development ultimately achieve levels of phonological, syntactic, semantic, and pragmatic skills on par with those of children who experience rich and continuous language input and responsiveness. There are no data to support such an assumption in the literature, and I predict that at least for the domains of semantic and pragmatic development there never will be. We simply have too much evidence of substantial effects of input and feedback variables on semantic and pragmatic development over the typical range of variation to expect that their virtual absence would have no effects.

## CHARACTERISTICS OF LANGUAGE DEVELOPMENT IN CHILDREN RAISED IN POVERTY

In this chapter, various subsets of data are described that have been collected from preschoolers from low-income families in Suffolk County, New York. This is the easternmost county of the two that constitute Long Island, with a population of 1.3 million. Although sections of the north shore of the county and the south fork are among the most affluent in the United States, the center of the county and some areas of the south shore include large groups of individuals living in conditions of poverty. Living costs, and particularly housing and utility expenses, are among the highest in the nation.

One of two principal groups of children, the child care cohort, consists of 73 three-year-olds who attend publicly subsidized child care centers in Suffolk

County. The limit on family income for this sample to qualify for subsidized child care was $25,000 for a family of four. Many parents were receiving welfare. (This sample is described in detail in Whitehurst, Arnold, et al., 1994.) The other principal group, the Head Start cohort, consists of 521 children who were first encountered when they were 4-year-olds attending Head Start in Suffolk County. The limit on family income to qualify for this program was approximately $14,000. These children were encountered in three different waves corresponding to 3 different years, and the oldest have been followed for 3 years, through the end of first grade. (The second wave of these children, which is similar to the other two waves, is described in detail in Whitehurst, Epstein et al., 1994.) This sample is from an affluent suburban county with high levels of social services. Seventy-one percent of the primary caregivers of the children in the Head Start sample had finished high school, and 46% had some college or trade-school coursework. In other words, although the economic poverty of this sample is quite real, and perhaps psychologically more pressing than usual because these are pockets of poverty within a region of highly visible affluence, the families in this sample do not, in general, have to contend with the levels of crime, drug abuse, lack of social and educational services, and disintegrating community institutions that are present in poverty areas in many urban centers.

Consistent with the previous point, there is no sense in which these children are an epidemiological sample of children from low-income backgrounds in the United States. They are, instead, a sample of convenience. However, my purpose here is not to produce a linguistic sociology of children reared in poverty, but rather to document how conditions of poverty can be associated with differences in the development of language skills. The present sample should serve that function.

The studies in which these children have been involved included interventions intended to influence language skills. These interventions and some of their effects will be described in a subsequent section. This section is descriptive, so I include only children who were randomly assigned to control conditions and thus never encountered an intervention, or children who had yet to encounter an intervention condition to which they had been assigned.

## Semantic Skills

The battery of language assessment devices that my colleagues and I administered included two widely used measures of semantic ability, the PPVT–R (Peabody Picture Vocabulary Test–Revised) (Dunn & Dunn, 1981a), a test of receptive vocabulary; and the EOWPVT (Expressive One-Word Picture Vocabulary Test) and the EOWPVT–R (Expressive One-Word Picture Vocabulary Test–Revised) (Gardner, 1981, 1990), tests of expressive vocabulary. In the PPVT–R children are asked in successive trials to choose a picture from among four pictures based on a label provided by the examiner. In the One Word, children are asked in successive trials to label a picture presented by the examiner. Figure 1 presents PPVT–R and EOWPVT scores in standard scores on an IQ-type scale where the population mean is equal to 100 and the population standard deviation is equal to 15. At the 3-, 4-, and 5-year-old levels, the performance of these children from low-income families averages approximately one standard deviation below the mean of 100 of the standardization sample. The upper whiskers in the graph, which extend one standard deviation above the mean of the sample and which seldom reach the population mean of 100, show that roughly 85% of the children in these samples score below average on both receptive and expressive semantics. The lower whiskers show that roughly 15% or more of children in these samples score within the mentally retarded range based on the typical IQ-based definition of mental retardation as a standard score below 70. This is five times the frequency of the mentally retarded–level *semantic* performance expected in the general population. Semantic performance is stressed in the previous sentence because tests that assess vocabulary skills, such as PPVT–R or the EOWPVT are not IQ tests and thus the data reported in Figure 1 are not IQ scores. However, because vocabulary subscales of IQ tests correlate more highly with full-scale IQ scores than any other subscales (e.g., Wechsler, 1974), and because the median correlation between the PPVT and the full-scale Stanford-Binet across a number of studies is .71 (Dunn & Dunn, 1981b), we should not simply assume that the data reported in Figure 1 are unrelated to the scores these children would obtain were they to be given a test said to measure IQ.

Is it possible that these findings are seriously distorted because the assessment devices are biased against the children's cultural backgrounds? Some depression in children's scores can be credited to this factor, but it seems unlikely that the general thrust of the findings could be discounted based on the presumed cultural insensitivity of the test materials or the testers. First, 90%–95% of the children represented in Figure 1 are from homes in which the primary caregiver was a native speaker of English, and no child is included in the data reported in Figure 1 who, in the judgment of teachers, had poor command of English as a second language. The data change very little if children from homes in which the primary caregiver was not a native speaker of English are excluded. Second, from 22% to 45% of the children represented in Figure 1, with the lower percentage at the age 3 level, are from homes in which the primary caregiver was European American. Although European American children as a group score higher than African American or Latin American children in these samples and typically come from homes in which the primary caregiver was better educated, the pattern in Figure 1 is the same for all groups, that is, scores significantly below range. Third, it is difficult to see the very basic semantic concepts that are represented in the PPVT–R and the One Word at the preschool level as incorporating much of a specific cultural bias. For example, objects that many children in the 4-year-old sample were unable to label on the One Word included chicken, triangle, ear, and leaf. Objects that many children

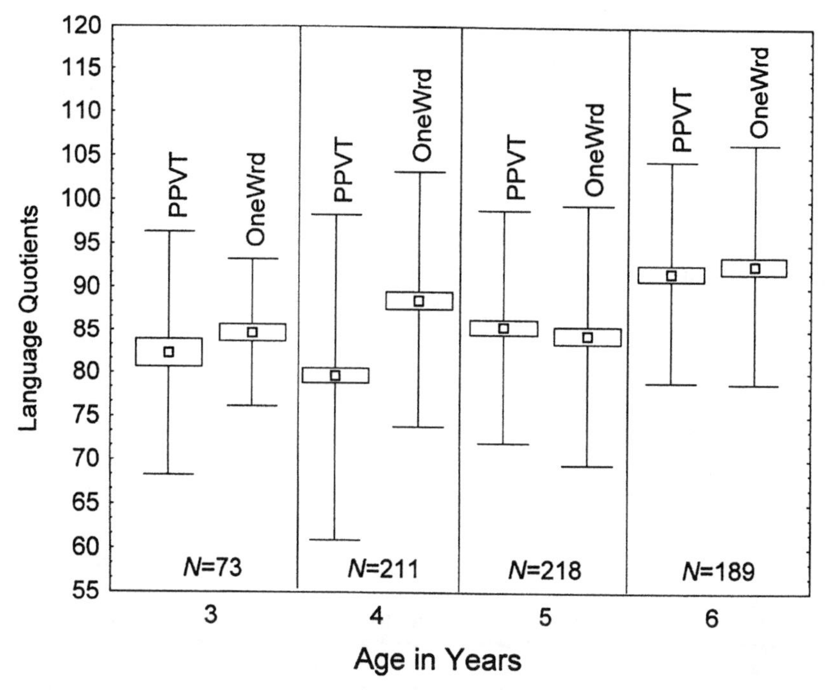


Figure 1. PPVT–R and EOWPVT (One Word) standard scores for children attending low-income child care (age 3) or Head Start (4–6) in a suburban county of New York. Through age 5, children are consistently one standard deviation below the mean for their age group (⊥ = ± standard deviation; ▭ = ± standard error; □ = mean).

in the 3-year-old sample were unable to point to on the PPVT–R included cow, lamp, drum, and knee. Although these tests are biased against children who do not have the opportunity to learn labels for such common objects, the objects themselves do not seem to favor one ethnic or racial group over another. Finally, the examiners who tested these children were experienced, advanced graduate students who were familiar figures in the children's schools.

Low levels of responding by minority group children on tests such as the PPVT have sometimes been attributed to test anxiety rather than low linguistic skill; however, retesting is supposed to eliminate these motivational problems (Zigler, Abelson, & Seitz, 1973). Therefore, the children at the age 5 level in Figure 1 had been tested twice on the same battery, and children at the age 6 level had been tested three times. Furthermore, comparison of children in these samples who were randomly assigned to experimental versus control conditions and given pretests and posttests has shown little or no positive change in language quotients for children in control conditions (Whitehurst, Arnold, et al., 1994; Whitehurst, Epstein, et al., 1994), as one would predict if their initial scores were depressed as a result of test anxiety. The apparent increase in scores with age in Figure 1 is not relevant to this point because these are different samples of children. When we have followed the same children longitudinally, we typically see a jump in scores after the first year of public school, but stable scores before and after that. In summary, I see no reason to believe that children in these samples had substantially higher semantic abilities than were indicated by their test scores.

## Syntax

Linguists frequently view syntactic ability as the sine qua non of language, as the invariant component that most directly reflects the underlying neurological structures that support language acquisition in humans. From that perspective, one should expect syntactic components of language to be most resistant to environmental effects. Our data provide some support for that view, depending on the degree to which particular measures of syntax are culturally loaded.

Table 1 presents the MLU (mean length of utterance) for the five longest utterances produced by 4-year-olds in the Head Start sample on the *Renfrew Bus Story* (BUS) (Cowley & Glasgow, 1994). The BUS consists of a short story about a bus, which is read aloud to a child who follows the storyline in a series of 12 pictures. The child then uses those pictures to retell the story. The child's narrative is transcribed and scored along a number of dimensions, including length. The mean length of the sample's five longest utterances at the age 4 and age 5 levels results in a standard score of approximately 100, which is at the norm.

A second syntactic measure derived from the BUS was each child's total number of complex sentences, defined as utterances with subordinate clause(s) linked to the main clause with conjunctions such as *when*, *because*, and *although*. As indicated in Table 1, children performed at a lower level on this measure than on MLU, with standard scores of approximately 90 at the two age levels, but this is still higher than the standard scores of 85 or lower on the tests of semantic ability.

A third test of syntactic ability focusing on morphosyntactic forms was the word structure subtest from the CELF–P (Clinical Evaluation of Language Fundamentals–Preschool) (Wigg, Secord, & Semel, 1992). In this assessment, the examiner provides a spoken model of a morphological form in response to a sample picture and then attempts to elicit the same form from the child in response to a new but related picture (e.g., "Here are three frogs. Here are

Table 1. Standard score means[a] and *SD*s for syntactic measures

| Measures | Length (BUS) | Complex Utterances (BUS)[b] | Word Structure (CELF–P) |
|---|---|---|---|
| Mean (SD) Age 4: | 97.95 (14.21) | 91.75 (9.61) | 91.30 (11.35) |
| Mean (SD) Age 5: | 101.95 (15.83) | 89.48 (11.85) | 90.35 (11.22) |

[a]All scores are reported on an IQ-type scale with normed mean=100 and *SD*=15.

[b]Standard scores for complex utterances are not provided in the BUS. They were derived here from tabled values of number of items correct by number of subjects for the normative sample reported in the BUS manual.

three ____" [bugs]). Although it is possible to score this test using different rules for children who are assumed to be from families speaking Standard English versus children from families who are assumed to be using a dialectical variation such as Black English, we applied the set of rules for Standard English to all children to maintain comparability of scores across children. As shown in Table 1, children in the Head Start sample performed with a mean standard score of approximately 90 at both age levels on this test, which is about the same level at which they performed on the measure of complex utterances. The concordance of the scores from the measure of word structure and the measure of complex utterances is reassuring because they are from different instruments, thus suggesting that the findings for syntax are not due to idiosyncracies in the standardization of the American version of the BUS.

One might summarize the results from the three measures of syntax by saying that an environment of poverty is least likely to affect the length of children's utterances, and moderately likely to affect the complexity of their utterances and their adherence to language-specific morphosyntactic rules.

### Narrative Abilities

To the extent that some of the subcultures of families living in poverty favor the social functions of language over the logical functions, as argued by Heath (1989), then children from poverty backgrounds should be relatively stronger on narrative tasks than on tasks that assess more abstract, formal characteristics of language (Feagans, 1982). To assess narrative skills, the BUS, previously described, allows scoring for information, which is the amount of story content that the child is able to relate in his or her own retelling of the story of the bus. Children's information scores on the BUS are, as with their other language abilities, approximately one standard deviation below the mean. The story sequence subtest from the Developing Skills Checklist (CTB, 1990) gives a child five picture cards, each with one scene representing part of the sequence of putting on and tying a shoe. The cards are shuffled and the child is asked to put them in order so that they tell a story. Children in the Head Start sample performed at very low levels, with only 5% of 5-year-olds able to perform the task successfully, compared with 49% of the normative sample. Only 43% of 6-year-olds were able to perform the task, compared with 79% of the normative sample. In summary, these children performed no better on narrative tasks than on semantic tasks. However, the BUS and the story sequence assessments are different from many everyday pragmatic interactions in that the motive for the child to produce a complex and coherent narrative is provided by the examiner's questioning. That motive may be more unusual and less compelling for a child reared in economic poverty than for a middle-class child. The effects of different pragmatic venues on children may vary with different social–cultural backgrounds, and require more research.

### Metalinguistic Awareness

Sensitivity to the metalinguistic structure of language (e.g., that a spoken word can be broken down into separate sounds; that a spoken sentence can be broken down into separate words) is thought to be an important linguistic precursor to reading and writing (e.g., Bradley & Bryant, 1983; Byrne & Fielding-Barnsley, 1991, 1993; Lundberg, Frost, & Petersen, 1988; Mann, 1993; Stanovich & Siegel, 1994). The auditory subscale of the Developing Skills Checklist was used to assess metalinguistic awareness. The auditory subscale includes four subtests: 1) identifying same/different words (e.g., "Are these two words, *sing–sink*, same or different?"), 2) segmenting sentences (e.g., "Pick out one block for each word in the sentence, *the dog ran*"), 3) segmenting words (e.g., "Pick out one block for each part in the word, *raincoat*"), and 4) rhyming ("These pictures are: car, fan, radio, TV. The man had a plan to buy a ____"). As with other tests of linguistic skills, children in the Head Start sample were approximately one standard deviation below children in the normative sample in metalinguistic awareness.

### Summary

Each dimension of linguistic development that has been examined in this sample of children from poverty backgrounds has been delayed compared with national norms. The degree of delay has generally been about one standard deviation below the mean of the normative sample, which corresponds to about the 16th percentile, except for measures of syntax, which have been closer to norms for age, or in the case of utterance length, at the norms for age. Significant numbers of children in these samples score more than two standard deviations below the mean on semantic, narrative, and metalinguistic awareness measures, which corresponds to about the 2nd percentile of the population. It is very unlikely that measured delays of this magnitude can be attributed substantially to culturally biased test materials. In that regard, even if one examines measures that generate separate norms for African American children, such as the metalinguistic measures, and compare performance of the African American children in this sample with those norms, there is still more than half a standard deviation of difference.

In interpreting these findings, it should be kept in mind the previous description of this sample as suburban and consisting of relatively well-educated mothers. To the degree that this sample is on the more favorable end of the environmental dimensions of economic poverty, the findings with respect to language skills and language delays are compelling.

## ENVIRONMENTAL EFFECTS ON LANGUAGE SKILLS OF CHILDREN IN POVERTY

The previous review of depressed levels of language skills in children from low-income families implies substantial social effects on language acquisition that might flow from sources such as low levels of language interaction, but it neither proves those effects nor indicates in any specific sense what they might be. It does not prove the effects because evidence suggests that the genetic variance in developing language skills is substantial (Hardy-Brown & Plomin, 1985; Plomin, DeFries, & Fulker, 1988). Any study that examines performance differences that correlate with social class must consider the possibility that some of those differences are genetically mediated. Scarr (1981) described the implications of genetic variation in the development of language and other skills for studies of the effects of social class as follows: "Social class groups . . . are subdivisions of races and represent different distributions of parental genotypes. . . . The genetic differences hypothesis, as it applies to social class groups within races, centers on the issues of assortative mating . . . and selective migration . . . within the social structure" (pp. 185–186). In other words, social class differences in verbal ability may partly reflect genetic differences among social class groups that occur because individuals with similar levels of ability are more likely to mate and because more able individuals will tend to migrate upward in social class. Relatively lower levels of language skill among children of low-income parents may reflect genetic as well as environmental effects associated with social class. Furthermore, environmental effects can be primarily social in nature (e.g., levels or forms of language interactions), or not (e.g., poor nutrition). For this reason as well as the need to understand specific effects of environment on language development, it is critical to go beyond descriptions of differences or deficits in language performance among children reared in poverty to a search for the specific causes of those differences and deficits.

### Effects of Literacy Environments on Language Development

We have focused our work on environmental effects on language development on children's literacy environments. Children's literacy environments vary across social class and may be a significant contributor to both between- and within-class differences in children's language development.

Several studies have demonstrated that children from low-income families are read to less frequently than children from higher socioeconomic groups. Adams (1990) estimated that a typical middle-class child in the United States enters first grade with 1,000–1,700 hours of one-to-one picture-book reading, while the corresponding child from a low-income family averages 25 hours. Ninio (1980) found that low-socioeconomic status mothers in Israel were less likely than middle-class mothers to engage in a number of potentially instructive behaviors during storytime. McCormick and Mason (1986) demonstrated large social class differences in the availability of printed materials in the homes of children in the United States. For example, 47% of parents of preschoolers who were receiving public assistance reported no alphabet books in the home compared with 3% of professional parents. Feitelson and Goldstein

(1986) found that 60% of the kindergartners in neighborhoods in Israel where children did poorly in school did not own a single book; in neighborhoods characterized by good school performance, kindergartners owned an average of 54 books each.

A growing literature finds significant correlations between the frequency of shared picture-book reading in the home and preschool children's language (e.g., Crain-Thoreson & Dale, 1992; Mason, 1980; Mason & Dunning, 1986; Rowe, 1991; Wells, 1985; Wells, Barnes, & Wells, 1984). This suggests that limited opportunities for literacy-related activities in the home may have significant effects on the language development of children from low-income families. The problems that may be associated with children's infrequent exposure to shared picture-book reading in low-income homes are compounded because book-reading interactions are known to attenuate social class differences in the forms of mothers' speech to children (Hoff-Ginsberg, 1991). Thus, children from low-income families, as a group, have infrequent exposure to the one setting for interaction during which maternal speech likely to stimulate language growth is most probable.

Most studies of the relation between social class and shared reading activity in the home have focused on how low-income or working-class families are different from families of higher SES (socioeconomic status) or have simply incorporated a measure of SES into a model of differences in literacy-related activities in the home (e.g., Hoff-Ginsberg, 1991; Ninio, 1980; Raz & Bryant, 1990; Wells, 1985). Adding to these studies is a nascent literature suggesting that there are substantial individual differences in the literacy practices within low-income families that may affect children's language and achievement outcomes. For instance, Teale (1986) found that book reading to children was very unevenly distributed across 22 low-income families in San Diego. Book reading occurred four or five times a week in 3 of the homes, while in the remaining 19 homes it occurred only about five times per year. Ricciuti, White, and Fraser (1993) also found a significant correlation between the home literacy environment and first-grade children's language and reading skills in a low-income sample.

### A Correlational Study of the Literacy Environment on Language Acquisition

My colleagues and I addressed the role of literacy environment in language acquisition in children from low-income families using what we hoped would be a more powerful method than had been used in other investigations. We employed a large *N*, used multiple indices of literacy environment and children's language, and allowed for separation of the effects of literacy environment and parental IQ and education (Payne, Whitehurst, & Angell, 1994). We included 323 four-year-olds attending Head Start and their mothers or primary caregivers. Children's literacy environment was measured using a questionnaire completed by each child's primary caregiver and included the following subscales:

overall frequency of shared picture-book reading, age at onset of picture-book reading, duration of shared picture-book reading during one recent day, number of picture books in the home, frequency of child's requests to engage in shared picture-book reading, frequency of child's private play with books, frequency of shared trips to the library, frequency of caregiver's private reading, and caregiver's enjoyment of private reading.

Using a primary subsample of 236 children, a composite literacy environment score was derived from the literacy environment measures and was correlated with a composite child language measure derived from two standardized tests of language skills, the PPVT–R and the EOWPVT. The canonical correlation between these two sets of measures was 0.43 ($p < .001$), which when squared produces an estimate that the literacy environment accounted for 18.5% of the variance in child language scores. Because canonical correlations capitalize on chance, we cross-validated the results by applying the canonical weights derived from the primary sample to a secondary sample of 87 children who had not been part of the initial analysis. The canonical correlation for the cross-validation sample was 0.42 ($p < .001$), which was virtually identical to the canonical correlation of 0.43 for the primary sample.

Literacy environment in the home may be a marker variable for genetic or other environmental differences among families. For example, homes in which children are exposed to more shared reading might be homes in which educational achievement is valued more or homes in which parents are more genetically advantaged in terms of verbal skills. It could be these other characteristics rather than emergent literacy experience per se that are causal. For that reason, we extended the simple canonical correlation procedure by conducting a forced-entry hierarchical regression in which primary caregiver IQ, measured using the Quick Test (Ammons & Ammons, 1962), and parental education, derived from parental report, were entered together in the first step of a stepwise regression, followed by the canonical literacy environment score. Again the dependent measure was a weighted average of the PPVT–R and the EOWPVT. After entering primary caregiver IQ and education in the first step of a stepwise regression (which together accounted for 11.6% of the variance in child language ability, $p < .001$), the canonical literacy environment score still added significantly to the multiple correlation. The squared increment to the multiple correlation indicated that the literacy environment accounted for 12.0% ($p < .001$) of the variance in canonical test scores after the influence of caregiver IQ and education was removed.

Because variables such as maternal IQ and education have sometimes been offered as explanations of the observed correlations between home literacy variables and child language development (e.g., Scarborough & Dobrich, 1994), it is instructive to reverse the hierarchical procedure described previously. Using the canonical language test score as the dependent variable, the canonical literacy environment score was entered in the first step of a stepwise regression, followed by primary caregiver IQ and education in the second step.

After removing the effect of the canonical literacy environment score, primary caregiver IQ and education produced a squared increment to the multiple correlation of 5.0% ($p < .001$). Thus, in equivalent hierarchical tests, literacy environment accounted for substantially more variance in child language scores than primary caregiver IQ and education combined.

In summary, literacy environment accounts for 18.5% of child language in a simple canonical correlation and 12.0% after the effects of caregiver IQ and education are removed in a hierarchical regression. Caregiver IQ and education are associated with biological factors and environmental factors unrelated to literacy environment. These factors influence children's language skills and should be removed from an estimate of the effects of literacy environment. However, caregiver IQ and education also are likely to be related to the nature of the interactions in which the caregiver engages the child during literacy-related events such as shared book reading. For example, because the measure of caregiver IQ used in this study was based on vocabulary and caregivers with more advanced vocabularies are likely to expose their children to more words during shared book reading, caregiver IQ should have a path of influence to child language that runs directly through literacy environment. Thus, removing all of the influence of caregiver IQ when estimating the effect of literacy environment probably leads to an underestimation of that effect.

## Experimental Studies of the Effects of Environment on Language Development

Correlational studies of environmental variation and language development can advance causal claims to the extent that competing causal variables are included in the design and analysis. However, although they may reduce causal ambiguity, they cannot eliminate it, nor do they typically allow very precise specification of the environment. Thus, in the previous study, literacy environment may have been confounded with third variables other than parental IQ or education that were not controlled statistically. Further gross estimates of variables such as the frequency of book reading in the home tell us little about the process or particulars of shared book reading. For causally unambiguous conclusions and more detailed specification of the environment, we need to turn to experimental methodologies. My colleagues and I conducted four separate experimental interventions in which children from low-income families were randomly assigned to treatment or control conditions, which varied in literacy environment.

The vehicle for intervening with children in each of these studies is a method of reading picture books called *dialogic reading* that we have demonstrated to be effective in increasing the language skills of middle-class children (Arnold, Lonigan, Whitehurst, & Epstein, 1994; Whitehurst et al., 1988). Dialogic reading differs substantially from how adults typically read picture books to children. A shift of roles is central: In typical book reading, the adult reads and the child listens, but in dialogic reading the child learns to become the storyteller. The adult then assumes the role of an active listener, asking questions about pictures in the book, adding information, and prompting the child to increase the sophistication of his or her descriptions. As the child becomes more skillful in the role of storyteller, the adult is encouraged to ask open-ended questions and to avoid yes/no or pointing questions. For example, the adult might say, "What is Eeyore doing?" or "You tell me about this page" instead of "Is Eeyore lying down?" As the child becomes older and cognitively more sophisticated, the open-ended category is expanded to include questions that distance the child from the book (e.g., "If you had your own donkey, what are some things that you and the donkey might do together?") or questions that require recall (e.g., "How does this story end? Can you remember?").

***The Mexican Child Care Study*** Valdez-Menchaca and Whitehurst (1992) conducted an experimental evaluation of the effects of dialogic reading using children attending a Mexican child care center. The families in this study had a mean income of $192 (U.S.) per month. Children were matched by language test scores and then assigned randomly to an experimental or control group. The intervention program consisted of 10-minute one-to-one dialogic reading sessions with each child and a graduate student teacher every weekday for 6 weeks, for a total of approximately 5 hours of intervention per child over the course of the intervention. Children in the control group engaged in a similar schedule of one-to-one activities with the teacher such as building with blocks and doing puzzles.

The effects of the dialogic reading intervention were first assessed through measures of children's spontaneous verbalizations while looking at a book with an unfamiliar female adult who asked specific and open-ended questions during a reading session. The intervention group produced significantly more utterances, longer utterances, and more complex utterances than the control group. It also used more diverse language than the control group and was more likely to provide answers, to initiate topics, and to continue conversations. These effects include the domains of syntax, semantics, and pragmatics and are perhaps the most general and extensive ever to have been demonstrated for a language intervention.

We also used standardized tests to evaluate the impact of dialogic reading. The experimental group was ahead of the control group by 29 language quotient points on the verbal expression subscale of the Illinois Test of Psycholinguistic Ability (Kirk, McCarthy, & Kirk, 1968), which measures the type of verbal fluency that was directly targeted by the intervention, and 7 points ahead on the PPVT–R. Two months after the intervention, the EOWPVT was given. The experimental group was 8 language quotient points ahead on this test. These results are both clinically and statistically significant.

***Low-SES U.S. Child Care Using Teachers and Parents*** Whitehurst, Arnold, et al. (1994) extended the procedures used in the Mexican study to children attending five government-subsidized child care centers in Suffolk County, New York. The children averaged 3.5 years old, but their language skills at pretest were much lower (i.e., their average EOWPVT score was 82 at pretest, which corresponds to 2 years, 8 months of language age). The children were randomly assigned to one of three groups: 1) a school-only group: these children were read to using dialogic reading by their teachers; 2) a combined school plus home group: these children were read to by their teachers and their parents; 3) and a control group: these children engaged in activities such as building with Lincoln Logs and Tinkertoys under the supervision of a teacher. We hypothesized that children who were read to by teachers in child care would show increments in language ability compared with a control group, and that children who were read to by teachers and parents would show even stronger effects, based on a greater frequency of shared reading and a synergistic interaction between shared reading experiences at home and at child care. Because dialogic reading requires frequent opportunities for a child to talk about a book with a responsive adult, teachers were asked to read to the children in small groups of three to four, in contrast to typical practice of reading to a class as a whole. The same small-group ratio was maintained for the activities of the children in the control condition.

Children's language skills were assessed following the 6-week intervention with the three standardized measures of language skill discussed previously in the context of the Mexican study, and with the Our Word, a nonstandardized expressive vocabulary test that we devised. The Our Word was in the same format as the EOWPVT. It consisted of black-and-white photocopies of 36 pictures from the books used in this study that were judged to call for novel vocabulary (e.g., a picture of a telescope). For each picture, the child was asked, "What is this?" or "What is this part of the picture?" The children were retested 6 months later on the same or alternate forms of the standardized tests used at pretest.

The results of this study are presented in Figure 2. There was substantial variability in the fidelity with which teachers followed the reading or activities schedule that was conveyed to them as part of training, as determined by the reading and activity logs that the teachers completed, with one center having extremely low levels of compliance. Consistent with these differences in program implementation, we found significant differences in the effects of the program across the centers. However, even including the least compliant center, significant effects of the reading intervention were obtained at posttest on the EOWPVT and the Our Word. Significant effects were found on the PPVT–R as well if the least compliant center was excluded. At the 6-month follow-up, overall effects of the intervention were found on the EOWPVT, and again effects of the intervention were found for the PPVT–R, excluding the least compliant center. The gains exhibited in the intervention groups were as large as 10 language quotient points. Where significant differences occurred between the

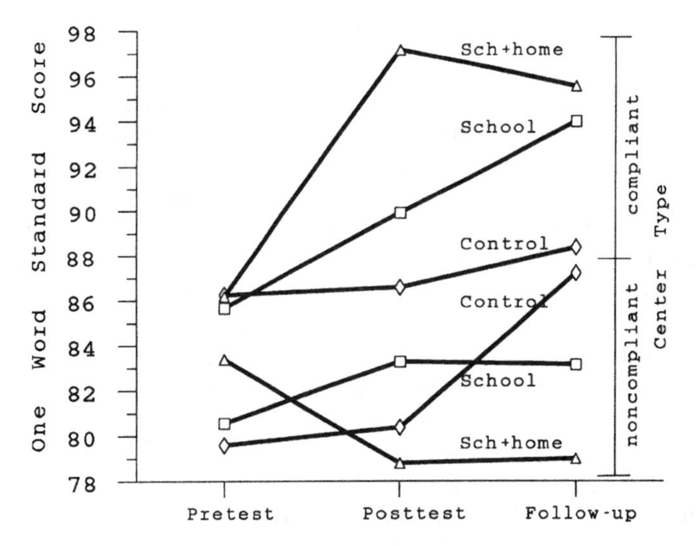


Figure 2. Pretest, posttest, and follow-up scores on the EOWPVT in each experimental condition of the child care intervention study described in the text. Illustrated are statistically significant main effects of experimental condition at posttest and at follow-up and effects for center at posttest. The two reading conditions are significantly different from the control at follow-up but are not significantly different from each other. The noncompliant center was significantly different from the other centers at posttest. It also had the lowest frequency of classroom reading sessions.

two reading interventions, they favored the school plus home group. Specifically, the school plus home group performed significantly better than the school only group on the posttest EOWPVT.

***An Intervention in Head Start Using Parents and Teachers*** The Head Start study differed from the U.S. child care study in that the children were 4 years old rather than 3 years old, the intervention lasted for 7 months rather than 6 weeks, and only two conditions were used, a control condition in which children received the regular Head Start curriculum and the intervention condition. The intervention was a school plus home program that combined about 10 minutes per day of classroom-based dialogic reading with an at-home component similar to that used in the child care study. Teachers in intervention classrooms also used a sound and letter awareness program that introduced children to the alphabetic and phonemic principles of reading. Classrooms of 4-year-olds were randomly assigned to intervention or control conditions. Children in control classrooms received a standard Head Start curriculum. Teachers and primary caregivers of children in intervention classrooms were taught to engage in interactive picture-book reading using training videos. Children were involved in interactive small-group shared picture-book reading several times each week in intervention classrooms over the course of the school year. These same children brought home the book that was being used in the classroom each week for use with their primary caregivers. Children were pretested and posttested on standardized tests of language and emergent literacy ability.

We published a report of the results from the first cohort of children who were involved in this study (Whitehurst, Epstein, et al., 1994). In this chapter, we report results on language measures from children from the second cohort of the study: the 182 children who were judged by their teachers to be very competent speakers of English at pretest. Children with moderate or poor English competence were excluded from the present analyses to allow a focus on environmental effects on the acquisition of a first language. The results from the second cohort of the study are more interesting for the purposes of this chapter than the results from the first cohort because the second cohort was given a more wide-ranging battery of language measures, including measures of syntactic ability.

Figure 3 displays differences between the control and intervention conditions at posttest (at the end of the Head Start year) in three domains of language: metalinguistic, semantic, and syntactic. The dependent variables are *z*-scores on the first unrotated principal component of three a priori groupings of language measures given as posttests. In deriving the first unrotated component in a principal components analysis, each test variable included in the composite measure is weighted to maximize the total variance in test scores that can be accounted for by the composite. In essence, a test that produces scores that are disparate from the scores produced by other tests in the composite will receive a lower weight than a test that is a good team player.

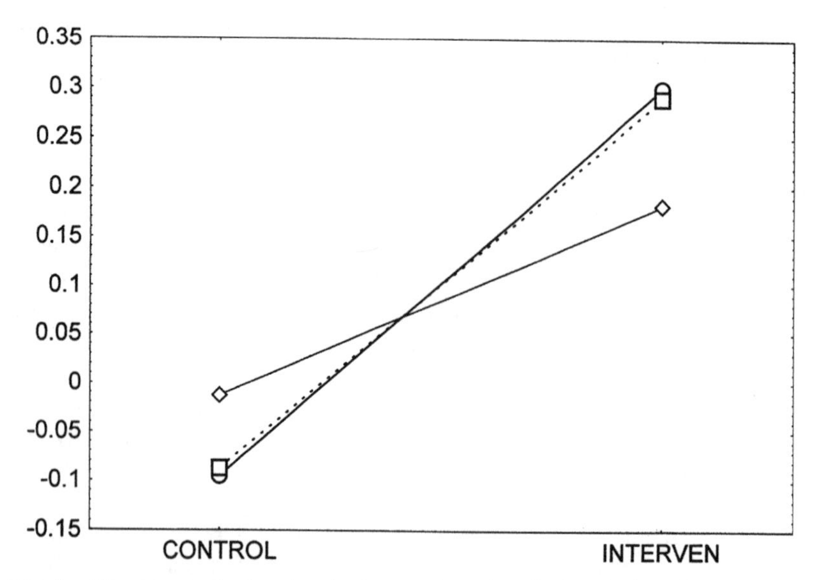


Figure 3. Outcome scores on the dimensions of syntax, semantics, and metalinguistics for the Head Start intervention study described in the text. Effects for semantics and metalinguistics are statistically significant; effects for syntax are not (○=metalinguistic; □=semantic; ◇=syntax).

The three a priori groupings of tests into metalinguistic, semantic, and syntactic composites were done on the basis of the stated target ability of the test instrument. The metalinguistic domain consisted of the first principal component of the letters, sound–letter, segmenting sentences, and segmenting words subtests of the Developing Skills Checklist. The semantic domain consisted of the first principal component of the EOWPVT, PPVT–R, information subtest score from the BUS, and basic concepts subtest score from the CELF–P. The syntactic domain consisted of the first principal component of the word structure subtest score from the CELF–P, the length subtest score from the BUS, and the complex utterance subtest score from the BUS.

The differences depicted in Figure 3 were investigated using an analysis of covariance in which each child's pretest scores on the PPVT–R and the CELF–P basic concepts subtest were covariants. Covariants were used to control for any differences between children in the two conditions of the study at pretest that occurred despite random assignment and to increase the precision of the analysis. The differences between the intervention and control conditions in the metalinguistic and semantic domains were each statistically significant ($ps < .025$), while the difference on the syntactic dimension was not significant ($p = .47$).

These results indicate that between 4 and 5 years of age, the semantic and metalinguistic skills of children from low-income backgrounds are still malleable as a result of relatively small changes in their environments (the school-based components of this intervention involved no more than 36 hours in total for any child). In contrast, and in keeping with the previous speculation, syntatic skills did not prove to be appreciably malleable.

### Structural Equation Modeling of Influences on Domains of Language Development

The research reviewed to this point has demonstrated that preschoolers from low-income families have depressed levels of semantic, narrative, and metalinguistic skills and that levels of performance in these domains can be affected by adult–child interaction with books. The domain of syntax was seen to be less affected by an environment of poverty than other language domains and less affected by interventions focused on interactive book reading. I believe these data are important and present significant theoretical challenges. One of those challenges is to understand what influences syntactic development and to understand if, when, and how individual differences in syntactic development, which seem to be relatively modular, affect development in other domains of language, such as semantics.

The data presented previously provide only a partial picture of social-environmental effects on language development, which surely involves more than the effects of literacy practices in school and home. Ultimately, progress in this field will depend on the development of causal models of social-environmental, nonsocial-environmental, and biological variables that affect the various domains of language in the child. These models should be consistent with data from large samples of children. At a mature stage in their development, these models should also account for proportions of variance in the language domains they address that approach the reliability coefficients of the assessment instruments that constitute the dependent variables. This would mean, at the very least, that we could predict with high accuracy individual differences in language development in children. Depending on how the predictor variables were constituted, it could also mean that we would have achieved considerable understanding of the processes of language development. As an example of the distinction between prediction and understanding in causal models, consider a model of language outcomes at 5 years of age that is based on predictors that are parallel measures of language outcomes collected at 2, 3, and 4 years of age. One might achieve high predictability in such a model because language skills at one age are strongly correlated with language skills at another age, without having identified any of the variables responsible for language development. A model that achieves its predictability from measures of variables other than the child's own language at earlier points in time would be more likely to involve processes that are explanatory.

Figure 4 includes diagrams of a structural equation model of language outcomes at age 5 for children in Head Start. The dependent variables in the model are the same three composites of metalinguistics, syntax, and semantics described in the intervention study in Head Start. These composites were derived from principal components analyses in the same manner stipulated for the analysis of the Head Start intervention. I use factors formed outside of the structural model rather than generating them as latent variables within the model because when working with correlated domains (e.g., semantic skills and metalinguistic skills) and when working with many correlated indicators within and across those domains (e.g., PPVT and BUS scores) a latent variable approach within the model typically generates a path of influence that is disorderly and uninterpretable. This is often not the case if sensible variable compositing is done outside of and before the structural equation model.

The $N = 137$ in Figure 4 includes all the children on whom data were reported in the previous section for whom there were complete data on all predictor and outcome variables. As in the intervention data, all children included in the analysis were reported by teachers to have no problems with English at the time they were pretested; that is, they were either native speakers of English or fluent speakers of English as a second language.

The structural model in Figure 4 includes five predictor variables: 1) siblings (the number of children in the child's family), 2) maternal IQ (the primary caregiver's IQ from the Quick Test), 3) classroom quality (the total score from the Early Childhood Environment Rating Scale [Harms & Clifford, 1980]),

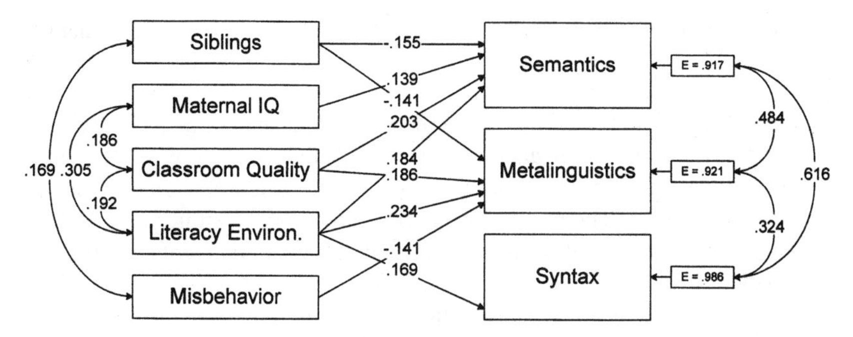


Figure 4. Structural equation model of process predictors of syntax, semantics, and metalinguistic outcomes at age 5 for 137 children attending Head Start. All paths are significant at $p<.05$ ($X^2_{(12)}=9.84$; $p=.63$; normed fit index=.95; comparative fit index=1.00)

4) literacy environment (the principal component factor score of questions related to home literacy practices from a questionnaire given to primary caregivers; see Payne et al., 1994), and 5) misbehavior (the sum of the asocial and hyperactivity scores on the *Conner's Rating Scales* [Conners, 1985]). Predictor variables that were considered but eliminated because they did not contribute independently to outcomes included primary caregiver's education, ratings by Head Start personnel of parental participation in Head Start, whether the primary caregiver's native language was English, and the primary caregiver's expectations for the Head Start child's grades in high school.

Consistent with the typical rules for graphic representation of structural equation models, and the particular rules for the EQS modeling software that was used here (Bentler, 1992), observed variables that have been entered explicitly into the model (as all were here) rather than being derived as latent variables by the model (as none were here) are represented in rectangles. Variables with lines having one-way arrows pointed to them are dependent variables in the model, while variables that are the sources of lines with arrows and have no arrows leading into them are independent variables. Lines with two-way arrows connecting variables represent covariance between variables, that is, correlation between variables that is not modeled as a causal influence. E terms in the model represent the residual variance in dependent variables that is not accounted for by the model. The numbers associated with each path (line) in the model are the beta weights that are generated for the data submitted to the model for that path of influence. Negative numbers represent negative correlations, while positive numbers represent positive correlations. The beta weights represent the independent influence of one variable on another, that is, variance accounted for once the influence of other independent variables has been removed. The test statistics include chi-square, which ideally should be nonsignificant, indicating that the tested model is not significantly different from the structure of the data to which it has been applied. Bentler's comparative fit index (CFI), also presented in the figure, adjusts for the biasing influence of sample size, as chi-square does not. It is the test statistic of choice and is generally viewed as representing adequate fit of a model to the data when it exceeds .90.

Figure 4 indicates a fit between the model and the data that is as high as one can obtain using the CFI, 1.00, and a nonsignificant chi-square. The variables that predict semantic and metalinguistic outcomes overlap substantially, with both sharing influence from number of siblings, classroom quality, and literacy environment. The difference between the paths of influence into these variables is that maternal IQ contributes only to semantic outcome while misbehavior contributes only to metalinguistic outcome. I believe these differences make sense under the assumption that metalinguistic skills such as understanding letter–sound correspondence are primarily a function of teaching activities in the classroom, while semantic skills are also a function of home activities. Thus, misbehavior, which is derived from teacher ratings, reflects children's inability to attend in instructional settings and should negatively affect metalinguistic skills that are imparted primarily in such settings. Semantic abilities, being in part a product of interactions with mother at home, are more likely to be influenced by maternal IQ, which is reflected in maternal verbal ability.

Consistent with previous discussions, the syntactic outcome has far fewer paths of influence into it, with only the literacy environment being significant in the present data. That influence is itself quite weak, with roughly only 3% of the variance in syntactic abilities accounted for by the model, contrasted with 15% for metalinguistic abilities and 16% for semantic abilities. This is not due to syntactic ability showing less variability among children than semantic or metalinguistic ability. The metalinguistic and syntactic outcomes have roughly the same variance, and both show more variance than the semantic outcome. For instance, on the measure of MLU on the BUS, which is obtained by taking the five longest utterances and dividing by five, the range MLUs across children is from 3 to 15, with a mean slightly above 8. Translating these raw scores to standard scores on an IQ scale generates a mean for the sample of 102 and a standard deviation of 15.8 (see Table 1). This degree of variation is not necessarily what one might expect from a nativistic theory. To the extent that the core of the language acquisition device is syntactic, one might expect much less variation across children on that dimension than on more environmentally loaded dimensions such as semantics and metalinguistics. One could have a nativistic theory consistent with large individual variation in syntactic skills by positing that the variation is genetic. A substantial portion of the unexplained variance in syntactic ability in Figure 4 may be genetically determined, a hypothesis that would have to be pursued with twin or consanguinity studies. However, the dominant psycholinguistic tradition that originated with Chomsky (1957) and that flows through Pinker (1994) has posited a common language acquisition device that is shared by all biologically typical children, and this position is incompatible with large genetic variation in the syntactic core.

I believe this is one of the major theoretical issues for developmental psycholinguistics that emerges from this chapter: Children vary substantially in syntactic abilities in the late preschool period. We have virtually no understanding of the genesis of those individual differences.

The structural model in Figure 4 has many limitations. Among them are that the *N* of 137 is marginal for this statistical approach, particularly because the model was bootstrapped rather than generated a priori. This means that a different sample might produce somewhat different results. There also may be artifacts in the data that belie the causal interpretation that one might be tempted to apply to the unidirectional arrows. The most likely artifact concerns the covariation among maternal IQ, classroom quality, and literacy environment. One reason for that covariation in this sample is that Head Start centers in better neighborhoods enroll higher-functioning children from more advantaged homes. Because more advantaged neighborhoods tend to have Head Start centers established at later points in time than neighborhoods with higher concentrations of families in poverty, facilities are newer and teachers are younger, have more formal education, and may find higher-functioning children more motivating to teach. This generates higher classroom quality scores. Thus, what looks like a causal link between classroom quality and semantic and metalinguistic skills in Figure 4 may be due in part to a confounding between children's skills and classroom quality at entry into Head Start.

The point of Figure 4 is not to defend a particular model of language outcomes in the late preschool period for children reared in poverty. It is to demonstrate that structural modeling of language outcomes is possible and that such exercises point both to clear causes of individual differences in language development and large gaps in our knowledge. It is relatively easy to build appealing theories of language acquisition based on observations of commonalities in behavior across selected children in selected situations. It is quite another matter to build theories and models that are sufficiently complete to account for substantial natural variation in language skills. I believe that formal attempts to account for variability in children's linguistic abilities should be the crucible in which any serious theory on language development is eventually tested.

## CONCLUSION

Children from low-income backgrounds develop language that is different in kind and degree from children in the general population. These differences were documented with tests of semantics, metalinguistics, narrative, and syntactics for a large sample of preschoolers in low-income child care or Head Start who have been involved in various research projects I have conducted since the 1980s. On all except measures of syntax, children in this research have averaged about one standard deviation below the mean of the general population of children their age.

Because discussion of language in children from low-income backgrounds has historically been embedded in the differences versus deficits debate, I reviewed some of its history and suggested that we need to distinguish between comparative differences, competitive deficits, and absolute deficits. Although many of the characteristics of the language of children reared in poverty might be described as no more than competitive deficits, the very low levels of basic semantic knowledge among some children, for example, not knowing the names for basic colors or body parts at age 4, might represent absolute deficits that would prevent these children from succeeding in any of the cultural settings available to them.

Moving from descriptive studies to correlational studies, and from broad characterizations of the environment to a focus on the literacy environment, I reported research showing that from 12% to 18% of the variance in semantic abilities among my low-income sample at 5 years of age could be attributed to literacy practices in their homes such as the availability of books, frequency of shared book reading, and trips to the library. Given that the measure of literacy environment was a parental questionnaire rather than a more direct measure, with the large degree of expected error in such a self-report instrument, and given that the dependent variables were standardized tests of language rather than more naturalistic samples of language, this represents a very large and significant environmental effect. One implication of this finding for theory in mainstream developmental psycholinguistics is that more attention is needed for differences in frequency and form of parent–child interaction as influences on language development.

Because correlational studies are always causally ambiguous and usually operate at a relatively abstract level in terms of environmental variables, I pursued the effects of literacy environment on the language development with experimental studies in which specific aspects of parent–child or teacher–child interaction around books was altered. Studies presented in this chapter focused on children from low-income backgrounds and demonstrated statistically and clinically significant effects on semantic and metalinguistic skills as a result of relatively minimal increases in the frequency of interactive book reading. Other research not presented here has demonstrated that it is primarily the interactive form of this book reading, rather than more frequent exposure to books per se, that is responsible for these gains in language skills (Arnold et al., 1994; Whitehurst et al., 1988). The implication of these findings for theories of typical language acquisition is that individual differences in children's rate of acquisition of language skills are strongly affected by variables in the areas of practice, feedback, and motivation that have often been written off by linguistic theorists (cf. Bohannon, MacWhinney, & Snow, 1990; Moerk, 1992; Pinker, 1994).

Work on literacy environment touches on only one of the many environmental influences on language development. Eventually researchers and theorists should move toward models that incorporate all major paths of influence on language development. In that spirit, I presented a preliminary structural equation model of semantic, metalinguistic, and syntactic skills at age 5. Significant sources of influence for individual differences included maternal IQ, literacy practices in the home, classroom quality, number of siblings in the home, and degree of misbehavior/inattention. The sources of influence accounted for about 15% of the variability in children's scores for semantic and metalinguistic skills, but only about 3% for syntactic skills. Causal models in other areas of development such as delinquency (Patterson, 1986) or early reading achievement (Wagner & Torgesen, 1987) routinely account for 30%–40% or more of variance in outcomes. Theorists and researchers of language acquisition have not tended to assess large samples of children or have an individual differences perspective. We have a long way to go to approach the level of prediction and understanding that exists for some other domains in the social-cognitive sciences. We are not likely to get there if we continue to avoid formal model building.

## REFERENCES


Adams, M.J. (1990). *Learning to read: Thinking and learning about print.* Cambridge, MA: MIT Press.

Ammons, R.B., & Ammons, C.H. (1962). *The Quick Test.* San Antonio, TX: Psychological Test Specialists.

Arnold, D.S., Lonigan, C.J., Whitehurst, G.J., & Epstein, J.N. (1994). Accelerating language development through picture book reading: Replication and extension to a videotape training format. *Journal of Educational Psychology, 84*, 235–243.

Austin, J.L. (1962). *How to do things with words.* Oxford, England: Oxford University Press.

Bates, E., Bretherton, I., Beeghly-Smith, M., & McNew, S. (1982). Social basis of language development: A reassessment. In H.W. Reese (Ed.), *Advances in child development and behavior* (Vol. 14, pp. 7–75). New York: Academic Press.

Bellugi, U., Marks, S., Bihrle, A., & Sabo, H. (1988). Dissociation between language and cognitive functions in Williams syndrome. In D.V.M. Bishop & K. Mogford (Eds.), *Language development in exceptional circumstances* (pp. 177–189). Edinburgh, Scotland: Churchill Livingstone.

Bentler, P.M. (1992). *EQS: Structural equations program manual.* Los Angeles: BMDP Statistical Software.

Bernstein, B. (1971). *Class, codes, and control: Vol. 1. Theoretical studies towards a sociology of language.* London: Routledge & Kegan Paul.

Bishop, D.V.M. (1992). The underlying nature of specific language impairment. *Journal of Child Psychology and Psychiatry, 33*, 3–66.

Bloom, L. (1993). *The transition from infancy to language: Acquiring the power of expression.* Cambridge, England: Cambridge University Press.

Bohannon, J.N., MacWhinney, B., & Snow, C. (1990). No negative evidence revisited: Beyond learnability or who has to prove what to whom. *Developmental Psychology, 26*, 221–226.

Bradley, L., & Bryant, P.E. (1983). Categorizing sounds and learning to read—a causal connection. *Nature, 301*, 419–421.

Brown, R. (1973). *A first language: The early stages.* Cambridge, MA: Harvard University Press.
Brown, R., & Herrnstein, R.J. (1975). *Psychology.* Boston: Little, Brown.
Byrne, B., & Fielding-Barnsley, R.F. (1991). Evaluation of a program to teach phonemic awareness to young children. *Journal of Educational Psychology, 82*, 805–812.
Byrne, B., & Fielding-Barnsley, R.F. (1993). Evaluation of a program to teach phonemic awareness to young children: A one year follow-up. *Journal of Educational Psychology, 85*, 104–111.
Chomsky, N. (1957). *Syntactic structures.* The Hague, The Netherlands: Mouton.
Clark, H.H., & Clark, E.V. (1977). *Psychology and language.* New York: Harcourt Brace Jovanovich.
Conners, C.K. (1985). *The Conners Rating Scales: Instruments for the assessment of childhood psychopathology.* Unpublished manuscript, Children's Hospital National Medical Center, Washington, DC.
Cowley, J., & Glasgow, C. (1994). *The Renfrew bus story—American edition.* Centreville, DE: The Centreville School.
Crain-Thoreson, C., & Dale, P.S. (1992). Do early talkers become early readers? Linguistic precocity, preschool language, and emergent literacy. *Developmental Psychology, 28*, 421–429.
CTB. (1990). *Developing skills checklist.* New York: McGraw-Hill.
Curtiss, S. (1977). *Genie: A psycholinguistic study of a modern-day "wild child."* New York: Academic Press.
Dunn, L.M., & Dunn, L.M. (1981a). *Peabody Picture Vocabulary Test–Revised.* Circle Pines, MN: American Guidance Service.
Dunn, L.M., & Dunn, L.M. (1981b). *Peabody Picture Vocabulary Test–Revised. Manual for Forms L and M.* Circle Pines, MN: American Guidance Service.
Feagans, L. (1982). The development and importance of narratives for school adaptation. In L. Feagans & D.C. Farran (Eds.), *The language of children reared in poverty: Implications for evaluation and intervention* (pp. 95–116). New York: Academic Press.
Feitelson, D., & Goldstein, Z. (1986). Patterns of book ownership and reading to young children in Israeli school-oriented and nonschool-oriented families. *Reading Teacher, 39*, 924–930.
Fodor, J. (1983). *The modularity of mind.* Cambridge, MA: MIT Press.
Gardner, M.F. (1981). *Expressive One-Word Picture Vocabulary Test.* Novato, CA: Academic Therapy Publications.
Gardner, M.F. (1990). *Expressive One-Word Picture Vocabulary Test–Revised.* Novato, CA: Academic Therapy Publications.
Gathercole, S.E., & Baddeley, A.D. (1990). Phonological memory deficits in language disordered children: Is there a causal connection? *Journal of Memory and Language, 29*, 336–360.
Hardy-Brown, K., & Plomin, R. (1985). Infant communicative development: Evidence from adoptive and biological families for genetic and environmental influences on rate differences. *Developmental Psychology, 21*, 378–385.
Harms, T., & Clifford, R.M. (1980). *Early Childhood Environment Rating Scale.* New York: Teachers College Press.
Heath, S.B. (1983). *Ways with words.* Cambridge, England: Cambridge University Press.
Heath, S.B. (1989). Oral and literate traditions among black Americans living in poverty. *American Psychologist, 44*, 367–373.
Hoff-Ginsberg, E. (1991). Mother–child conversation in different social classes and communicative settings. *Child Development, 61*, 782–796.

Hunt, J.M., Kirk, G.E., & Lieberman, C. (1975). Social class and preschool language skill: IV. Semantic mastery of shapes. *Genetic Psychology Monographs, 91*, 115–129.

Hunt, J.M., Kirk, G.E., & Volkmar, F. (1975). Social class and preschool language skill: III. Semantic mastery of position information. *Genetic Psychology Monographs, 91*, 317–337.

Kirk, G.E., Hunt, J.M., & Lieberman, C. (1975). Social class and preschool language skill: II. Semantic mastery of color information. *Genetic Psychology Monographs, 91*, 299–316.

Kirk, G.E., Hunt, J.M., & Volkmar, F. (1975). Social class and preschool language skill: V. Cognitive and semantic mastery of number. *Genetic Psychology Monographs, 91*, 131–153.

Kirk, S.A., McCarthy, J.J., & Kirk, W.D. (1968). *Illinois Test of Psycholinguistic Abilities.* Urbana: University of Illinois Press.

Labov, W. (1972). *Sociolinguistic patterns.* Philadelphia: University of Pennsylvania Press.

Lundberg, I., Frost, J., & Petersen, O. (1988). Effects of an extensive program for stimulating phonological awareness in preschool children. *Reading Research Quarterly, 23*, 263–284.

MacWhinney, B. (1993). Connections and symbols: Closing the gap. *Cognition, 49*, 291–296.

Malakoff, M.E., Mayes, L.C., & Schottenfeld, R.S. (1994). Language abilities of preschool-age children living with cocaine-using mothers. *American Journal on Addictions, 3*, 346–354.

Mann, V.A. (1993). Phoneme awareness and future reading ability. *Journal of Learning Disabilities, 26*, 259–269.

Mason, J.M. (1980). When children do begin to read: An exploration of four year old children's letter and word reading competencies. *Reading Research Quarterly, 15*, 203–227.

Mason, J.M., & Dunning, D. (1986, April). *Toward a model relating home literacy with beginning reading.* Paper presented at the American Educational Research Association, San Francisco.

McCormick, C.E., & Mason, J.M. (1986). Intervention procedures for increasing preschool children's interest in and knowledge about reading. In W.H. Teale & E. Sulzby (Eds.), *Emergent literacy: Writing and reading* (pp. 90–115). Norwood, NJ: Ablex.

Moerk, E.L. (1992). *A first language taught and learned.* Baltimore: Paul H. Brookes Publishing Co.

Ninio, A. (1980). Picture-book reading in mother–infant dyads belonging to two subgroups in Israel. *Child Development, 51*, 587–590.

Olson, D.R., & Hildyard, A. (1981). Assent and compliance in children's language. In W.P. Dickson (Ed.), *Children's oral communication skills* (pp. 313–336). New York: Academic Press.

Patterson, G.R. (1986). Performance models for antisocial boys. *American Psychologist, 41*, 432–444.

Payne, A.C., Whitehurst, G.J., & Angell, A. (1994). The role of home literacy environment in the development of language ability in preschool children from low-income families. *Early Childhood Research Quarterly, 9*, 427–440.

Pinker, S. (1984). *Language learnability and language development.* Cambridge, MA: Harvard University Press.

Pinker, S. (1994). *The language instinct.* New York: William Morrow.

Plomin, R., DeFries, J.C., & Fulker, D.W. (1988). *Nature and nurture during infancy and early childhood.* Cambridge, England: Cambridge University Press.

Raz, I.S., & Bryant, P. (1990). Social background, phonological awareness and children's reading. *British Journal of Developmental Psychology, 8*, 209–225.

Ricciuti, H.N., White, A.M., & Fraser, S.M. (1993). Maternal and family predictors of school readiness and achievement in black, Hispanic, and white 6- and 7-year-olds. *Society for Research in Child Development Abstracts, 9*, 567.

Rowe, K.J. (1991). The influence of reading activity at home on students' attitudes towards reading, classroom attentiveness and reading achievement: An application of structural equation modelling. *British Journal of Educational Psychology, 61*, 19–35.

Ruder, K., & Smith, M. (1984). *Developmental language intervention: Psycholinguistic applications.* Baltimore: University Park Press.

Rymer, R. (1994). *Genie: A scientific tragedy.* New York: HarperPerennial.

Scarborough, H.S, & Dobrich, W. (1994). On the efficacy of reading to preschoolers. *Developmental Review, 14*, 245–302.

Scarr, S. (1981). *Race, social class, and individual differences in I.Q.* Hillsdale, NJ: Lawrence Erlbaum Associates.

Schiff-Myers, N. (1988). Hearing children of deaf parents. In D. Bishop & K. Mogford (Eds.), *Language development in exceptional circumstances* (pp. 47–61). Edinburgh, Scotland: Churchill Livingstone.

Searle, J.R. (1969). *Speech acts.* Cambridge, England: Cambridge University Press.

Stanovich, K.E., & Siegel, L.S. (1994). Phenotypic performance profile of children with reading disabilities: A regression-based test of phonological-core variable-difference model. *Journal of Educational Psychology, 86*, 24–53.

Teale, W.H. (1986). Home background and young children's literacy development. In W.H. Teale & E. Sulzby (Eds.), *Emergent literacy: Writing and reading* (pp. 110–121). Norwood, NJ: Ablex.

Valdez-Menchaca, M.C., & Whitehurst, G.J. (1992). Accelerating language development through picture book reading: A systematic extension to Mexican day-care. *Developmental Psychology, 28*, 1106–1114.

Wagner, R.K., & Torgesen, J.K. (1987). The nature of phonological processing and its causal role in the acquisition of reading skills. *Psychological Bulletin, 101*, 192–212.

Watkins, R.V., & Rice, M.L. (Eds.). (1994). *Communication and language intervention series: Vol. 4. Specific language impairments in children.* Baltimore: Paul H. Brookes Publishing Co.

Wechsler, D. (1974). *Wechsler Intelligence Scale for Children–Revised.* New York: The Psychological Corporation.

Wells, G. (1985). *Language development in the preschool years.* Cambridge, England: Cambridge University Press.

Wells, G., Barnes, S., & Wells, J. (1984). *Linguistic influences on educational attainment.* Bristol, England: University of Bristol, Department of Education and Science.

Whitehurst, G.J., Arnold, D.H., Epstein, J.N., Angell, A.L., Smith, M., & Fischel, J.E. (1994). A picture book reading intervention in daycare and home for children from low-income families. *Developmental Psychology, 30*, 679–689.

Whitehurst, G.J., & DeBaryshe, B.D. (1989). Observational learning and language acquisition. In G.E. Speidel & K.E. Nelson (Eds.), *The many faces of imitation in language learning* (pp. 251–276). New York: Springer-Verlag.

Whitehurst, G.J., Epstein, J.N., Angell, A., Payne, A.C., Crone, D., & Fischel, J.E. (1994). Outcomes of an emergent literacy intervention in Head Start. *Journal of Educational Psychology, 84*, 541–556.

Whitehurst, G.J., Falco, F.L., Lonigan, C., Fischel, J.E., DeBaryshe, B.D., Valdez-Menchaca, M.C., & Caufield, M. (1988). Accelerating language development through picture book reading. *Developmental Psychology, 24*, 552–558.

Whitehurst, G.J., & Fischel, J.E. (1994). Early developmental language delay: What, if anything, should the clinician do about it? *Journal of Child Psychology and Psychiatry, 35*, 613–648.

Whitehurst, G.J., Fischel, J.E., Lonigan, C.J., Valdez-Menchaca, M.C., Arnold, D.S., & Smith, M. (1991). Treatment of expressive language delay: If, when and how. *Topics in Language Disorders, 11*, 55–68.

Wigg, E.H., Secord, W., & Semel, E. (1992). *Clinical Evaluation of Language Fundamentals—Preschool.* San Antonio, TX: The Psychological Corporation.

Zigler, E., Abelson, W.D., & Seitz, V. (1973). Motivational factors in the performance of economically disadvantaged children on the Peabody Picture Vocabulary Test. *Child Development, 44*, 294–303.

# 11

# The Facilitative Effects of Input on Children's Language Development

## Contributions from Studies of Enhanced Milieu Teaching

Ann P. Kaiser,
Mary Louise Hemmeter, and Peggy P. Hester

The disciplines of child development, speech-language pathology, and special education share an interest in the development of children's social-communication skills. Differences in the primary paradigms of inquiry used within these disciplines and each discipline's relative emphasis on development versus intervention have contributed to a pattern of isolated discipline-based knowledge that is frequent among related human science disciplines (Gottleib, 1991; Kaiser & Warren, 1988). Fragmentation of knowledge along disciplinary lines occurs for a variety of reasons, including differences in the primary training of professionals as well as specialization of theory, research methodology, and practice. In addition, specific characteristics or histories of individual disciplines may further increase the barriers to shared knowledge.

Research on early language intervention can be examined for the barriers to shared knowledge and the potential contributions of an applied science to theories of child language and social communication development. Both language intervention and developmental child language research have long traditions of empirical study (Bricker, 1993). Both are concerned with describing the behavior of children using observational methods and analytical models

Research reported in this chapter was supported by grants from the National Institute of Child Health and Human Development (#HD27583 and #HD15051) and the Office of Special Education Programs (#H023C10031).

that focus on the development of linguistic and social pragmatic aspects of language. Furthermore, much intervention research has been influenced by findings in the area of child language (Kaiser & Warren, 1988) and by the methods of description developed by child language researchers (MacWhinney, 1991; Miller & Chapman, 1983). The barrier between these two disciplines should be extremely permeable because of shared interests and methods. In fact, there has been a regular transfer of knowledge in one direction: The findings from developmental child language research, which have changed in emphasis from syntax to semantics to pragmatics, have consistently influenced the methods, content, and developmental perspectives of language intervention research.

This chapter begins with an overview of the existing barriers between language intervention and developmental child language research. An alternative approach for the mutual sharing of knowledge between the disciplines is proposed. Next, we describe research on a specific early language intervention, EMT (enhanced milieu teaching), as an example of how intervention research might contribute to the understanding of language development. We describe the theoretical basis of EMT, noting the blending of developmental and behavioral theories at the base of this intervention model. We describe the intervention model and the results of its application in two studies involving children in the early stages of language learning. Finally, we return to the proposed paradigm for integrating knowledge from intervention research and developmental research into theories of child language development.

## BARRIERS TO SHARED KNOWLEDGE

Since systematic research on early language intervention began in the 1970s, intervention researchers have articulated a theoretical base that shared many tenets with child language development (Bricker & Bricker, 1974). The notable influence of behaviorism on early language intervention (e.g., Guess, Sailor, & Baer, 1976) was not echoed in the typical developmental literature, however. After a relatively brief period of intense debate about the mechanisms of language learning in the late 1950s and 1960s (Chomsky, 1959; Premack, 1970; Skinner, 1957), the field of child language moved away from behavioristic models of development and began a period of study marked primarily by interests in the cognitive mechanism underlying development and descriptions of the syntactic and semantic development of young children (Cromer, 1988). Although researchers and practitioners in language intervention continued to be influenced by findings in the child language literature, the influence between the disciplines became largely unidirectional: Information from the study of child language in a developmental perspective flowed into applications in early language intervention, but the reverse did not occur.

There were several reasons for the unidirectional pattern of influence between developmental and intervention research. The first reason concerns the characteristics of behavioral theory and its manifestations in applied behavior analysis. Applied behavior analysis emphasizes the functional relationship between behavior and its antecedents and consequences (Baer, Wolf, & Risley, 1968). Although behaviorism is not atheoretical (Morris, 1992), its emphasis on function rather than structure of human behavior sets it apart from many other theories of child development and human behavior. This difference was greatly magnified by applied behavior analysts working within a strictly functional paradigm to study the effects of interventions on language learning and performance. Second, the evolution and practice of single-subject designs consistent with the applied behavioral framework (Baer et al., 1968; Tawney & Gast, 1984) further differentiated the paradigm of inquiry from the mainstream of developmental psychology and child language. Although intervention researchers embraced single-subject research methodology because it allowed a focus on individual differences in response to intervention, developmental researchers continued to use case studies and descriptive and comparative group designs to track the natural course of development. In addition, because language intervention researchers were primarily concerned with children who experienced difficulties in learning language, the children with mental retardation and language delays whom these researchers studied further differentiated them from the mainstream of developmental psychology and child language research. In sum, as a natural evolution of application in science, early language intervention research became associated with a behavioral, and presumably atheoretical, approach to language as behavior, single-subject methodology, and atypical populations.

Many researchers in early language intervention continued to be influenced by the emergent theory and findings in the literature on child language development. Thus, theoretical basis of language intervention did not remain extricably linked to behaviorism. Use of group designs to evaluate treatment outcomes became more common in intervention research as interventions were developed, larger populations of children were identified, and comparisons of treatment became more relevant to understanding the efficacy of early intervention (e.g., Yoder, Kaiser, & Alpert, 1991). Developmental child language research concurrently became more focused on dyadic interaction as a condition of typical language development (Goldberg, 1977a; Moerk, 1972; Ratner & Bruner, 1978). The focus on social interaction, partner input variables, and a more comprehensive explanatory model of development appeared to offer an opportunity for the convergence of theoretical interests between applied intervention research and developmental perspectives. Citation of developmental literature in support of naturalistic and socially based intervention strategies is common as intervention researchers bridge theory and practice in early language intervention (Kaiser & Warren, 1988; Snyder-McLean & McLean, 1978). Even with these developments, the transfer of knowledge has remained largely unidirectional.

Research on intervention continues to be published largely in journals addressing atypical populations, intervention, and therapy, while publication of research on child language development occurs in journals primarily addressing typical development. Although there has been crossover between journals, most crossover articles report comparative studies contrasting typical and atypical development rather than the effects of interventions. In general, separation by population is consistent with the separation of mental retardation research from typical child development research and with the separation of educationally oriented studies from their developmental, sociological, and ethological counterparts.

## RETHINKING THE RELATION BETWEEN THEORY AND PRACTICE

Implicit in this pattern of separated disciplines is an assumption that there is a hierarchy of knowledge. In this hierarchy, basic science is valued most highly and viewed as the root discipline for more applied areas of research and practice (MacMillan & Schumacher, 1984). The findings of basic science are viewed as more generalizable than those of applied science, and theory derived or tested in conjunction with basic science is viewed as more comprehensive and more broadly descriptive than theory derived from research that is intervention oriented, occurs in applied contexts, or includes individuals who are deviant from typical individuals. Thus, although the study of typical child language frequently relies on the same methods as intervention research, the focus on typical children and on theory-driven research questions is presumed to place developmental research relatively low in the hierarchy of knowledge.

An alternative and potentially more useful view of the relationship between applied and basic research and, in this instance, between theoretically driven developmental research and the findings of applied studies of early language intervention, might encompass a circular or cybernetic view of research and theory. Figure 1 provides a contrast between a hierarchical arrangement of empirical knowledge with information and theory flowing in only one direction (with Jacob's ladder as a metaphor for this arrangement; Shepherd, 1993) and a cybernetic model where both theory and specific information may flow in either direction and all types of inquiry are influenced by valid empirical knowledge from related inquiry (Sarah's circle is an apt metaphor for this arrangement; Shepherd, 1993). These contrasting views of the pathways for sharing knowledge are consistent with emergent feminist models of inquiry (Noddings, 1984; Shepherd, 1993) and with more qualitative and interpretivist methods (Bogdan & Biklen, 1992; Denzin & Lincoln, 1994).

The responsibility for bidirectional sharing of knowledge resides with both disciplines. Researchers in early language intervention have not presented their findings as informing the development of theory or as having relevance to

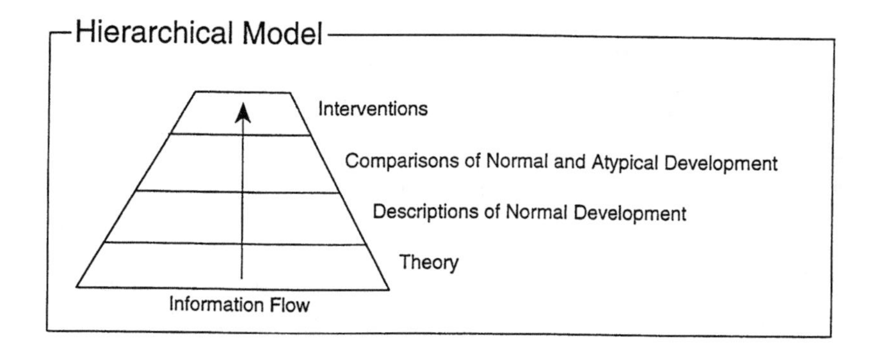


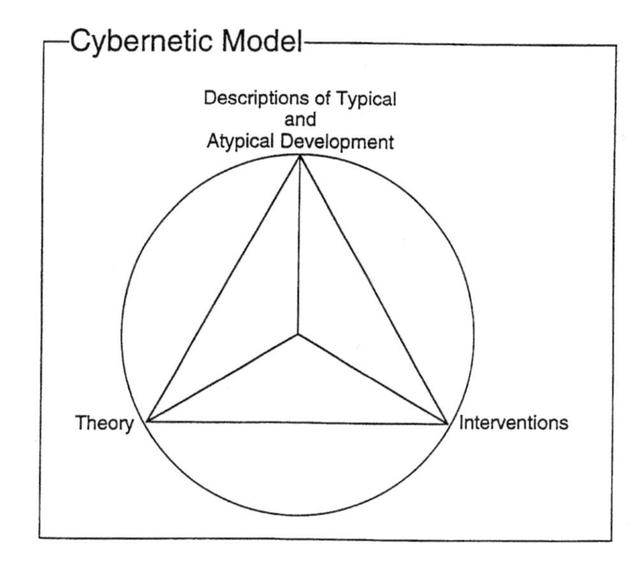


Figure 1. Hierarchical and cybernetic models of information flow across research domains.

our understanding of typical development. Many intervention researchers, although well trained in the scientific method, are uncomfortable in discussing theory because it is not an integral part of their disciplinary training or the practice of their discipline. This book is an important step toward opening the circle of knowledge and theory so that knowledge gained from intervention research can inform theory. The next section in this chapter provides an example of how science and practice have contributed to the development of a naturalistic language intervention model in ways that have benefited both disciplines.

## ENHANCED MILIEU TEACHING

EMT is a model of early language intervention that systematically combines milieu teaching (Hart & Rogers-Warren, 1978) with adult language modeling and interactional strategies that appear to support children's language development. Specifically, EMT combines incidental teaching (i.e., the least intrusive of the milieu teaching procedures), responsive interaction strategies (e.g., expanding the child's language, modeling language at the child's level, responding contingently to the child), and strategies for creating a context in which children want and need to learn language (e.g., following the child's lead, responding positively to children's behavior). Selected elements of responsive interaction in EMT provide frequent models of appropriate language, increase the semantic contingencies provided by the conversational partner, and make the intervention more child centered. Incidental teaching (Hart & Risley, 1968, 1975) ensures high-quality opportunities for the child to practice functional language and to receive systematic feedback.

## Roots of EMT in the Processes Shaping Typical Development

EMT is grounded in research describing typical language development as well as research comparing parent–child interactions when the child has a disability with parent–child interactions when the child is developing typically. Research on typical child language development and the input variables that affect it provides a theoretical foundation for this model of language intervention. We assume that effective strategies should reflect the same processes or input variables that support typical language development. Research suggests that parent–child interactions are both qualitatively and quantitatively different when the child has a disability and that these differences appear to be the result of both parent behavior and child skills in the interaction (Cardoso-Martin & Mervis, 1985; Kaiser & Blair, 1987; Mahoney, 1988). Adult input depends on and is affected by the language and communication skills of the child.

Four specific aspects of parent input appear to be associated with language development: 1) joint attention, 2) contingent responsiveness and topic maintenance, 3) social routines, and 4) modeling and expansions. Joint attention refers to instances in which two people are attending to and acting upon the same object, activity, or topic (Schaffer, 1989). Joint attention is assumed to facilitate language development by enhancing children's understanding that their behavior is having some effect on their environment and by mapping nonverbal communication with language to help them establish and maintain the interaction (Tomasello & Farrar, 1986). Naturalistic observations of parents and children have documented a significant positive relationship between time spent in joint attention and vocabulary acquisition (Goldberg, 1977b; Smith, Adamson, & Bakeman, 1988; Tomasello, Mannle, & Kruger, 1986), time spent in joint attention and frequency of communicative utterances and length of conversation (Tomasello & Farrar, 1986), and the proportion of joint attention preceding adult models and rate of language development (Nelson, 1973).

A second characteristic of adult language that appears to facilitate child language development is the extent to which the adult responds contingently to the child's communication. Contingent responsiveness refers to parental input that occurs shortly after a child's communicative attempt and is related to the topic and content of that attempt. This type of semantically contingent speech ensures that parent and child messages have some meaningful relationship to one another (McDonald, 1985). The most important element of contingent responsiveness appears to be the semantic contingency (i.e., the close match of parent meaning to child's intended meaning) (Cross, 1978). There is empirical evidence of the relationship between contingent responsiveness and child linguistic development (Cross, 1978), verbal imitation (Snow, 1989), and vocabulary (Olson, Bayles, & Bates, 1986). Yoder, Davies, and Bishop (1992) suggested that continuing a child's topic is likely to elicit further conversation from the child because the child's interest in the topic serves as an incentive for communication. It may be easier for the child to understand the adult's speech when it is related to the child's own topic.

A third aspect of parent input related to child language development is the use of social routines (Ratner & Bruner, 1978; Snow, Perlman, & Nathan, 1987; Snyder-McLean, Solomonson, McLean, & Sack, 1984). Social routines are hypothesized to facilitate language by setting up a situation in which the child is familiar enough with the activity to attend to the adult's language models; the number of semantic meanings and utterances are limited and familiar, making the adult models more salient; and a predictable sequence is provided in which appropriate language responses can be inserted (Ratner & Bruner, 1978). Research on child language learning in the context of social routines provides evidence of the specific effects of routines. Data have indicated that children use more complex language (Conti-Ramsden & Friel-Patti, 1987; Snow et al., 1987), make more initiations, and take longer turns in routines than in nonroutines (Conti-Ramsden & Friel-Patti, 1987).

The fourth component of parent input that appears to facilitate child language development is the use of models, which are utterances that provide the child with examples of appropriate language responses. Language models are assumed to be effective because they assist the child in understanding the relationship between form, content, and use; provide the child with linguistic stimuli that are meaningfully related to the child's interest; and provide the child with language that is slightly more advanced than the child's current language skills (Snow, 1984; Tannock & Girolametto, 1992). Expansions (including descriptive talk) are the most common form of models. Adult use of expansions has been associated with frequency of child imitations (Folger & Chapman, 1978; Scherer & Olswang, 1989), gains in MLU (mean length of utterance) and semantic complexity of child speech (Barnes, Gutfreund, Satterly, & Wells, 1983), and spontaneous object labels (Scherer & Olswang, 1989).

Although each of these aspects of parent input has been described, researched, and discussed as individual components of parent behavior, it is likely that the interaction of these variables with each other and with characteristics of the child provides the foundation for language learning (Hoff-Ginsberg, 1990). The extent to which parents use these variables depends at least in part on the child's ability to process the information and the extent to which the child provides communicative behaviors to which the parent can then respond. Parent input to the child is modified in response to the amount of child feedback and participation (Bohannon & Marquis, 1977) and to the content of the child's utterances. Information on parent input variables, the interaction of these variables, and the input of the child provides a foundation for developing an intervention designed to facilitate children's language development.

## Evolution of EMT

The current form of EMT evolved as our research group conducted studies comparing milieu teaching, responsive interaction, and didactic language interventions. Using both single-subject methodology and comparative group designs, we implemented milieu teaching and responsive interaction in a series of studies (Kaiser et al., in preparation; Yoder et al., 1991; Yoder et al., 1995) and found that both had positive effects on children's language use over time in training sessions and in generalization sessions across persons (another adult partner) and across settings (at home).

Milieu language intervention, which is grounded in research in typical language development, teaches functional language in the context of naturally occurring interactions between children and significant others (Hart & Rogers-Warren, 1978). It focuses on individual child and parent differences to the intervention and to each other over time. The milieu model incorporates several of the components of parent input previously discussed. All milieu teaching episodes begin with joint attention to the topic or object in which the child is interested. Child responses are followed by expansions that provide models for future language use. All prompts and reinforcers are based on the child's focus. A fundamental component of the milieu teaching model is incidental teaching (Hart & Risley, 1968, 1975). Opportunities for the child to practice functional language and to receive systematic feedback are provided by having the adult respond to child requests, both verbal and nonverbal, and using these opportunities to elicit and/or model more complex child language. This procedure not only models more elaborate language but also teaches turn-taking and topic continuation skills and improves conversation skills as well.

Responsive interaction interventions are designed to facilitate parent–child interactions in which the primary focus is communication (Tannock & Girolametto, 1992). In these types of communicative interactions, natural opportunities for learning language can occur regularly. Adults are taught to follow the child's lead; to respond contingently to child communication using repetitions, models, and expansions; to provide opportunities for the child to take a turn; and to provide natural consequences that are related semantically to the child's interest in the context of naturally occurring interactions and daily routines (Girolametto, 1988; Mahoney & Powell, 1988; Tannock & Girolametto, 1992).

From our research comparing milieu teaching and responsive interaction interventions, it became apparent that an intervention that combined elements of both models would more fully address the range of language-learning needs of young children. Responsive interaction strategies and incidental teaching represent aspects of parent input identified as facilitative of children's language development.

The extent to which adult–child interactions are facilitative of language learning depends on the presence of three relational components: 1) the child must engage with the environment, 2) the child and the caregiver must interact contingently with one another, and 3) the caregiver must mediate the physical environment for the child. Child engagement with the environment ensures that there is a topic of interest to the child and a focus of communication. Contingent interactions provide a context in which the child can determine the meaning of communication. Although milieu teaching alone addresses these relational aspects of interaction, it provides the conversational partner with only one strategy (i.e., prompting elaborated language) for responding to the child. The addition of responsive interaction strategies provides conversational partners with multiple options for responding to the child's language and for mapping the child's communication and environmental context in which the child is attempting to communicate. Combining responsive interaction with milieu teaching results in an intervention that permits the conversational partner to prompt language at highly salient moments and to use expansions, models, and descriptive talk to establish joint attention and to respond to the child's verbal and nonverbal communicative attempts. In sum, EMT is an intervention model that facilitates interactions characterized by joint attention and mutual enjoyment and that provides meaningful and functional opportunities for adults to prompt and model language. Table 1 provides a summary of the components of EMT.

## Studies of EMT

This section reviews the results of two studies (Hemmeter & Kaiser, 1994; Kaiser & Hester, 1994) that examined the effects of EMT on children's language performance in training and generalization contexts. In these studies, we focused on the systematic implementation of the hybrid model as a means of changing the behavior of key conversational partners (i.e., parents and teachers) and then examined changes with other untrained partners.

***Study 1: Effects of Parent-Implemented Language Intervention*** The Hemmeter and Kaiser (1994) study sought to determine if parents could learn

Table 1. Components of EMT

| Training content | Child skills trained |
|---|---|
| I. **Environmental arrangement**<br>Selecting materials<br>Arranging materials<br>Mediating the environment<br>Use of specific strategies to manipulate the environment | Facilitates: 1) child interest in the environment; 2) sustained attention to the environment; 3) verbal and nonverbal communicative initiations, including requests and comments; 4) engagement between the child and adult |
| II. **Responsive interaction strategies**<br>Principles of conversational interactions<br>Following the child's lead<br>Balancing turns<br>Maintaining child's topic<br>Parallel and self-talk<br>Matching child's complexity level<br>Expanding and imitating child utterances<br>Latency, pausing, and sustained attention | Facilitates: 1) engagement between the child and adult; 2) turn taking; 3) sustained interactions; 4) topic continuation; 5) comprehension of spoken language; 6) spontaneous communicative imitations to the adult |
| III. **Milieu teaching techniques**<br>Child-cued modeling<br>Mand-modeling<br>Time delay<br>Incidental teaching | Facilitates: 1) responsiveness to adult speech; 2) generalized imitation skills; 3) requesting behavior; 4) production of elaborated lexical and syntactic skills (and targets); 5) turn-taking skills; 6) topic continuation skills; 7) communicative initiations to the adult; 8) improved conversational skills |

to use EMT and to examine the effects of the parents' use of EMT on the children's productive language skills and global language development. The study involved four preschool children with disabilities and their mothers. The children (three boys and one girl) ranged in age from 25 to 49 months at the beginning of the study. Each of the four children was in the early stages of language learning and was verbally imitative. A summary of the four dyads is shown in Table 2.

Parents were taught to use the three components of EMT: environmental arrangement, responsive interaction strategies, and incidental teaching. Parents were trained during 20 sessions using a variety of training strategies, including modeling, feedback, coaching, lectures, written materials, and videotapes. Fifteen-minute parent–child play sessions were videotaped in a clinic setting, with generalization probes conducted in the home with the parent and in the clinic with trained interactors who were not otherwise involved in the study. A multiple-probe design across two families replicated across two additional families was used to assess the effects of the intervention on the children's social-communicative skills. Specific language targets were identified for each child. In addition, pre- and postassessments of children's language development were made. Table 3 summarizes the contexts and measures used in this study.

Table 2. Subject characteristics

| Dyad | Parent | Child | Disabling condition | Language age of child | Language targets |
|---|---|---|---|---|---|
| A | MBA<br>Electrical engineer<br>Father | 25 mo<br>Male | Down syndrome | RCA[a] - 16mo<br>ECA[b] - 12mo | more<br>help<br>verbs (e.g., go, roll, kick) |
| B | BS in nursing<br>Not employed<br>Mother | 25 mo<br>Female | Language delay<br>Behavior problems | RCA - 8 mo<br>ECA - 16 mo | want + noun<br>more + noun<br>verbs (e.g., blow, jump, go) |
| C | BS in nursing<br>Not employed<br>Mother | 45 mo<br>Male | Pervasive develop-mental disorder | RCA - 8 mo<br>ECA - [c] | nouns (e.g., toy, music)<br>verbs (e.g., blow, jump, bounce)<br>more |
| D | BS in education<br>Not employed<br>Mother | 49 mo<br>Male | Cerebral palsy<br>Seizure disorder | RCA - 24 mo<br>ECA - 24 mo | more<br>want<br>verbs (e.g., draw, go, drive) |

[a]Receptive language age as measured by the Sequenced Inventory of Communication Development (SICD; Hedrick, Prather, & Tobin, 1975).

[b]Expressive language as measured by the Sequenced Inventory of Communication Development (SICD; Hedrick et al., 1975).

[c]Not able to compute.

Table 3. Study 1: Contexts and measures

| Condition | Context | Measures | Effects |
|---|---|---|---|
| Baseline/training (child with teaching adult) | Clinic | Use of targets[a]<br>Frequency of intentional communication[a]<br>MLU[b]<br>Diversity of vocabulary[b] | Primary effects of intervention |
| Home generalization (child with teaching adult) | Home | Use of targets<br>Frequency of intentional communication<br>MLU<br>Diversity of vocabulary | Generalization of training effects across settings |
| Clinic generalization (child with three different nonteaching adults) | Clinic | Use of targets<br>Frequency of intentional communication<br>MLU<br>Diversity of vocabulary | Generalization of training effects across people |
| Pre-/Postassessments | Clinic | SICD–E, SICD–R[c]<br>MLU<br>Diversity of vocabulary | Development/generalization of child's language skills |

[a]As measured by the Combined Milieu Teaching/Responsive Interaction Code (CMT/RIC; Alpert, Tiernan, Hemmeter, & Fischer, 1989).
[b]Derived from verbatim transcriptions using the Systematic Analysis of Language Transcripts (SALT) protocol (Miller & Chapman, 1983).
[c]Expressive and receptive scores from the Sequenced Inventory of Communication Development (SICD; Hedrick, Prather, & Tobin, 1975).

Each parent learned to use all three components of the intervention in the clinic setting and generalized the use of the strategies to the home generalization setting. All four children learned their language targets and used them productively in the training setting as shown in Figure 2. Moreover, each of the children showed increases in spontaneous communication (although Child C's increases were not as marked as the other three) as a result of their parents' use of the intervention strategies. These data are shown in Figure 3. Three of the four children generalized their use of language targets to the home setting and demonstrated increases in their spontaneous communication as shown in Figure 4. Similar changes were observed in the clinic generalization sessions.

Children A and B showed the most consistent changes across all five measures of global language development (SICD–E, SICD–R, MLU, longest utterance, and number of different words in a language sample). Changes were observed for Children C and D on two measures. Children A and B were developmentally younger, and the discrepancy between their chronological age and their linguistic age was smaller than for Children C and D.

The results of this study suggest that systematic changes in parent input to children can result in positive changes in children's productive language in both training and generalization settings and across conversational partners. The individual graphs of the children and their partners in the single-subject de-

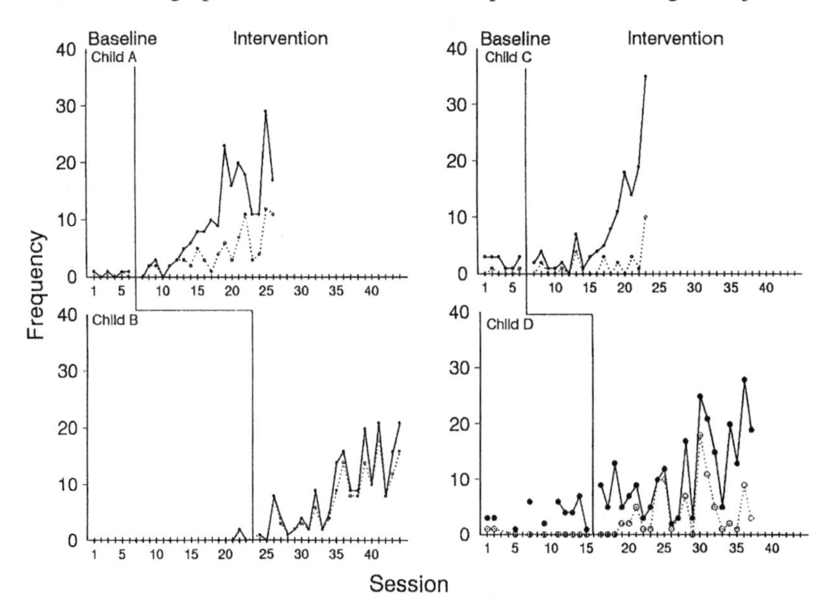


Figure 2. Frequency of spontaneous use of targets and total use of targets by children in the training setting. (-●- = total use of targets; --○-- = spontaneous use of targets.) (From Hemmeter, M.L., & Kaiser, A.P. [1994]. Enhanced milieu teaching: Effects of parent-implemented language intervention. *Journal of Early Intervention, 18*[3], 280; reprinted by permission.)

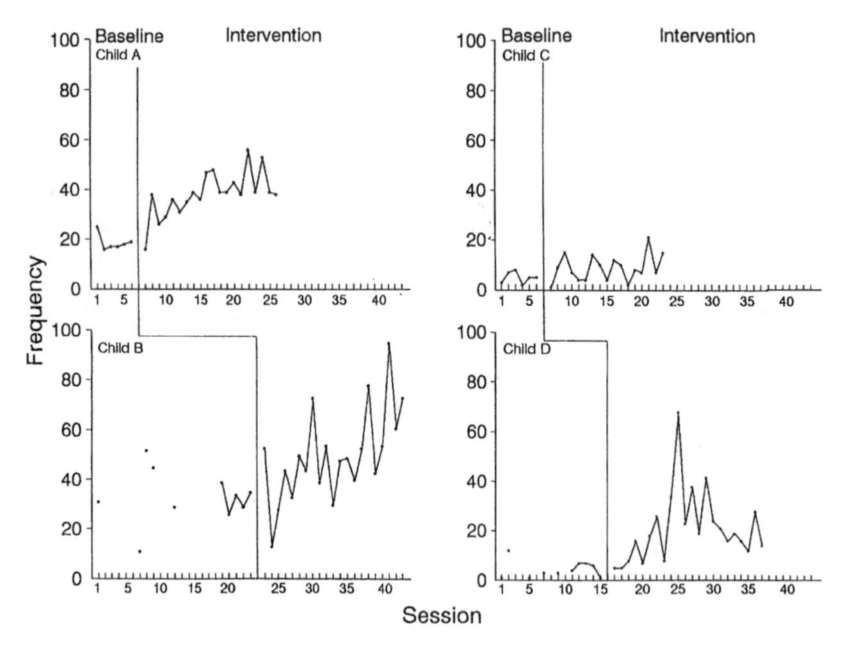


Figure 3. Frequency of spontaneous communicative utterances by the children in the training setting. (From Hemmeter, M.L., & Kaiser, A.P. [1994]. Enhanced milieu teaching: Effects of parent-implemented language intervention. *Journal of Early Intervention, 18*[3], 281; reprinted by permission.)

sign highlight the variability and similarities in the children's language development. Changes in at least two measures were observed for all subjects. The most consistent effects across children were in the use of targets in the training setting. Although the generalization data are more varied, they provide evidence of generalization beyond what has been observed in previous studies of parent-implemented interventions. In parent-implemented studies where generalization has been assessed, it has typically been in the context of the parent–child interaction. Thus, these studies have demonstrated that changes in child language skills generalized to other situations or activities that involved the parent and the child and that modest generalization occurs outside of the parent–child interaction.

***Study 2: Analysis of the Generalized Effects of EMT*** The Kaiser and Hester (1994) study involved six preschool children in the early stages of language learning. The characteristics of the children are shown in Table 4. This study sought to systematically analyze the generalized effects of the intervention on the children's interactions across conversational partners: their teachers in the classroom, parents at home, and peers in their classroom. Three generalization assessments were conducted with each partner before and after the intervention training condition. Table 5 summarizes the contexts and measures in the current study.

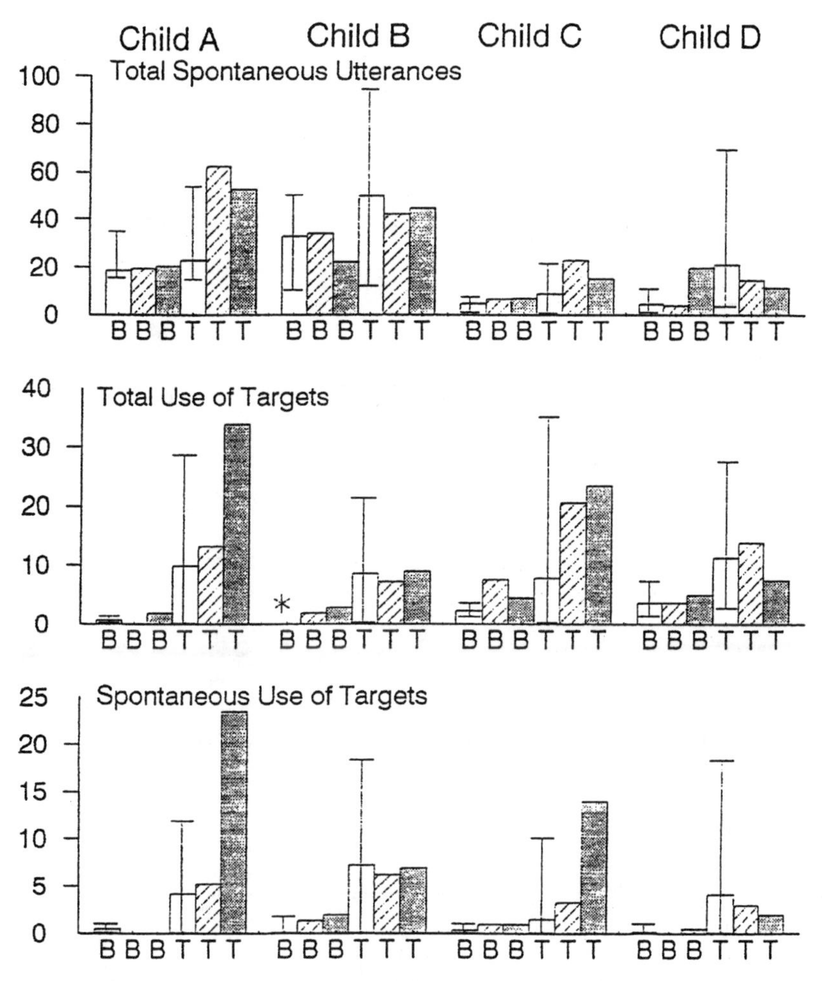


Figure 4. Child spontaneous utterances, total use of targets, and spontaneous use of targets in training, home generalization, and clinic generalization settings. (☐=training setting; ▨=home generalization setting; ▩=clinic generalization setting; B=baseline; T=training; * =mean and range were zero.)

In a multiple baseline design across three dyads of children, trainers implemented the EMT procedures during interactions with the target children in a classroom free-play setting. Each play session lasted 15 minutes. The training was in a small area inside or immediately adjacent to the children's preschool classrooms, which was equipped with dramatic play, art, and manipulative materials.

All six children showed systematic increases in their use of intentional communicative utterances and use of their targets (Figure 5) in the training setting when the EMT procedures were introduced. Generalization across communicative partners was determined on the basis of four measures of child lan-

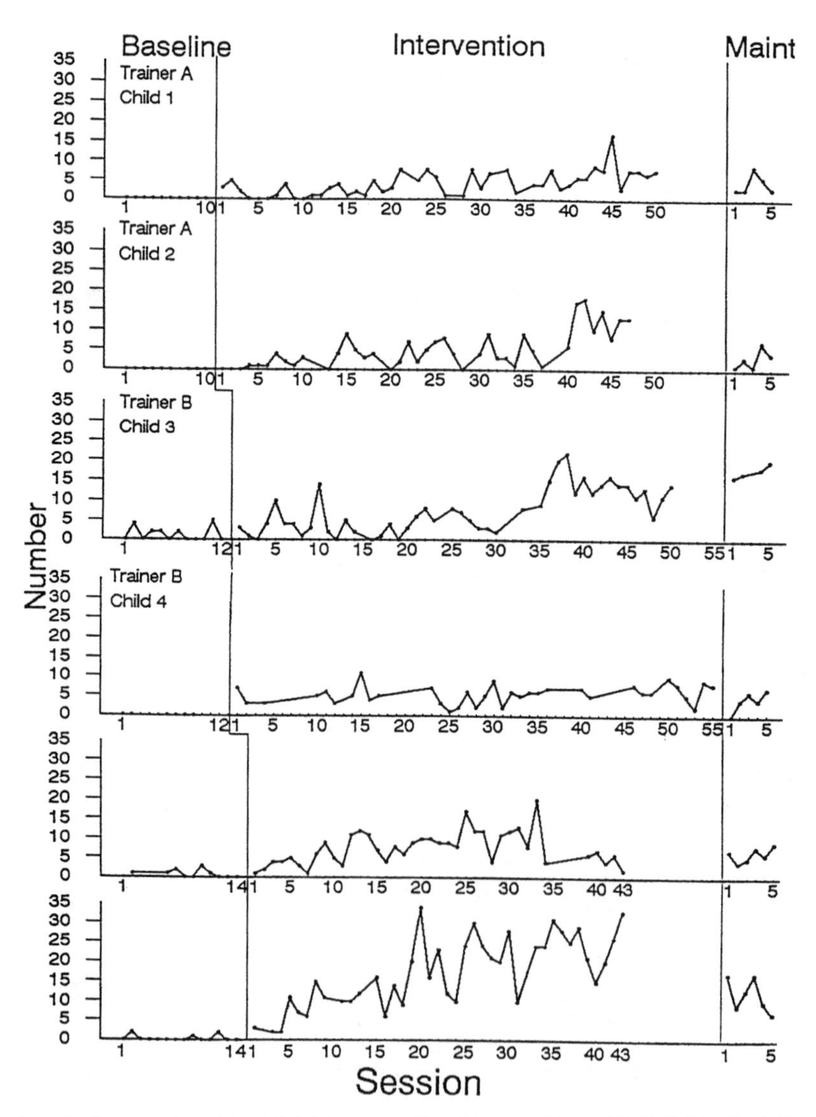


Figure 5. Frequency of use of targets in training sessions. (From Kaiser, A.P., & Hester, P.P. [1994]. Generalized effects of enhanced milieu teaching. *Journal of Speech and Hearing Research, 37*[6], 1331; reprinted by permission.)

guage collected in each setting: 1) total communicative utterances, 2) use of targets, 3) diversity of vocabulary, and 4) MLU. All six children showed some level of generalization to interactions with their teachers. All six children showed generalization on one or more measures observed in interactions with their parents at home. These effects were judged to be modest to minimal for

Table 4. Child–participant characteristics

| Child | Disabling condition | Language age of child | | | | Language targets |
|---|---|---|---|---|---|---|
| | | | | SICD* | | |
| | | IQ | MLU | EXP | REC | |
| Child 1<br>5.1 yr. Male | Language delayed<br>Articulation disorders | 64 | 1.53 | 28 | 36 | agent + action + object<br>noun + preposition + noun |
| Child 2<br>6.8 yr. Male | Language delayed<br>Autistic-like | 51 | 1.3 | 20 | 28 | agent + action<br>action + object<br>preposition + noun |
| Child 3<br>4.1 yr. Male | Autistic-like<br>General developmental delay | 68 | 1.12 | 16 | 16 | agent + action<br>action + object<br>functional requests |
| Child 4<br>3.1 yr. Male | Cerebral palsy<br>General developmental delay | 86 | 2.79 | 28 | 28 | present progressive use of conjunction *and* (minimum of four-word utterances) |
| Child 5<br>3.5 yr. Male | Down syndrome | 70 | 1.41 | 28 | 28 | agent + action<br>action + object<br>adjective + noun |
| Child 6<br>4.5 yr. Female | Apraxia<br>General developmental delay | 63 | 1.12 | 36 | 28 | agent + action<br>action + object<br>adjective + noun |

*Expressive (EXP) and receptive (REC) scores from Sequenced Inventory of Communication Development (SICD; Hedrick et al., 1975).

Table 5. Study 2: Contexts and measures

| Condition | Context | Measures | Effects |
|---|---|---|---|
| Baseline/training/maintenance | Classroom | Use of targets[a]<br>Frequency of intentional communication[a]<br>MLU[b]<br>Diversity of vocabulary[b] | Primary effects |
| Teachers (pre/post) | Classroom | Use of targets<br>Frequency of intentional communication<br>MLU<br>Diversity of vocabulary | Generalization across people |
| Parents (pre/post) | Home | Use of targets<br>Frequency of intentional communication<br>MLU<br>Diversity of vocabulary | Generalization across settings and people |
| Peers (pre/post) | Classroom | Use of targets<br>Frequency of intentional communication<br>MLU<br>Diversity of vocabulary | Generalization across people |
| Pre-/Postassessments | Testing room adjacent to classroom | PPVT[c], EOWPVT[d], SICD-E, SICD-R[e], MLU<br>Diversity of vocabulary | Development generalization |

[a]Measured by the Combined Milieu Teaching/Responsive Interaction Code (CMT/RIC; Alpert et al., 1989).

[b]Derived from verbatim transcriptions using the Systematic Analysis of Language Transcripts (SALT) protocol (Miller & Chapman, 1983).

[c]Peabody Picture Vocabulary Test–Revised (PPVT; Dunn & Dunn, 1981).

[d]Expressive One Word Picture Vocabulary Test (EOWPVT; Gardner, 1981).

[e]Sequenced Inventory of Communication Development (SICD; Hedrick et al., 1975).

four of the six children (Children 1, 2, 4, and 5) and strong for the remaining two children (children 3 and 6).

Four of the six children demonstrated generalized changes from pre- to posttraining assessments in their interactions with peers. Two of these children (Children 1 and 5) showed strong effects while the remaining two showed modest effects (Children 2 and 3). A post hoc correlational analysis of child performance with partner behavior during the pre- and postintervention generalization assessments revealed that child performance at both periods (before and after the intervention) was associated with specific partner communication behaviors—number of questions to the child and total amount of partner talk to the child. The strongest evidenced generalization was observed with parents who asked questions and talked with the child most frequently. The second strongest generalization was observed in small-group interactions that included the child's teacher and two peers from his or her classroom. In this generalization setting, teacher questions and talk to the target child were constrained by the presence of other children; teachers distributed their attention across the three children during the session. The least generalization was observed with peers who talked at the lowest rates and asked few, if any, questions. Because the peers in this study were also children with developmental delays (although demonstrating better language skills than the target children), the competency of the peers as conversational partners was limited. Three children (Children 1, 2, and 3) showed robust changes on at least four of the six global measures of language development (SICD–E, SICD–R, PPVT, EOWPVT, MLU, and diversity of vocabulary in a standardized language sample). All children showed changes on at least one measure that were greater than expected based on their rate of development before the intervention.

As depicted in the graphs of the individual children and their partners in the single-subject design, across all settings and measures, a pattern similar to that observed in Study 1 emerged. All children showed systematic changes in the training setting when EMT was implemented and partner input was altered to increase the aspects of adult input and adult–child interaction believed to be facilitative of the children's language. These changes generalized to untrained partners for most children; however, the specific measures showing change, the amount of change, and the consistency of change across partners varied by child. Some changes in measures of global language were observed for all children; however, only three of the six children showed consistent changes across measures. In this study, the children who showed relatively clear generalization across partners were the same children who demonstrated consistent changes on global measures of language.

### Implications of These Findings for Understanding Typical Development

The data from these two intervention studies suggest several important findings about the influence of partner input on child language. First, altering the language and interactional style of a conversational partner to include those components of partner input associated with accelerated language development in typical children results in systematic changes in the frequency and complexity of the communication of children with language delays in interactions with that partner. That is, as a result of implementing the EMT procedures, we consistently achieved effects on child language performance in the training setting by manipulating partner input variables associated with accelerated language performance. The results confirm findings in the developmental literature that conversational partner behavior is a powerful factor in children's daily use of language (Moerk, 1977).

Second, the effects of this systematic change in one partner's input generalized to children's subsequent interactions with other partners, including unfamiliar adults, teachers, parents, and peers. Thus, facilitative changes in input by a primary partner may be sufficiently powerful to teach language skills that will be used with other partners who may not provide input that is highly supportive of language learning. Regular interactions with an effective conversational partner, particularly a primary caregiver, might be sufficient (and possibly necessary) for some children to learn communication skills that can be used with other partners.

Third, the evidence of differential effects across generalization partners, however, supports the first finding that conversational partner input is closely associated with language performance. It further suggests that generalization from training may be, at least in part, dependent on partner input. When new partners use input strategies that support child talk in general (e.g., asking questions, talking to the child), the child's generalization from training is facilitated.

Fourth, for some children, optimal input from a conversational partner may result in changes in global measures of their language. For the children in these studies, effective partner input in the form of the EMT intervention may have been facilitative of their development or might have had generalized effects on their use of language in contexts far removed from that of the partners providing optimal input. Thus, the effects of effective partner input may extend outside of immediate conversational context and affect children's use of language separate from the context in which it was learned. Because changes on global measures reflect language learning in addition to the acquisition of specific targets, it is possible that effective partner input may have broad as well as specific effects on children's learning. The nature of a conversational or naturalistic intervention is such that many aspects of language are modeled in addition to the specific targets of the intervention. This broad base of modeling parallels naturally occurring input and may be facilitative of overall development.

In both of these studies, it is essential to note the variability across children and across measures in this sample of preschool children with disabilities. These individual variations suggest that different aspects of input may be more or less useful for children, and unmeasured child characteristics may determine the extent to which input will affect more distal or global changes in child language. Variability of effects across children in the training setting was less than the variability observed in the generalization settings and in the global assessments of development. Changes in input appear to produce consistently robust, immediate, in-context effects and more variable effects as the context for assessment becomes more removed from the primary setting and the measures become more divergent from the supported conversational use of language. Partner behavior in the generalization setting continued to exert a direct effect on child performance, even though performance improved after the intervention. This finding is consistent with a strong contextual effects model of verbal performance; thus, these findings parallel what has been observed in typically developing children. The facilitative effects of partner behavior influence both learning and generalization behavior (Keetz, 1994; Ostrosky & Kaiser, 1995). When partner behavior is viewed as a variable that potentially affects child communication in all settings, the examination of generalization must be reframed to describe the contributions of assessment. Tests of global language development represent a unique set of conditions of partner behavior in terms of typical experience with language use. Frequency and duration of the intervention (i.e., the length of time in which the child is exposed to optimized partner input) may also affect the generalized and global effects observed on children's language outside the training setting.

These findings provide support for a model of child language development that posits that the social-communicative style (e.g., amount of talk, use of questions, following the child's conversational lead) and linguistic input of a conversational partner (e.g., talk at the child's level of understanding and production, modeling of targets, expansions of child utterances containing models) support child performance of more complex language (i.e., a potential context effect of partner behavior) and facilitate children's learning of new forms (i.e., a generalized effect or a developmental effect). The consistency of these findings with children with language delays might be interpreted in one of two ways. First, it might suggest that partner-input variables are particularly robust in their influence over child language performance. Because language learning and use are presumed to be relatively more difficult for children with developmental delays, optimal partner input may be especially powerful to produce this pattern of results. Alternatively, children with language delays may be more sensitive to or dependent on partner input and communication style. The differential language performance across communication partners exhibiting different levels of supportive social-communication style suggests such sensitivity. Further research comparing children with and without developmental delays, who are at the same level of current language skill, would be needed to determine such differential sensitivity to optimal partner behavior.

The potential contribution of such research, regardless of the findings, would be a better understanding of how partner input and social-communicative style interact with child characteristics to support language development.

### Contributions of Intervention Research Using Naturalistic Interaction Models

Beyond the specific implications of the findings of these two studies, studies of naturalistic interventions such as EMT might contribute to theory and understanding of developmental processes in other ways. First, interventions based on principles derived from studies of typically developing children in interactions with their caregivers offer an opportunity to test these developmental principles in experiments. True experiments, when constructed to ensure high levels of internal validity, can offer stronger evidence of causal relationships than is possible to obtain in descriptive, correlational studies of development. Potentially, such experiments might be conducted with typically developing children, as well as with children exhibiting language delays of different degrees and etiologies. A set of experiments, carefully constructed to examine the effects of an intervention based on developmental principles and including systematic replications across a range of individuals with different entry language skills, could greatly contribute to understanding the influence that partner behavior has on children's language development.

Second, intervention studies where the components of the intervention are applied systematically or where two or more naturalistic interventions that contrast on a critical theoretical dimension are compared can elucidate how particular aspects of social interaction style and linguistic input influence development. Again, the use of experimental designs offers a unique opportunity to extend information obtained in correlational developmental studies and to refine social interactionist theories of language development.

Third, using designs that incorporate the systematic analysis of generalization across partners and communication contexts can provide an empirical basis for understanding the influence of contextual factors on child performance. The basic design of a generalization study includes multiple preintervention assessments in the generalization setting or with the generalization task, implementation of the intervention in the treatment setting, and concurrent assessments in the generalization setting that continue after the intervention phase. Although many studies use only before- and after-intervention generalization assessments, continuous monitoring of generalization allows examination of its process. Using a gradient of increasingly difficult tasks, settings, or partners makes it possible to test developmental sequences by predicting the pattern of generalization and to assess the parameters of communicative competence at a given stage of development. Although across-setting and across-partner generalization might be studied in a descriptive design without an intervention, examining patterns of generalization for newly learned behaviors (i.e., those with a known learning history) provides greater experimental control, increases the specificity of questions that can be asked, and allows the possibility of extremely well-controlled systematic replication across subjects. The use of generalization analysis designs in combination with a primary intervention design offers the opportunity to study both naturally occurring and facilitated development in ways that cannot be easily done in a nonintervention design.

Fourth, intervention studies challenge researchers to examine language and communication from an integrative perspective addressing the relationship among the cognitive, linguistic, and social-pragmatic aspects of development. Informally, intervention studies are potentially rich opportunities for examining the "real" effects of theoretically driven intervention. As researchers observing the effects of an applied intervention, we were confronted with the limits of our understanding of the complexity of the language system. Theoretical arguments about the relative dominance of one subsystem over another might be resolved through experiments targeting specific dimensions of the system, but only if a holistic analysis of the outcomes, based on social use of appropriate language in context, is integral to the experiment. Using social validation strategies (Wolf, 1978), clinical performance evaluations, multiple assessments, or qualitative methods to examine the functional use of communication in addition to systematic measures of target intervention outcomes provides an extended empirical basis for theories relating to development of subcomponent systems.

For the most part, the preceding discussion argues for true experimental designs as a basis for strengthening causal arguments offered in theories of child language development. Single-subject designs can contribute to the knowledge base in other ways. Single-subject designs rely on multiple samples of an individual's behavior in two or more experimental conditions (e.g., baseline, treatment). These designs allow the tracking of performance, if not development, over time and permit examination of the shifts in level and trend associated with the introduction of procedures posited to support language learning and use. Potentially, single-subject designs have the advantages of a case study (e.g., focus on an individual, measurement over an extended period of time, opportunity to quantify the behavior of others as they interact with the child) combined with the rigor of a quasiexperiment in which the reliability and internal validity can be evaluated against a set of scientific standards. The interest in growth curve or hierarchical linear modeling (Byrk & Raudenbush, 1992) in combination with interventions suggests that studying individual development over time, especially before, during, and after an intervention, is of interest to developmental researchers. Use of microgenetic experiments (Orihara, 1983) with some of the same characteristics as single-subject designs has been very informative in understanding children's development of math reasonings with changing levels of support for learning, for example. Interest in dyadic interactions over time requires multiple data points as a basis for examining process and evolution in social interactions. The design of single-subject studies allows the examination of the effects of interactional variables (e.g., interaction strategies of the adult and the child's responses to these strategies) before, immediately after, and across time after the intervention is introduced. Time-series designs incorporating an intervention are especially valuable for studying trends in secondary variables that reflect dyadic interaction (e.g., changes in turn ratio, mutual responsiveness, complexity of language addressed to the other) and for determining who leads such shifts in the dyadic interaction.

## CONCLUSION

Future studies of EMT and other naturalistic communication interventions offer a unique opportunity to understand the influences of social and linguistic input on children's communication across contexts. The explicitly social nature of the intervention bridges language and communication into more broadly defined social behaviors of both the adult and the child. This bridging of language and behavior, in turn, provides a new opportunity to study the linkages between communication and behavior in development. For example, it is well established that many children with behavior disorders also present language and social-communication difficulties (Baker & Cantwell, 1987; Baltaxe & Simmons, 1988; Fujiki & Brinton, 1994). The theoretical and practical connections between these two aspects of social-interactional behavior in early development are not well understood but early co-occurrence of language and behavior problems appears to predict later significant conduct disorders, poor academic performance, and difficulty in forming positive peer relationships (Hadley & Rice, 1991; Stevens & Bliss, 1995). By examining the effects of early language intervention on the social-behavioral repertoires and interactions of young children, it may be possible to expand both theories of early social development and approaches to preventative interventions. The potential outcome is a more holistic view of how communication interfaces with other aspects of development and how the course of development is affected by changes that address any of the component systems.

For intervention research to enter into the circle of empirical information and theory that forms our understanding of early development, several steps must be taken. First, as intervention researchers, we must continue to read the developmental literature and listen to our colleagues with developmental and theoretical interests. Second, we must point out the explicit contributions of intervention research to developmental theory. We must acknowledge where theory may be incomplete, inadequate for explaining atypical development or intervention effects, or where we find existing theory to be wrong. We must think in terms of theory and place the findings of intervention research in a theoretical context. Third, we must challenge loosely constructed or poorly conceived directions for intervention provided by our colleagues with traditionally stronger theoretical orientations. Although it is important to consider recommendations seriously for intervention research and practice that come from theory and typical development, it is also important that we examine them systematically, challenge them when we disagree, and engage in dialogue about the strengths and limitations of the recommendations. Intervention researchers must take responsibility for responding to the offerings of our more theoretical colleagues and for refining theory to encompass intervention findings and children with atypical development. In doing so, we take responsibility for promoting a cybernetic, holistic, and multivoiced discussion of theory, development, and intervention practice. We move the metaphor of our field from Jacob's ladder to Sarah's circle, and we seek to build bridges in ways that will ultimately benefit both science and practice.

## REFERENCES

Alpert, C.L., Tiernan, M., Hemmeter, M.L., & Fischer, R. (1989). *Combined milieu/responsive interaction code.* Unpublished manuscript, Vanderbilt University, Nashville, TN.

Baer, D.M., Wolf, M.M., & Risley, T.R. (1968). Some current dimensions of applied behavior analysis. *Journal of Applied Behavior Analysis, 1*, 91–97.

Baker, L., & Cantwell, D.P. (1987). Comparison of well, emotionally disordered, and behaviorally disordered children with linguistic problems. *Journal of the American Academy of Child and Adolescent Psychiatry, 26*, 193–196.

Baltaxe, C.A.M., & Simmons, J.Q. (1988). Communication deficits in preschool children with psychiatric disorders. *Seminars in Speech and Language, 8*, 81–90.

Barnes, S., Gutfreund, M., Satterly, D., & Wells, G. (1983). Characteristics of adult speech which predict children's language development. *Journal of Child Language, 10*(1), 65–84.

Bogdan, R.S., & Biklen, S.K. (1992). *Qualitative research for education: An introduction to theory and methods* (2nd ed.). Needham, MA: Allyn & Bacon.

Bohannon, J., & Marquis, A. (1977). Children's control of adult speech. *Child Development, 48*(3), 1002–1008.

Bricker, D. (1993). Then, now, and the path between: A brief history of language intervention. In A.P. Kaiser & D.B. Gray (Eds.), *Communication and language intervention series: Vol. 2. Enhancing children's communication: Research foundations for intervention* (pp. 11–31). Baltimore: Paul H. Brookes Publishing Co.

Bricker, W.A., & Bricker, D.D. (1974). An early language training strategy. In R.L. Schiefelbusch & L.L. Lloyd (Eds.), *Language perspectives: Acquisition, retardation, and intervention* (pp. 431–468). Baltimore: University Park Press.

Byrk, A.S., & Raudenbush, S.W. (1992). *Hierarchical linear models: Applications and data analysis methods.* Beverly Hills: Sage Publications.

Cardoso-Martin, C., & Mervis, C.B. (1985). Maternal speech to prelinguistic children with Down syndrome. *American Journal of Mental Deficiency, 89*(5), 451–458.

Chomsky, N. (1959). A review of Skinner's *Verbal Behavior Language, 35*, 26–58.

Conti-Ramsden, G., & Friel-Patti, P. (1987). Scriptedness: A factor in children's variation in language use? In K. Nelson & A. Van Kleek (Eds.), *Children's language* (Vol. 6, pp. 108–123). Hillsdale, NJ: Lawrence Erlbaum Associates.

Cromer, R.F. (1988). Differentiating language and cognition. In R.L. Schiefelbusch & L.L. Lloyd (Eds.), *Language perspectives: Acquisition, retardation, and intervention* (2nd ed., pp. 91–124). Baltimore: University Park Press.

Cross, T. (1978). Motherese: Its association with the rate of syntactic acquisition in young children. In N. Waterson & C. Snow (Eds.), *The development of communication* (pp. 199–216). New York: John Wiley & Sons.

Denzin, N.K., & Lincoln, Y.S. (1994). Introduction: Entering the field of qualitative research. In N.K. Denzin & Y.S. Lincoln (Eds.), *Handbook of qualitative research* (pp. 1–17). Beverly Hills: Sage Publications.

Dunn, L.M., & Dunn, L.M. (1981). *Peabody Picture Vocabulary Test—Revised.* Circle Pines, MN: American Guidance Service.

Folger, J.P., & Chapman, R.S. (1978). A pragmatic analysis of spontaneous imitations. *Journal of Child Language, 5*(1), 25–38.

Fujiki, M., & Brinton, B. (1994). Social competence and language impairment in children. In R.V. Watkins & M.L. Rice (Eds.), *Communication and language intervention series: Vol. 4. Specific language impairments in children* (pp. 123–143). Baltimore: Paul H. Brookes Publishing Co.

Gardner, M.F. (1981). *Expressive One-Word Picture Vocabulary Test.* Novato, CA: Academic Therapy Publications.

Girolametto, L.E. (1988). Improving the social-conversational skills of developmentally delayed children: An intervention study. *Journal of Speech and Hearing Disorders, 53*(2), 156–167.

Goldberg, S. (1977a). Social competency in infancy: A model of parent–infant interaction. *Merrill-Palmer Quarterly, 23*(3), 163–177.

Goldberg, S. (1977b). Talking to children: Some notes on feedback. In C.E. Snow & C.A. Ferguson (Eds.), *Talking to children: Language input and acquisition* (pp. 199–218). Cambridge, England: Cambridge University Press.

Gottlieb, G. (1991). Experimental canalization of behavioral development: Theory. *Developmental Psychology, 27*(1), 4–13.

Guess, D., Sailor, W., & Baer, D.M. (1976). *Functional speech and language training for the severely handicapped.* Lawrence, KS: H & H Enterprises.

Hadley, P.A., & Rice, M.L. (1991). Conversational responsiveness of speech and language impaired preschoolers. *Journal of Speech and Hearing Research, 34*(6), 1308–1317.

Hart, B.M., & Rogers-Warren, A.K. (1978). A milieu approach to teaching language. In R.L. Schiefelbusch (Ed.), *Language intervention strategies* (Vol. 2, pp. 192–235). Baltimore: University Park Press.

Hart, B.M., & Risley, T.R. (1968). Establishing the use of descriptive adjectives in the spontaneous speech of disadvantaged preschool children. *Journal of Applied Behavior Analysis*, 1, 109–120.

Hart, B.M., & Risley, T.R. (1975). Incidental teaching of language in the preschool. *Journal of Applied Behavior Analysis, 8*, 411–420.

Hedrick, D.L., Prather, E.M., & Tobin, A.R. (1975). *Sequenced Inventory of Communication Development.* Seattle: University of Washington Press.

Hemmeter, M.L., & Kaiser, A.P. (1994). Enhanced milieu teaching: Effects of parent-implemented language intervention. *Journal of Early Intervention, 18*(3), 269–289.

Hoff-Ginsberg, E. (1990). Maternal speech and the child's development of syntax: A further look. *Journal of Child Language, 17*(1), 85–99.

Kaiser, A.P., & Blair, G. (1987). Mother–child transactions in families with normal and handicapped children. *Upsala Journal of Medical Sciences, 44*, 204–207.

Kaiser, A.P., & Hester, P.P. (1994). Generalized effects of enhanced milieu teaching. *Journal of Speech and Hearing Research, 37*(6), 1320–1340.
Kaiser, A.P., & Warren, S.F. (1988). Pragmatics and generalization. In R.L. Schiefelbusch & L.L. Lloyd (Eds.), *Language perspectives: Acquisition, retardation, and intervention* (2nd ed., pp. 397–442). Austin, TX: PRO-ED.
Kaiser, A.P., Yoder, P.J., Fischer, R., Keefer, M., Hemmeter, M.L., & Ostrosky, M.M. (in preparation). *A comparison of milieu teaching and responsive interaction implemented by parents.*
Keetz, A. (1994). *Effects of a naturalistic social communicative intervention on the peer interactions of preschool children with disabilities.* Unpublished dissertation, Vanderbilt University, Nashville, TN.
MacMillan, J.H., & Schumacher, S. (1984). *Research in education: A conceptual introduction.* Boston: Little, Brown.
MacWhinney, B. (1991). *The CHILDES project: Tools for analyzing talk.* Hillsdale, NJ: Lawrence Erlbaum Associates.
Mahoney, G. (1988). Maternal communication style with mentally retarded children. *American Journal of Mental Deficiency, 92*(4), 352–359.
Mahoney, G., & Powell, A. (1988). Modifying parent–child interaction: Enhancing the development of handicapped children. *Journal of Special Education, 22*(1), 82–96.
McDonald, J.D. (1985). Language through conversation: A model for intervention with delayed persons. In S.F. Warren & A.K. Rogers-Warren (Eds.), *Teaching functional language* (pp. 89–122). Austin, TX: PRO-ED.
Miller, J., & Chapman, R. (1983). *SALT: System analysis of language transcriptions.* Baltimore: University Park Press.
Moerk, E. (1972). Principles of dyadic interaction in language learning. *Merrill-Palmer Quarterly, 18*(3), 229–257.
Moerk, E. (1977). *Pragmatic and semantic aspects of early language development.* Baltimore: University Park Press.
Morris, E.K. (1992). The aim, progress, and evolution of behavior analysis. *The Behavior Analyst, 18*(1), 3–29.
Nelson, K. (1973). Structure and strategy in learning to talk. *Monographs of the Society for Research in Child Development, 38*(1-2, Serial No. 149).
Noddings, N. (1984). Awakening the inner eye: Intuition in education. In N. Noddings & P.J. Shore (Eds.), *Awakening the inner eye.* New York: Teachers College Press.
Olson, S.L., Bayles, K., & Bates, J.E. (1986). Mother–child interaction and children's speech progress: A longitudinal study of the first two years. *Merrill-Palmer Quarterly, 32*(1), 1–20.
Orihara, S. (1983). The effects of repetitive presentation and of I. S. I. in microgenetic experiment with Rorschach cards. *Journal of Child Development, 19*, 23–28.
Ostrosky, M.M., & Kaiser, A.P. (1995). The effects of peer mediated intervention on the social communicative interactions between children with and without special needs. *Journal of Behavioral Education, 5*(2), 151–171.
Premack, D.A. (1970). A functional analysis of language. *Journal of the Experimental Analysis of Behavior, 14*, 107–125.
Ratner, N., & Bruner, J. (1978). Games, social exchange and the acquisition of language. *Journal of Child Language, 5*(3), 391–401.
Schaffer, H.R. (1989). Language development in context. In S. von Tetzchner, L.S. Siegel, & L. Smith (Eds.), *The social and cognitive aspects of normal and atypical language development* (pp. 1–22). New York: Springer-Verlag.

Scherer, N.J., & Olswang, L.B. (1989). Using structured discourse as a language intervention technique with autistic children. *Journal of Speech and Hearing Disorders, 54*, 383–394.

Shepherd, L.J. (1993). *Lifting the veil: The feminine face of science.* Boston: Shambhala.

Skinner, B.F. (1957). *Verbal behavior.* New York: Appleton-Century-Crofts.

Smith, C.B., Adamson, L.B., & Bakeman, R. (1988). Interactional predictors of early language. *First Language, 8*, 143–156.

Snow, C.E. (1984). Parent–child interaction and the development of communicative ability. In R.L. Schiefelbusch & J. Pinker (Eds.), *The acquisition of communicative competence* (pp. 69–107). Baltimore: University Park Press.

Snow, C.E. (1989). In G.E. Speigel & K.E. Nelson (Eds.), *The faces of imitation in language learning* (pp. 84–117). New York: Springer-Verlag.

Snow, C.E., Perlman, R., & Nathan, D.C. (1987). Why routines are different. In K. Nelson & A. van Kleek (Eds.), *Children's language* (Vol. 6, pp. 281–296). Hillsdale, NJ: Lawrence Erlbaum Associates.

Snyder-McLean, L.K., & McLean, J.E. (1978). *A transactional approach to early language training.* Columbus, OH: Charles E. Merrill.

Snyder-McLean, L.K., Solomonson, M.A., McLean, J., & Sack, S. (1984). Structuring joint action routines: A strategy for facilitating communication and language development in the classroom. *Seminars in Speech and Language, 5*(3), 213–228.

Stevens, L.J., & Bliss, L.S. (1995). Conflict resolution abilities of children with specific language impairment and children with normal language. *Journal of Speech and Hearing Research, 38*, 599–611.

Tannock, R., & Girolametto, L. (1992). Reassessing parent-focused language intervention programs. In S.F. Warren & J. Reichle (Eds.), *Communication and language intervention series: Vol. 1. Causes and effects in communication and language intervention* (pp. 49–79). Baltimore: Paul H. Brookes Publishing Co.

Tawney, J.W., & Gast, D.L. (1984). *Single subject research in special education.* Columbus, OH: Charles E. Merrill.

Tomasello, M., & Farrar, M.F. (1986). Joint attention and early language. *Child Development, 57*(6), 1454–1463.

Tomasello, M., Mannle, S., & Kruger, A.C. (1986). Linguistic environment of 1- to 2-year-old twins. *Developmental Psychology, 22*(2), 169–176.

Wolf, M.M. (1978). Social validity: The case for subjective measurement or how applied behavior analysis is finding its heart. *Journal of Applied Behavior Analysis, 11*(2), 203–214.

Yoder, P.J., Davies, B., & Bishop, K. (1992). Getting children with developmental disabilities to talk to adults. In S.F. Warren & J. Reichle (Eds.), *Communication and language intervention series: Vol. 1. Causes and effects in communication and language intervention* (pp. 255–275). Baltimore: Paul H. Brookes Publishing Co.

Yoder, P.J., Kaiser, A.P., & Alpert, C.L. (1991). An exploratory study of the interaction between language teaching methods and child characteristics. *Journal of Speech and Hearing Research, 34*, 155–167.

Yoder, P.J., Kaiser, A.P., Goldstein, H., Alpert, C., Mousetis, L., Kaczmarek, L., & Fischer, R. (1995). A comparison of milieu teaching and responsive interaction in classroom applications. *Topics in Early Childhood Special Education, 14*(4), 218–242.

# 12

# Theoretical and Applied Insights from Multimedia Facilitation of Communication Skills in Children with Autism, Deaf Children, and Children with Other Disabilities

Keith E. Nelson, Mikael Heimann, and Tomas Tjus

This chapter discusses the authors' studies of advances in reading and writing under multimedia literacy instruction by children with varied disabilities. The children in the studies ranged in age from 5-year-olds beginning to read to 10- to 16-year-olds with serious delays in reading and writing skills. Their disabilities included autism, deafness, motor disabilities, dyslexia, and ADHD (attention-deficit/hyperactivity disorder). Regardless of age and disability, these children worked with multimedia computer software designed to facilitate skills in the text mode by patterning text sentences together rapidly with other media channels—graphics, voice, and sign language. Although the findings from this research might appear to have little bearing on understanding

Research reported in this chapter was supported in part by grants from the Swedish Council of Social Research, Stockholm (#90/0090 and #92-0173), to Mikael Heimann. Portions of this chapter have been presented at the sixth Biennial Conference of the International Society for Augmentative and Alternative Communication, Maastricht, the Netherlands, October 1994, and at the IV European Congress of Psychology, Athens, Greece, July 1995. In the United States, research was supported by the Hasbro Children's Foundation and Grants G008300361 and G008302959.

The authors gratefully acknowledge the assistance of Mats Lundälv, Margareta Kärnevik, Eva Lundälv, Lisbeth B. Lindahl, and Katarina Mühlenbock in conducting portions of the research. Special thanks are also due all the participating children, their families, and their schoolteachers.

how communication advances occur in children without disabilities, there are rich connections at the theoretical level among acquisition of different communication modes at different ages by very differently abled children. These theoretical connections arise in part because the design of the multimedia materials and their placement in the social context of teaching were grounded in developmental theory and in part because observations of children with widely varying disabilities making excellent progress in acquisition have generated refinements in theory. In addition, across many years of research effort one can discern further mutual effects, with advances in theoretical accounts of communicative progress in children with disabilities influencing refinements in theoretical accounts for language-typical children, and vice versa.

The first section in this chapter provides the theoretical basis for the multimedia procedures. The next section reviews results of field research for children's advances in reading and writing and for related teacher and child variables. Most of the results involve deaf children and children with autism, but there are important additional data on children with other disabilities and children without disabilities. This chapter also presents significant elaborations and revisions of the initial theoretical base and integrative conclusions.

## FROM THEORY TO PRACTICE: RARE EVENT LEARNING THEORY AND THE DESIGN OF MULTIMEDIA INSTRUCTION

Theoretically we framed our initial work in multimedia with the concepts of REL (Rare Event Learning) theory. According to REL theory, a key to improving learning is to recognize that episodes of significant learning typically are rare because it is difficult to bring together multiple relevant conditions (Nelson, 1980, 1987, 1989, 1991). "Tricky mixes" of conditions must co-occur (Nelson, Perkins, & Lepper, 1996). Challenges must be combined with appropriate preparedness of the learner and complex feedback and regulation conditions. Especially if a child is far behind in skills, such as first-language or literacy skills, then finding new ways to create more effective convergence of multiple learning conditions could be of great importance. Children developing typically and those with disabilities both present a theoretical challenge of providing better, more differentiated accounts of what combinations of learning conditions support slow, moderate, and rapid rates of development. For example, if excellent mixes of conditions are brought together, a child whose learning is typically rare and slow may be able to shift into rapid, sustained rates of learning in the same domain over many months or years.

As our observations of varied children's learning in several cultures grew more differentiated, so too has REL theory. Here we summarize the stable core of ideas in REL theory and present some themes and implications directly influencing the multimedia literacy research. Updates on the theory, including further differentiations of learning conditions, are given in the final two sections of this chapter.

## Overview of REL Theory

REL theory is summarized according to multiple conditions required for significant developmental steps forward, for acquisition of significant new "structures" of comprehension and/or expression. Significant new structures are those that represent definite additions to the complexity and flexibility of the child's repertoire. Across domains and across developmental levels, the broad terms *performance* or *deployment* of a significant new structure are used to allow for a variety of advances in literacy, first-language communication in speech or sign language, problem solving, mathematics, music, art, and other complex domains. The central characteristics of the REL theory have been presented in previously published presentations of the model (Heimann, 1992; Nelson, 1980, 1982, 1987, 1989, 1991; Nelson, Heimann, Abuelhaija, & Wroblewski, 1989). Five categories of learning conditions, abbreviated as *LEARN*, are organized under REL theory, as defined below.

1. *L: Launching Conditions* lead to initial engagement with new challenges. These conditions include paying attention to challenging structures, priming of multiple relevant prior representations, and storing some information in long-term memory, however incomplete, about the challenges. For example, learners might encode into long-term memory some partial representation of structures that challenge their current developmental levels; for beginning readers these might include relative clauses in text, such as "The monkey with the white foot rode the pony."
2. *E: Enhancing Conditions* include some catalysts (e.g., challenge-carrying recasts, rapid interplay of multiple information channels) that limit competing processing demands and that specifically scaffold comparison and abstraction processes in working memory. Other examples of enhancers are learner strategies that fit the current context of learning.
3. *A: Adjustment Conditions* concern ongoing adjustments during learning so that emotion, self-esteem, and motivation converge with other conditions. The learner and supporting partners often will need to take regulatory steps to ensure that emotional, motivational, and attentional levels support sustained processing and learning.
4. *R: Readiness Conditions* are illustrated by preparedness (prior knowledge, interest, and motivation) for new challenges and by degree of intactness of learning mechanisms, which is often hard to estimate for children with autism and many other disabilities.
5. *N: Network Conditions* refer to the need for representations of new structures to be integrated into representational networks. Convergent learning conditions that support such integration often will include multiple modes

of representation and at least a few separate occasions of active processing before newly abstracted structures are consolidated. In addition, powerful effects on developmental progress can be seen if particular episodes of learning stimulate multiple levels of processing of challenging new structures.

In comparison with related developmental theories, REL theory provides more emphasis than most on understanding the conditions under which new structures are initially acquired and then consolidated. It is one variety of cognitive information-processing theory and thus has many commonalities with cognitive orientations in accounts of growth of language and conceptual knowledge (Bohannon & Stanowicz, 1989; Bowerman, 1985; Maratsos & Chalkley, 1980; Slobin, 1985). However, because REL theory stipulates that social, emotional, and self-concept conditions integrally mix with traditionally more cognitive and linguistic components of learning, it has the heuristic value of suggesting new kinds of observations on how learning is hindered or supported. In this respect, REL theory has much in common with dynamic systems accounts of how multiple systems (perceptual, motor, emotional, social, linguistic) couple or interact to support skilled performance and learning (e.g., Csikszentmihalyi, 1990, 1993; Thelen, 1988; Thelen & Smith, 1994). Left open is the possible identification of maturationally based neural components specific to language, but any such components would affect language progress only when other conditions in the child's actual interactions with conversational partners are favorable. In common with cognitive theorizing by Siegler (1991), REL theory suggests that the path to eventual mastery of new complex skills can be highly varied across individual children.

## REL Theory in Multimedia Literacy Design

In the context of first-language learning, the framework of REL theory has helped to identify specific growth recast discourse events that carry syntactic challenge and make such challenge highly processable. *Growth recasts* in conversation are adult replies that maintain a child's basic meaning but that recast sentence structure to incorporate a challenge to that child's current syntax. Processability and learning of the challenge is aided by the convergence of primed meaning and syntax from the child's own sentence with the recast challenge and with additional conditions that limit processing demands overall in working memory. Empirically, findings from naturalistic as well as experimental work have shown that adult uses of syntactic recasting outside computer contexts have promoted children's acquisition of new syntactic structures (e.g., Camarata & Nelson, 1992; Camarata, Nelson, & Camarata, 1994; Nelson, 1977, 1987, 1989, 1991).

Design of our multimedia communication procedures was directly influenced by this framework in three ways. First, multimedia teachers were trained to employ side conversations that incorporated growth recasts, both to boost the child's first-language foundation (sign or speech) for literacy and to provide additional cognitive-social *enhancer* conditions that could aid in engaging the child's processing of the challenging text material on the computer.

Second, the multimedia event sequences were designed to direct the child's limited active processing capacity toward comparisons of new text to already known representations of graphic events and of voice or sign. Table 1 gives some examples of the possible interactive sequences among child, computer, and teacher. As viewed from the REL theory, such intermodal comparisons were expected to contribute rapidly to learning if multiple processing facilitators were built into the multimedia (MM) interactions. One such *catalyst* was the one-to-one nature of the modes used in the multimedia materials ALPHA and Delta*Messages*, where each sentence in text corresponds closely to the animated graphic and first-language (speech or sign) sentences, as for "THE DINOSAUR FEEDS THE PENGUIN" example in Table 1. Such close correspondence is not typical in instructional sequences with books and with many other MM programs. In addition, rapid creation of a sentence followed by animations and voice or sign also was considered another potentially strong *catalyst* for effective processing. Within about 20 seconds all three modes of representation for a single complex event can be entered into active processing arenas and used to support explicit comparisons between text structure and the information carried by the other modes. Furthermore, after the child "launches" his or her completed sentence, there are no demands for response (and thus no processing capacity demanded to support such responses) occurring while the child processes the graphic and first-language modes of presentation. In combination, the sequence of events provides *multiple processing opportunities for building new representational networks.*

The third direct influence of REL theory on the multimedia procedures was design to support three *adjustment conditions*: emotional, self-esteem, and motivational levels. The MM was designed so that the child's successful initia-

Table 1. Examples of interactive sequences

| |
|---|
| *Hearing children with autism or other disabilities* |
| Child enters text, "THE DINOSAUR FEEDS THE PENGUIN" |
| MM[a] animation, The dinosaur feeds the penguin |
| MM voice says, "The dinosaur feeds the penguin" |
| Child comments in voice |
| Teacher recasts or elaborates in voice |
| *Deaf children using sign language* |
| Child enters text, "THE DINOSAUR FEEDS THE PENGUIN" |
| MM animation, The dinosaur feeds the penguin |
| MM signs, THE DINOSAUR FEEDS THE PENGUIN |
| Child comments in sign |
| Teacher recasts or elaborates in sign |

[a]MM (multimedia).

tion and control of exploratory MM sequences would promote high self-esteem and high motivation to explore many sequences. In addition, colorful, rapid, animated graphics as well as teacher–child interactions were expected to support positive emotions and continued motivation to explore.

REL theory oriented us to look for new observations on how multiple converging conditions can trigger effective learning of new reading and writing skills. From the outset the research program sought to adapt patterns of multimedia and teacher presentation of challenges to children with different disabilities. For example, switch versions would make navigation of multimedia possible for children with motor impairments. Similarly, sign language "in" the multimedia and "beside" the multimedia (teacher sign recasts) would give deaf children processing opportunities for directly comparing their first language to graphics and text. However, as production and field testing of the multimedia design proceeded, practice has also driven theory, making REL theory increasingly differentiated.

## PRACTICE: FIELD TEST RESEARCH RESULTS

All results are from studies in which children worked with multimedia along with a teacher who used specific social-interactive strategies. The multimedia materials provided the ALPHA teaching series to children using Apple II computers and Delta*Messages* teaching series to children using Macintosh computers. Table 2 describes key features of ALPHA and Delta*Messages* including sign language options and single- or double-switch options for children with motor disabilities.

Within ALPHA or Delta*Messages*, each child creates text sentences by selecting written words or phrases. This selection varies by the child's disability and the available hardware, with children selecting from a standard keyboard; a programmable keyboard; or on-screen interfaces controlled by head switches, breath switches, or a keyboard mouse. The children spend most of their time in an interactive exploratory activity in which the computer offers choices of words for making sentences, and each child interacts with these choices to create a sequence of text sentences. The child's interactive choices also determine whether graphics only or additional modes (sign or speech) are triggered when a text sentence is completed. In these exploratory periods, children are expected to learn new reading and writing skills based on the cognitive comparisons they make between text and other representational modes. Some sequences of events typical in these exploratory periods were shown in Table 1 for deaf children and for hearing children with disabilities such as autism and cerebral palsy.

Field tests exploring the impact of ALPHA and Delta*Messages* on literacy and other communication skills revealed important shared characteristics for the multiple studies reviewed in the following sections. In each, multimedia

Table 2. Brief descriptions of the ALPHA and Delta*Messages* programs

| | ALPHA[a] | Delta*Messages*[b] |
|---|---|---|
| Lessons | A total of 112 lessons and 180 words (mostly nouns and verbs) in either English or Swedish | A total of 10 lessons and 60 words |
| Working modes | One of the following: Individual Words (IW), Creating Sentences (CS), Testing Words (TW), and Testing Sentences (TS) | Selection of one of the following: Pretest 1, Pretest 2, Creating Sentences, Posttest 1, Posttest 2 |
| Type of sentences | The central learning activity is Creating Sentences by combining words in simple noun-verb-noun sequences such as "The bear"-"jumps over"-"the horse." When the sentence is complete the computer triggers an animation showing the action the child has described. | Lessons 1–6 make it possible to construct noun-verb-noun sequences. Lessons 7 and 8 add prepositions, and lessons 9 and 10 make use of conjunctions and adjectives; 190 different sentences can be constructed in the 1995 version of the program. |
| Options | The child and his or her teacher had the options of 1) American Sign Language; 2) scanning for single-switch users; and 3) a basic computer keyboard (arrow keys) version. Speed adjustment of animations was also possible. | Three versions of the program exist: 1) Swedish Sign Language, 2) scanning for single-switch users, and 3) a basic mouse version. Speed adjustment of animations was also possible. |
| Procedure | After having explored a lesson in CS mode twice, the teacher switched to the TS mode for that lesson. At any given level, a child was judged to have reached mastery if he or she achieved a score of or above 80% correct in the TS mode. | Depending on the needs of the individual learner, particular combinations of language modes can be employed (e.g., graphics and speech can be presented after the child writes a sentence such as "The panda puts the pizza on the gorilla's table"). Alternatively, children who have motor disabilities use specially adapted controls for the computer enabling them to complete all multimedia explorations and tests that other children experience. |
| System requirements | Apple IIe, 128K RAM, 2 5¼" disk drives, and color monitor with an optional videodisc player | Macintosh (68020 or faster processor), 8 MB RAM, and a CD-ROM drive or an external SyQuest 22MB drive. |

[a] Nelson & Prinz (1991).
[b] Nelson & Heimann (1995).

exploration was the primary activity to promote text learning, and side conversations with teachers assisted with literacy and promoted first-language skills (in speech and sign). In a typical ALPHA or Delta*Messages* study, schools have provided fairly brief instruction (approximately 10–30 hours over 2–4 months) as a supplement to an extant reading and writing curriculum. Multimedia pretests and posttests have been one gauge of student progress in literacy. In addition, individual studies have examined additional aspects of gains in first language, generalized literacy gains outside the multimedia, details of what specific literacy gains have been made, and student and teacher characteristics associated with rates of student progress.

## Introduction to Research in Sweden on Children with Autism

Because language skills are considered a core factor for later functioning, and for prediction of outcome in adulthood, we were motivated to try our MM strategy with children with autism. Yet autism presents special challenges for multimedia instructional strategies. In one study of the effect of multimedia procedures for promoting language learning among children with autism, Colby (1973) reported positive effects on language and motivation for 13 out of 17 participating nonspeaking children with autism. Overall, the few published results tend to report some positive effects of computer-based instruction for children with autism (e.g., Bernard-Optiz, Ross, & Tuttas, 1990; Chen & Bernard-Optiz, 1993; Coldwell, 1991a,b; Jordan & Powell, 1990a,b; Panyan, 1984). In addition, several studies have also found that computer instruction might be beneficial for children with other types of developmental disabilities (e.g., Green & Clark, 1991; Light, 1988; Nelson, Prinz, Prinz, & Dalke, 1991; Romski & Sevcik, 1989, 1991; Underwood & Underwood, 1990). However, the studies show large variations in subject selection, length of training, and type of program used, making it difficult to compare results across studies. Romanczyk, Ekdahl, and Lockshin (1992) noted that children with autism who had explicitly expressed their preference for the computer actually performed better with the teacher instead. Thus, viewed in whole, the literature suggests the need for more carefully documented studies to sort the advantages and disadvantages of particular kinds of computer instruction with or without multimedia procedures for children with autism.

Children with autism, however, typically possess two characteristics that might seem to contradict their "fit" with the multimedia literacy approach just described. First, because they show relatively low skill and low interest in language, their engagement with the speech and text channels of multimedia presentations could be limited. Second, because children with autism often have a relatively low interest in social interaction, this could blunt the effectiveness of side conversations between teacher and child. Children with autism have severe problems in establishing any interaction that requires mutuality or understanding intentions (e.g., Caparulo & Cohen, 1983; Frith, 1989), and approximately half the population of children with autism fail to acquire even rudimentary spoken language (Lotter, 1978; Tager-Flusberg, 1989, 1994).

Despite these potential difficulties, we decided to use our approach of multimedia plus teacher instruction with children with autism as well as with children with other disabilities. As long as the program included appropriate text challenges for an individual child and some method of basic communication existed between teacher and child, we were willing to try our procedures with any child after obtaining parental consent. This optimism was based on the theoretically guided features of the multimedia procedures that were intended to support motivational engagement as well as cognitive processing of new levels of text complexity. In addition, some observations stress that many children with autism are visual thinkers and might need strong visual input to learn new material (Grandin, 1995).

Swedish ALPHA and Delta*Messages* studies will be considered first, followed by observations made within a series of studies carried out in the United States and Belgium.

## Swedish ALPHA Research: Design and Methods

In Sweden, ALPHA software (Nelson & Prinz, 1991) was first offered to children with autism who had displayed some ability to communicate in spoken sentences (Heimann, Nelson, Gillberg, & Kärnevik, 1993; Heimann, Nelson, Tjus, & Gillberg, 1993). We reasoned previously that if enough positive adjustments of emotion and motivation could be provided by the MM strategy, then the convergence of these conditions with multiple processing and abstraction catalysts embedded in the program would make learning more efficient for new text challenges as suggested by REL theory. The theory also stipulates that any obvious progress made by a child would in turn feed the child's motivation for further interaction and learning. A key task for the teachers, accordingly, was to use as many attentional facilitators and self-esteem supports and individually adjusted growth recasts as possible to help engage the children with autism. For other groups of children—children with deafness, motor problems, and/or mental retardation—the theoretical underpinnings remained the same, but the teachers adapted their side conversations to the children's quite diverse attentional and language patterns. In REL terms, the combined teacher strategies and software characteristics were melded to try to achieve a convergence (i.e., tricky mix) of multiple conditions favorable for learning and motivation for each child.

Three groups of children participated in the Swedish ALPHA research program (Heimann, 1995; Heimann, Nelson, Gillberg, & Kärnevik, 1993; Heimann, Nelson, Tjus, & Gillberg, 1995; Heimann, Tjus, & Nelson, 1995):

1. Children with autism: nine boys and two girls with a median CA (chronological age) of 7:11 years (range: 6:9–13:8) and a median MA (mental age) of 6:11 years (range: 3:0–9:5)

2. Children with mixed disabilities: four boys and five girls with cerebral palsy and/or mental retardation and a median CA of 15:7 years (range: 6:11–20:9) and a median MA of 5:6 years (range: 5:0–6:6)
3. Preschool children: 10 typical preschool children (2 boys and 8 girls) with a median CA of 6:1 years (range: 5:0–7:6) and a median MA of 6:2 years (range: 5:6–8:0)

The children worked weekly with the ALPHA program ($M=1.5$ times per week; $SD=0.9$) over a period of 2–4 months ($M=13.6$ weeks; $SD=8.3$), and each session lasted up to 30 minutes. All children were tested for reading (word and sentences) and phonological awareness at the onset (Start-test), at the end of the intervention (Post 1), and at a follow-up approximately one semester later (Post 2). In addition, each dyad was videotaped for 9 minutes during one initial and one final lesson with ALPHA to allow coding of varied teacher and child behaviors. The most relevant behavior categories, coded by 10-second intervals and incorporating both nonverbal and verbal behavior, for the child were "off task," "relevant verbal expressions," "asks for help," and "enjoyment"; and for the teacher (see Table 3), "enjoyment," "elaborates" (on child verbal expression), and "directs verbally" (directing attention to multimedia).

## Swedish ALPHA Research: Results

***Abstractions of New Text Skills*** Both the children with autism and mixed disabilities displayed a significant increase in reading gains (on mea-

Table 3. A brief description of categories for coding the teacher's interactive behavior while working with ALPHA

| Category | Brief description or example |
|---|---|
| Procedural comments | "Click on the green button, move the cursor." |
| Content comments | "Did you see what the man did?" |
| Directs verbally | "Look at the screen!" |
| Solves problem | The teacher helps the child to move the cursor when the child has problems handling the mouse. Or, the teacher takes control of the mouse and moves the cursor to its appropriate area on the screen. |
| Explains | The teacher explains why something is happening (e.g., why the printer is working after a certain command). |
| Elaborates | The student is saying something and the teacher picks up the meaning and gives it back in a new frame (e.g., the child says, "The egg is eating the window" and the teacher responds, "Yes, that doesn't happen in real life, but here we can see magic things!"). |
| Praises | "Well done!" |
| Scolds | "Don't be foolish!" |
| Helps | This variable was only scored if the student asked specifically for help (otherwise the solves problem category was used). |
| Enjoyment | Both verbal and nonverbal expressions or comments indicating a positive affect |

sures made outside the MM computer setting) during the intervention. On average, the children with autism increased their reading levels 11% and the children with mixed disabilities, 5%. Only the children with autism continued to display significant gains after the intervention had ended: The follow-up (Post 2) test revealed an additional gain of 5% on reading. A different pattern was detected for the typically developing preschool children: Significant gains were observed at all three data points (Start, Post 1, and Post 2), which suggests that the employed intervention had a more specific effect on reading for the children with communicative disabilities than for the preschool group.

***Abstraction of New First-Language Skills*** The combined results for the children with autism and mixed disabilities reveal a significant gain on a sentence imitation measure of overall skill in spoken Swedish as a result of the intervention.

***Verbal and Motivational Clues to Children's Engagement*** The intervention succeeded in promoting an increase in relevant interaction between children with autism and the teacher. An increase of 75% was observed for the child variable "relevant verbal expressions" ($t(10)=2.89$; $p<.01$). In contrast, the "off task" category remained unchanged from early to late in the lesson series. Furthermore, the children with autism also asked for help more frequently (an increase of 108%) during the final lesson than during the initial intervention phase, which might be a positive side effect caused by the observed increase in verbal expression or because the children felt more comfortable with the MM computer environment toward the end of the intervention. Furthermore, a significant increase in "enjoyment" ($t(10)=2.19$; $p<.03$) was observed for the children with autism, indicating that the children increased their tendencies to express positive feelings as an effect of working with the ALPHA program. These changes over time in children's verbalizations and enjoyment seem to reflect the rich and engaging teaching environment created by the combined triadic interaction among the child, teacher, and program. Reading gains and child-controlled exploratory choices by the children may have contributed to the emotional climate during instruction and also may have aided in *self-esteem regulation, enhancement of motivation*, and *confidence*.

Data on the teachers also give insights into the instructional dynamics. For example, the teachers' "enjoyment" as coded from the videos correlated positively ($r=.55$, $p<.03$, $n=17$) with observed gains in reading scores from start to follow-up when data from the children with autism and the children with mixed disabilities were combined. In contrast, the category "directs verbally" displayed a negative relationship with gains in reading ($r=-.56$; $p<.02$, $n=17$). Another almost significant positive correlation was noted between the teachers' use of elaborations and gains in reading, although this was only significant for the children with autism ($r=.57$, $p<.08$, $n=10$).

In combination, these findings on teachers' interactive styles indicate that a highly supportive atmosphere (e.g., a lot of enjoyment) and nonintrusive demeanor promote a learning environment that increases the children's motivation, independence, and self-esteem, thus enhancing the chances of learning. These conclusions arising from the field-test data are reflected in the Revised Theory section later in the chapter. In addition, they also fit conclusions put forward by Koegel and Koegel (1995) and Prizant and Wetherby (1989), who believe that a facilitative teaching style is more advantageous than a directive style. That is, a more responsive, less directive teacher in a context of child-controlled exploration of multimedia might promote more relevant interaction and more communicative eye gaze and might stimulate the student to ask more questions.

Clues to *motivational engagement* can be seen also in the active choices made by children. The only rule that ALPHA imposes on the child is that the sentence has to be grammatically correct; the content is decided by the child. This can be exemplified by the words included in ALPHA Lesson 14: *the horse, the apple, the banana, the lion, the crocodile, the girl, eats*, and *jumps over*. These words make it possible to construct both realistic sentences such as "The girl eats the apple" and fantasy sentences such as "The apple eats the lion." This program flexibility is important for conveying to the child that language is created in the mind and can be used to describe all kinds of events, whether they are possible in the real world. In the Swedish ALPHA study, all three groups of children increased their observed means of fanciful sentences (see Table 4). The children's use of realistic sentences, however, showed a different pattern (see Table 4): The children with autism and mixed disabilities displayed a significant decrease over time in the use of realistic sentences while the typical preschool children displayed no change. Thus, the program motivates all children to create new and fanciful events, regardless of whether the child has a disability or not. The fantasy sentences also seem to be so interesting for children with autism or mixed disabilities that the proportion of fantasy sentences rises relative to realistic sentences.

Table 4. Mean frequencies of fanciful and realistic sentences created by three different groups of children while working with the Swedish version of the ALPHA program

| | Start | | Post | | |
|---|---|---|---|---|---|
| | *M*[a] | *SD* | *M*[a] | *SD* | *p*-level |
| *Fanciful sentences* | | | | | |
| Autism | 3.2 | 2.3 | 8.3 | 5.5 | <.05 |
| Mixed disabilities | 6.7 | 6.6 | 13.2 | 10.6 | ns |
| Preschool | 1.8 | 1.5 | 6.5 | 2.7 | <.02 |
| *Realistic sentences* | | | | | |
| Autism | 7.2 | 3.6 | 4.7 | 3.0 | <.07 |
| Mixed disabilities | 13.2 | 10.6 | 8.3 | 7.6 | <.05 |
| Preschool | 6.5 | 2.7 | 6.9 | 1.8 | ns |

[a]Reported means are based on the three first and three final ALPHA sessions when the child used the Creating Sentences mode.

Children with autism ($n=9$), mixed disabilities ($n=9$) and preschool children ($n=8$).

One specific case illustration helps convey the motivational effects on literacy of the multimedia instruction. Mats, a 19-year-old man with autism (MA: 9:6 years), used ALPHA although he was almost too good a reader to be included in the study. But he greatly enjoyed the program and constantly asked his teacher if he could continue to work with ALPHA. This boy did not show strong gains on our tests because he began already close to the ceiling, but following his entry into the ALPHA procedures he did start to combine words into two- and three-word sentences when asked to write down simple descriptions. For example, Mats provided written descriptions when asked by his teacher to write a short note on what he did during the weekend. To his teacher and his parents, this breakthrough in his development was a major achievement. He always had written his messages in telegraphic one-word sentences, and his teacher had struggled for years with Mats' inability to write sentences. For Mats, "writing" ALPHA sentences to produce graphic animations on the computer may have provided *multiple opportunities to enrich* representational networks. These new representations in turn may have helped him to consolidate his awareness of written expression and to move toward more flexible use of his text skills (Nelson & Nelson, 1978).

Children's *readiness* for learning also influenced reading progress. There was a strong prediction to reading gain from the initial willingness and success of the child in imitating sentences verbally. This very simple sentence imitation test displayed a correlation of .78 with gains in reading scores measured at the follow-up. Also, as expected, estimation of the children's MA proved predictive ($r = .53$) as did the receptive (Reynell Developmental Language Scales; Reynell, 1985) language score ($r = .45$). Summarizing these results with the information on the teachers, from a REL theory perspective, higher rates of progress during literacy instruction may be a dynamic mix of learner *readiness*, social-emotional *adjustments* by both the child and teacher, and *multimedia-enhanced abstractions* of new text structures.

### Swedish Delta*Messages* Research: Introduction and Design

Delta*Messages* provides a powerful new multimedia learning station for communicative development. The system takes advantage of the skills of the teacher in providing rich conversational models and in helping to motivate the child's learning from the multimedia material. Thus, regardless of the particular child's initial literacy and general communication skills, the multimedia teaching project aims to help each child move forward through higher levels of reading, writing, and general communication skills (e.g., from simple noun-verb-noun sentences to more complex events that include both adjectives and conjunctions).

Delta*Messages* for Macintosh is a newer program (Nelson & Heimann, 1995) than the ALPHA program for Apple II that allows an even faster pace of events and increases both the number of language modes that can be employed and the complexity of the sentences that can be constructed. For instance, a deaf child may construct a sentence in text and then see the appropriate meaning a few seconds later in sign language along with video clips and/or graphics of the relevant events, and a child with cerebral palsy might use specially adapted controls for the computer enabling him or her to complete all multimedia explorations and tests that other children experience. In cognitive processing terms, combinations of presentation modes are chosen so that each child finds it easy to process his or her best modes (e.g., graphics, speech) and uses these modes to learn new modes and new levels of communication.

Based on experience with ALPHA, researchers expected Delta*Messages* to provide new, expanded research insights into learning processes and to be a flexible and motivating tool for supporting communicative development among both children with disabilities and typically developing children. Some support for this can be found in our first preliminary analysis of the reading data from 31 boys and 18 girls who had used the program before May 1996. These children had a median CA of 9:5 years (range: 5:1–13:8) and a median MA of 8:6 years (range: 5:0–13:8) and belonged to four main groups:

1. Children with autism: 10 boys and 3 girls with a median CA of 9:10 years (range: 5:1–11:11) and a median MA of 6:6 years (range: 5:6–10:9).
2. Children with learning disabilities (dyslexia and/or ADHD): 12 boys and 2 girls with a median CA of 8:8 years (range: 7:3–13:8) and a median MA of 8:8 years (range: 7:3–13:8).
3. Deaf children (all of whom use Swedish Sign Language as their main mode of communication): four boys and seven girls with a median CA of 7:5 years (range: 5:10–8:0) and a median MA of 8:6 years (range: 5:0–11:0).
4. Children with motor disabilities (e.g., cerebral palsy): five boys and six girls with a median CA of 10:2 years (range: 9:5–12:11) and a median MA of 5:6 years (range: 5:6–9:0).

The children who participated used a Swedish version of Delta*Messages* and received instruction during 3–4 months ($M=3.4$ months; $SD=1.4$). Comparison data were collected also during baseline and follow-up periods ($M=1.6$ months, $SD=0.7$ and $M=2.1$, $SD=0.6$). All children received training more than once weekly and each session lasted between 15 and 30 minutes.

Multiple assessments were carried out for all children (during baseline, at start, during the intervention, at the end, and in follow-up). In addition, teachers were given questionnaires, and the software itself builds in brief but effective assessment activities as a part of every session with the computer and teacher. However, only the data on the children's reading gains per month have been analyzed.

Three different tests were used to measure progress in reading: Flashcard A or B (sentences), Flashcard C (words), and Umesol (letter identification and word reading). Flashcards A, B, and C were developed within the project

(Heimann, Nelson, Tjus, & Gillberg, 1995), while the Umesol reading test (Taube, Tornéus, & Lundberg, 1984) is a recognized instrument in Sweden. The reading score measured gain in readings based on a combined score from all three tests.

### Swedish Delta *Messages* Research: Results

Our analyses show almost no gain in reading during the initial baseline period ($M = 1.4$; $SD = 5.8$), but a significant increase during training with Delta*Messages* ($M = 4.8$; $SD = 5.6$; $t\ (48) = 3.5$, $p < .001$) was noted. Of the 49 children, 35 showed an increase in reading as a result of the MM computer strategy. Specifically, positive gains were displayed by 10 of the 13 children with autism, 10 of the 14 children with learning disabilities, 7 of the 11 deaf children, and 8 of the 11 children with motor disabilities. However, in these initial findings, neither the results from the follow-up nor the data from letter identification tests, in-built tests within the computer program, or teacher questionnaire reports are incorporated.

### Integrative Conclusions from Swedish Studies

The ALPHA and Delta*Messages* findings from Sweden suggest two conclusions. First, progress in literacy and other communicative modes can be triggered by teacher plus computer instructional programs if both the multimedia (sign, voice, text, graphics) and the teacher's strategies and styles are well adapted to the child's cognitive, language, socioemotional, and perceptual-motor levels. Second, concepts from the REL theory have relevance for children with autism, deafness, and other disabilities. They help us to understand why learning sometimes has not taken place and provide analytic tools that can help in the design of teaching strategies and multimedia event patterns so that there are greatly enhanced chances that learning will take place.

### Field-Test Research in the United States and Belgium: The ALPHA Program and Deaf Children

Deaf children between 6 and 18 years of age in every country studied have shown on average very substantial delays in their progress in literacy. Many studies have found reading ability at age 18 to be only at the second- to fourth-grade level for the majority of high school students (Nelson, Loncke, & Camarata, 1993). Our research has focused on students with moderate to profound hearing impairments who read below grade level and who know and use sign language, but with varying levels of mastery. For these students, creating favorable learning conditions consistent with REL theory often is complicated without the use of multimedia because there is a shortage of teachers who have fluent sign language skills. Abstracting new text skills according to REL theory should be supported by rapid entry into working memory of the child's best conversational language (here it is sign) together with nonverbal meaning and text. The sign-text-graphics multimedia in ALPHA plus specially chosen teachers with fluent sign skills as the child's partner for the multimedia sessions comprise one theoretically motivated approach to facilitating text and sign alike through the same teaching sessions.

Varied test trials have generated six sets of related outcomes. First, Nelson et al. (1989) found that all 63 deaf children taught with ALPHA performed in the range of 87%–100% correct on the ALPHA test sentence assessments built in to ALPHA for assessing mastery after lesson exploration. On independent paper-and-pencil reading tests, gains were 14.8% from preinstruction to postinstruction.

Second, deaf and hearing children alike need to learn to deal with text in the "formal" sense that a written sentence means whatever it says, even if the message is fanciful (e.g., "The dinosaur feeds the girl"). Two studies examined children's handling of such sentences, and they concurred that with ALPHA materials deaf children reach equal mastery on fanciful sentences and on highly realistic sentences (Nelson, Carter, & Prinz, in review; Nelson et al., 1991). These results complement the findings reported on active engagement with fanciful sentences by Swedish children.

Third, in Belgium, a program used a variation on ALPHA that organized the sentences examined during exploratory activity into stories. Deaf children received instruction either in French or in Dutch, depending on their best prior text language. Evaluation completed on the Dutch material demonstrated gains of more than 50% after 10 weeks of instruction (Prinz, Nelson, Loncke, Geysels, & Willems, 1993).

The fourth related outcome is that generalized reading gains averaging 19% were shown when 16 deaf students received computer-based ALPHA materials supported by videodisc graphics and sign language (Nelson et al., 1991).

Fifth, in a direct comparison of high-frequency use of optional sign language graphics and low-frequency use of such graphics, Nelson et al. (in review) observed a substantial learning bonus for the deaf students opting for high-frequency comparisons of the sign language to the text and event-graphics channels explored during ALPHA interactions.

The sixth related outcome concerns deaf children using ALPHA who made gains in general communication skills that appear to have been supported by the combination of multimedia language channels and the side conversations (with teacher recasting). In particular, sign language skill gains, compared with children only receiving traditional literacy instruction, were made at the level of sentence complexity and in terms of flexible referential communication messages that clearly described pictures.

### Conclusions for Studies in the United States and Belgium

These studies show extensive replication of literacy gains by U.S. and Belgian deaf children who explored ALPHA multimedia programs. As predicted theoretically, reliance on sign language as one representational channel within the multimedia boosted rates of learning to read and write. Writing is directly involved because within the multimedia the children write text to create sentences (both in tests and in exploration), with accurate test performance dependent on the child reading and selecting the appropriate text chunks from the interface (monitor or special keyboard). Moreover, it is clear that the successful abstraction of new text skills for deaf children can be achieved through many variants on multimedia details: fanciful sentences as well as realistic ones, diskette-stored computer graphics versus film and video clips on videodisc, sentence-level exploration, or sentences embedded in story contexts. Abstraction of new sign language skills depended primarily on the recasting side conversational behavior of the teachers, but the multimedia sign presentations probably also played a positive role. Finally, it is of theoretical relevance to observe that deaf learners are as efficient in their literacy gains per hour of ALPHA multimedia instruction as children with no disabilities. This outcome is fully in line with many theoretical arguments and empirical observations indicating that cognitive mechanisms for deaf students match those for hearing students. To apply intact cognitive abilities successfully to literacy and in turn to academic achievement is notably harder and less frequent for the deaf students because it has been much harder to set up equally supportive learning conditions for the deaf (Clark, 1993; Marschark, 1993; Nelson et al., 1993).

The following sections address theoretical refinements influenced by the full set of these field-test outcomes. The discussion also covers potential ways of further enhancing processing and learning through modifications of the multimedia software and the interlinked teacher activities.

## FROM PRACTICE TO REVISED THEORY: TRICKY MIX ELABORATIONS OF THE REL THEORY

Theoretically, how the children in the ALPHA and Delta*Messages* projects progressed in literacy and other skills holds insights concerning learning processes and instructional design for children without disabilities. This section offers a newly differentiated account of the many "tricky mix" conditions that need to converge in multimedia teaching to produce significant learning and elaborates on key components of REL theory presented previously in this chapter. The revised theory is discussed for typical language acquisition as well as for varied communicative modes in children with disabilities.

The revised theory claims that it is indeed "tricky" to achieve sufficiently appropriate and supportive conditions to trigger sustained, significant learning in any child, but that the five central factors making up the tricky mixes are basically the same for children with and without disabilities. What varies substantially across individual children are the moves by interacting teachers or interacting multimedia that bring particular realizations of these central factors into effective tricky mixes.

Based on work by Nelson, Perkins, and Lepper (1996) and reflections on the data just given, we present some of the most salient conditions that seem to work together to facilitate children's learning of significant new skills. The REL framework stresses that any one of these conditions is insufficient for learning. Instead, the conditions need to be woven together in a dynamic fashion to form richly scaffolded occasions of learning. Table 5 uses the five LEARN categories explained previously in this chapter but elaborates with more specific conditions that contribute to tricky mixes.

## Launching Conditions in Tricky Mixes

Learning any new level of literacy must begin by somehow challenging a child's current skill levels. In ALPHA and Delta*Messages*, challenges to literacy occur only if the lesson selected is appropriate; sometimes the student may

Table 5. Tricky mixes for learning: Dynamically contributing conditions within five central categories

| | |
|---|---|
| L | Launching conditions |
| | Challenges to learner |
| | Prior primes |
| | Settings |
| | Initial expectancies |
| E | Enhancers: Strategies and catalysts |
| | Attentional catalysts |
| | Motivational catalysts |
| | Abstraction catalysts |
| | Background processing strategies |
| | Foreground mindfulness and monitoring |
| | Feedback elicitors |
| | Fun, humor, and entertainment |
| A | Adjustment processes |
| | Inhibition regulation |
| | Emotional regulation |
| | Self-esteem regulation |
| | Expectancy/confidence regulation |
| | Cultural–social processes |
| | Motivational cycles |
| | Attributional processes |
| R | Readiness: Learner conditions |
| | Domain engages learner identity |
| | Motivational and attributional dispositions |
| | Intactness of learning mechanisms |
| | Initial learner strategies |
| | Learner preparedness for challenge |
| N | Networks: Multiple networked representations |
| | Parallel processing and multiple buffers |
| | Multiple recasting-facilitated comparisons |
| | Follow-through opportunities |
| | Sustained processing rounds until new structures are consolidated |
| | Redundant and "overlearned" networks |

not object if lively multimedia without challenge is presented. A child and adult may have a smooth, enjoyable conversation that offers no challenge. In working with deaf children, drills may be selected that are too simple to introduce needed complexities and that preclude full exposure to a written language (de Villiers, de Villiers, & Hoban, 1994). Thus, it is far from routine to ensure that challenges are available to a child, either at home or at school. There also is the complex issue of what particular levels or zones of challenge are needed to allow processing and learning by a child at a particular stage of acquisition in speech, text, sign language, or other skill domains (e.g., Nelson, 1991; Olswang, Bain, & Johnson, 1992; Salomon, 1993; Salomon, Globerson, & Guterman, 1989).

Analyzing the structure of new text material such as "The dinosaur feeds the lion" within Delta*Messages* may be substantially easier as an episode of interaction proceeds. Long-term memory primes will become increasingly rich as the child progresses from the first sentence to a fifth or tenth sentence dealing with overlapping content, just as priming becomes increasingly rich when a series of recasts tied to one central sentence event is produced. These prior primes retrieved from long-term memory are likely to allow more powerful and complete abstraction processes than teaching instances in which a challenge previously unseen is initially placed before the learner.

## Enhancers: Strategies and Catalysts in Tricky Mixes

The rapid timing, animation or video motion, color, and learner control and navigation are central ALPHA and Delta*Messages* features, which can serve as attentional catalysts and motivational catalysts for learners both with and without disabilities. In the multimedia research reviewed in this chapter, recasts are central techniques employed within the software and also by the child's teacher. Single recasts and multiple recast sequences are among the best-established catalysts of comparisons between challenges and already retrieved current language structures. These comparisons in turn will lead in many instances to the abstractions of new structural representations that are crucial to significant learning. However, many new techniques and procedures are needed that also serve as catalysts for comparison, abstraction, and learning of new communicative structures.

Beyond single occasions of effective processing of some aspects of a new text challenge, fully learning the challenge requires a powerful long-term memory. Central to learning most complex new challenges in language (speech, sign, or text) is the build-up in long-term memory of a set of examplars and related information that never co-occurred in any brief episode for the learner. When selective retrieval assembles multiple examplars for a type of word, sentence, or narrative that represents a challenge for the child, then abstraction and comparison processes can go to work on this examplar set. This timely retrieval in turn depends on selective storage in long-term memory of processed challenges and "tags" for later retrieval. We have seen some children with autism and developmental delays whose immediate memory was intact but whose retrieval of challenge information later from long-term memory was markedly impaired compared with peers' memory. Within the multimedia framework of Delta*Messages*, the tricky mix perspective suggests that specific retrieval cue bonuses can be provided as a scaffold for long-term memory efficiency by such children.

Even if all these other conditions are met, unless a match in strategies occurs for the learner relative to the learning context, there may be frequent disruptions of the learner's processing and learning of available challenges. For example, if a child who seldom finds direct imitation useful is asked by a teacher, parent, or therapist to produce such imitative responses, he or she may react with lower affective engagement and then lower attention and learning (Haley, Camarata, & Nelson, 1994; Nelson, Camarata, Welsh, Butkovsky, & Camarata, 1996). Or too much directiveness by a teacher may disrupt the learning of a child who prefers independence in exploring multimedia challenges.

Similar notions apply in research by Lepper, Woolverton, Mumme, and Gurtner (1993) on children's progress in mathematics when they receive remedial tutoring. Analysis of videotapes of highly effective versus less-effective tutors indicates that they often teach by indirect means, such as focusing their comments more on encouragement, self-esteem support, the child's own experience and reflection, and humor than on direct steps needed to solve a problem correctly.

## Adjustment Processes in Tricky Mixes

As Fox (1994) argued, successful action and decision sequences depend as much on inhibition processes at both cortical and subcortical levels as on focused activation. Especially in children with autism, there is considerable evidence that failures to engage and learn material are often a result of breakdowns in patterns of inhibition. More broad, for most children at some times, it is likely that learning will not proceed until inhibition processes are more strongly invoked. Within multimedia efforts, the combination of the child's active motor selection of keys or buttons that control event navigation along with rapid pace and multimodality presentations could play a role in supporting appropriate inhibitory process. However, much remains to be learned about appropriate inhibition of competing actions, comparisons, and searches (Campos, Mumme, Kermoian, & Campos, 1994; Cole, Michel, & Teti, 1994).

Attention, inhibition, arousal regulation, and emotional regulation are all related processes. They are intertwined with the complex processes of retrieval, comparison, abstraction, and storage that are central in the extraction and encoding into long-term memory of new text or speech structures. The rapid, multivariate, and nonlinear nature of these co-occurring strands of the tricky mix invites application of theoretical notions of dynamic systems theory, or "chaos theory" (Fogel, 1993; Thelen, 1988; Thelen & Smith, 1994). These emotional and arousal regulation factors have not been seriously considered in theories of skill acquisition or multimedia literacy programs. In children with autism, there appears to be a need for software and interacting teachers to be attuned to the child's emotional and arousal states. For example, Kinsbourne (1987) argued that in many children with autism there is an uneven, oscillating dysregulation that produces swings between hyperarousal, with shallow processing (as in echolalia) or constricted focus on just a few aspects of a sentence or other stimulus, and underarousal, with no or low responsiveness to any cues. The child's emotional states may also be affected by the swings in processing and responsiveness. Multimedia instruction could be adjusted to the child's emotional and arousal states, including sometimes postponing presentation of any complex challenges.

The ALPHA and Delta*Messages* results suggest that greater reading gains are made when both child and teacher enjoy the interaction and when the teacher's limited directiveness allows the child to attribute his or her success to his or her own efforts and thinking. Over repeated episodes of learning, higher self-esteem could be expected to develop for such children, which may allow even more independent actions by the child in new learning episodes and a positive "spiral" of higher learning, enjoyment, confidence, and self-esteem (Malone & Lepper, 1987).

### Readiness: Learner Conditions in Tricky Mixes

Another crucial factor from the REL theory perspective is that the domain of instruction should engage the learner's identity. In multimedia work, there are differences in how readily boys as compared with girls have made computer activities and computers savvy parts of their identity (Schofield, Evan-Rhodes, & Huber, 1990). Effective literacy instruction is far more likely to succeed if the child initially or after a period of multimedia activity personally values both computer use and literacy. Future software and teacher scaffolding could personalize many aspects (e.g., choices of favorite pets, friendship vs. competition, age/nationality/gender/hobbies of characters on screen) of the multimedia experience to better connect with the self-concepts of individual girls and boys (Lepper et al., 1993) as well as incorporate language-specific matches to the learner (as with our multimedia sign language for deaf children).

Within the studies previously reported there is a substantial (more than 50%) subset of children who are deaf or have autism and motor disabilities who match the learning rates in the multimedia shown by children without disabilities. The degree to which these children have many intact REL mechanism components is underestimated by their levels of learning under prior literacy instruction conditions and by tests of intelligence. Thus, when new tricky mixes are created that produce new rates of acquiring and generalizing skills, insights are gained simultaneously into relevant learning conditions and the cognitive preparedness of the learners.

Learner preparedness and learner strategies for the multimedia plus teacher interactions varied somewhat by disability type. Within the program the child is allowed to write anything he or she likes, and this freedom is more of a change for a child with disabilities compared with a typically developing 5- to 7-year-old child. It is quite common for programs aimed at children with autism to focus on a narrow, concrete, and very structured language environment because these children often have severe difficulties in organizing their language and separating relevant and irrelevant information. Children with mixed disabilities, especially those with cerebral palsy, often have to struggle to communicate even the simplest message, and fantasy and joking mostly have to be expressed nonverbally. However, it is possible that this limitation in language use often imposed on these varied groups might obscure the possible positive impact on language learning that new, fun, and challenging interactions can have. Thus, it is important to make teaching and learning as enjoyable as possible, as often as possible. As Durand (1992) stated in his discussion of educational programming for children with autism:

> Too often, many good teachers are pressured into teaching so many useful skills in such a short amount of time that they forget that the *process* should be enjoyable. . . . The challenge of our field will be to design environments that teach functional skills within a context that encourages play, humor, and friendship. It will be important to keep the *fun* in functional. (p. 284)

## Networks: Multiple Processing Opportunities in Tricky Mixes

For an already-fluent reader, reading a story requires considerable parallel processing to keep track of all the lexical, syntactic, and discourse information comprising the story. For a nonfluent reader trying to learn new text skills along with enjoying and understanding as much of the story as possible, the demands for extended parallel processing are much higher. For new abstractions and storage into long-term memory to occur, the learner's cognitive system may need to devote extra buffers (Calvin, 1990) or other forms of multiple parallel processing beyond those that would be recruited in less complex performance situations. Experimental on-line probes are needed by researchers to provide data on how and when additional processing resources are recruited for analysis of communicative challenges.

Here we consider additional possibilities of how richly scaffolded complex processing may underlie learners' literacy progress within the multimedia plus teacher interactions of our instruction. In part, the success of children who are deaf, have autism, or have mental retardation in matching text-learning rates of typical children led us to question theoretically the adequacy of our previous discussions. Rather than focusing on one narrow framing of a challenge and an immediate recast in another multimedia mode, a revised REL theoretical account looks at longer event sequences and at the overall richer set of converging conditions we call tricky mixes.

In the ALPHA and Delta*Messages* multimedia material, the multiple modes of information presentation could support parallel processing of more than one structural comparison. There could be a competition for the best new abstractions of text structure when text is compared with sign language (or speech) in two or three processing buffers. In other buffers, there could be a simultaneous competition to see if new text structure abstractions emerge from text or graphic-event comparisons.

***Recasting Processes at Multiple Levels*** Initially, recasts were considered at the level of speech or sign recasting by the teacher. After the child expressed a sentence referring to prior MM events, the teacher would pick up on the child's meaning and recast it into a new and challenging sentence structure. For example, "That lion was big!" could be recast into "Yes, that lion is really big, isn't he?" These recasts within a language mode are viewed theoretically as facilitators of processing and learning new language structures (e.g., the tag sentence structure in the recast example here). However, the MM sequences themselves meet the definition of recasting as well, if one considers cross-mode comparison processes (e.g., a meaning expressed first in a text sentence immediately followed by expression of the same meaning in either a spoken sentence or signed sentence). Once multiple representations of the same meaning enter active processing space, the child may abstract new structural elements from any mode regardless of where the new structural information was placed in the interaction and presentation sequence. From this theoretical perspective, processing enhancers for abstraction of new text structures may occur in each of the kinds of multimedia–child–teacher recast sequences that occur when ALPHA or Delta*Messages* has been employed in teaching (see Table 6).

***Sustained Processing Rounds Until New Structures Are Consolidated*** Mere presence in multimedia or conversational input of a new, challenging language structure—in text, sign, speech. L1 (first language) or L2 (second language)—does not guarantee the learner's abstraction or uptake of the challenge. The authors have encountered deaf adolescents whose reading skills reflected uptake from 6 to 8 years of literacy instruction of only a few extremely frequent but isolated fragments of English, such as recognizing the word *the* but not any content noun (Nelson et al., 1991). Good application of multimedia tools should include close monitoring of attention not only through teacher judgment but also through built-in documentation of the learner's speed of reaction and speed of navigation through the instructional material.

### Further Elaborations and Implications

There are many contributing conditions to learning, and launching, enhancer, adjustment, readiness, and network (LEARN) categories overlap and interact.

Table 6. Multiple processing opportunities

| |
|---|
| Graphic events establish meaning 1<br>child constructs text sentence (recast 1 of meaning 1)<br>teacher acknowledges and says sentence (recast 2 of meaning 1[a]) |
| Child constructs text sentence, creates meaning 1<br>graphic events give one-to-one recast 1 of meaning 1<br>MM gives sign language (recast 2 of meaning 1)<br>child paraphrases sentence (recast 3 of meaning 1)<br>teacher recasts the child's sign (recast 4 of meaning 1) |
| Child constructs text sentence, creates meaning 1<br>graphic events give one-to-one recast 1 of meaning 1<br>MM gives sign language (recast 2 of meaning 1)<br>child signs a new comment, creates meaning 2<br>teacher recasts the child's sign (recast 1 of meaning 2) |
| Child constructs text sentence, creates meaning 1<br>graphic events give one-to-one recast 1 of meaning 1<br>MM expresses spoken language (recast 2 of meaning 1)<br>child speaks a new comment, creates meaning 2<br>teacher recasts the child's speech (recast 1 of meaning 2) |

[a]*Note*: This sequence is common in test sentences and implies learning during the testing is probable.

The particular ways in which dynamic patterns occur that produce learning will vary by the learner, the challenge, and the context. Future work should provide coordinated monitoring of all five LEARN categories to ensure empirical identification of how more conditions interact.

Similarly, the tricky mixes and REL theory frameworks hold implications for future work in first-language acquisition and literacy for children without disabilities. Close monitoring of multiple LEARN conditions in relation to acquisition should better specify how children learn in naturalistic contexts. There are already clues from ALPHA literacy results that learners without disabilities benefit from the multimedia instruction and benefit more when the computer multimedia events are scaffolded by enhancement and adjustment conditions in the accompanying teacher–child interactions. Keeping the same theoretical base, Delta*Messages* software could be adapted to spoken first-language teaching. Further suggestive evidence comes from an experimental treatment study examining progress in recasting language therapy by language-typical children (Newby, 1994). Analysts examined details of behavior in relation to language targets that were strongly acquired (multiple spontaneous uses at home and clinic) versus targets with weak or no acquisition. These behaviors were analyzed during the first treatment session and before any acquisition by any child and thus were potential predictors of degree of acquisition. Predictors of strong acquisition were nonverbal activities related to the recast, positive affect, normal or animated voice (versus a flat voice contour), and more frequent pauses before replying (thus potentially allowing processing of the recast to proceed further than if an immediate reply was produced). These results fit with the notions that high rates of processing and learning may depend on a mix abstraction enhancers (pauses, verbal–nonverbal relationships, challenging recasts) and facilitative social-emotional states.

## CONCLUSION

This chapter reviewed the influence of REL theory on the design of multimedia instruction for children with disabilities and the relevance of the revised theory for children without disabilities. ALPHA and Delta*Messages* multimedia software were documented to produce literacy gains and related communication gains along with enjoyment of the interactions by both students and teachers. In addition, many of the children in this research further demonstrated an interesting cluster of significant outcomes: Not only did they make gains in reading and writing, but they matched the pace of learning of children with no disabilities and also learned new sign language structures (deaf children) or spoken language structures. Together these findings indicate reasonably high levels of *learner readiness.* The children with disabilities frequently demonstrated sufficiently *intact cognitive and linguistic* mechanisms to support efficient abstracting of multiple levels of communication structures from teaching episodes that are complex and multimodal. Note, however, that these "successes" in learning occurred in settings where theoretically-based structuring of multimedia events and teacher–child side dialogues were employed. Many *catalysts* for attending to and abstracting new language structures were mixed into the instructional interactions.

For children with disabilities who demonstrated efficient learning under ALPHA or Delta*Messages* or in similar circumstances, there are some strong implications. If, as has been typical in our research, we are working with children who are 8–16 years of age but who are many years behind in literacy, in academic subjects generally, and in achieved level of first-language comprehension and expression, there is the daunting task of trying to create a high frequency of high-quality learning conditions. If that goal could be met, then catching up to their peers without disabilities (Caparulo & Cohen, 1985) would be expected, perhaps even fully catching up, if the demonstrated high cognitive potential of many of these children with disabilities is taken at face value. Multimedia could be adapted to incorporate sign language and spoken language more fully, so that the same theoretically driven timing and patterning of events used so far with a stress on reading and writing could facilitate and assess progress in the child's first language. The teacher and the multimedia would thus challenge the child more regularly at the first language as well as the text level. Similar multimedia could also be tested as intervention tools in first language for preschool children who have not yet shown any language delay but who have been identified as at risk.

Our theory-driven design of the software and the computer plus teacher interactional contexts has evolved as has the initial theory. Even if one focuses exclusively on the interactional events that might contribute most directly to cognitive challenge presentation and processing, we now hold that theoretical descriptions must take into account many interrelated events and their sequential patterning. Thus, within REL theorizing, abstraction and learning of a challenging language structure can be facilitated by event sequences ranging from two steps (platform sentence followed by recast of that sentence) to 6, 7, or more steps in multiple modes. Beyond this, the cognitive elements relevant to abstraction of a new language structure (in text, sign, or speech) are embedded in an ongoing mix of social and motivational processes. Successful processing and learning is even trickier than earlier versions of REL theory claimed. Social and motivational conditions require equal consideration with cognitive-linguistic details in planning instruction with or without multimedia. Accordingly, we described how the multimedia ALPHA and Delta*Messages* projects not only present challenges to learning but also help arrange other learning conditions that may contribute to significant learning of new communication skills. From the tricky mix perspective, these multiple conditions should be more often measured and used to guide individualized contextual adjustments.

One unusual example of such individualization occurred for a boy named Lars in the ALPHA field research. Lars was an 11:4-year-old boy with autism whose IQ was within the normal range. His ability to write and read Swedish was already well above the levels that ALPHA could provide. Therefore his teacher suggested that the English version of ALPHA be used. This proposal was easily accepted by the parents because Lars already had a little knowledge of the language. It was obvious that Lars was strongly attracted by the rewarding animations he could create by constructing sentences "telling" the computer what animations to show. Lars made rapid progress with ALPHA over 13 weeks, covering almost all of the 144 lessons included in English ALPHA. Furthermore, his ALPHA text skills generalized well beyond the multimedia environment. Such rapid progress supported by convergences of excellent motivational regulation, challenges in a second language, and multiple catalysts is not typical of language-learning contexts for children with autism.

The theoretical framework emphasized in this chapter applies equally to children with and without disabilities. REL theory and its associated tricky mix perspective are expected to help further develop tools and techniques that facilitate communication skill development in a variety of children. As further research proceeds, we expect that increasingly differentiated accounts will be given of how individual children and adult partners find learner preparedness, motivational engagement, personal relevance, emotional regulation, cognitive challenges, and processing catalysts productively mixed together within the contexts of effective multimedia instruction and first-language conversational contexts.

## REFERENCES

Bernard-Optiz, V., Ross, K., & Tuttas, M.L. (1990). Computer assisted instruction for autistic children. *Annals of the Academy of Medicine, 19*(5), 611–616.

Bohannon, N., & Stanowicz, L. (1989). Bidirectional effects of imitation and repetition in conversation: A synthesis within a cognitive model. In G.E. Speidel & K.E. Nelson (Eds.), *The many faces of imitation in language learning* (pp. 121–150). New York: Springer-Verlag.

Bowerman, M. (1985). Beyond communicative adequacy: From piecemeal knowledge to an integrated system in the child's acquisition of language. In K.E. Nelson (Ed.), *Children's language* (Vol. 5, pp. 369–398). Hillsdale, NJ: Lawrence Erlbaum Associates.

Calvin, W.H. (1990). *The cerebral symphony.* New York: Bantam.

Camarata, S., & Nelson, K.E. (1992). Treatment efficiency as a function of target selection in the remediation of child language disorders. *Clinical Linguistics and Phonetics, 6*, 167–178.

Camarata, S., Nelson, K.E., & Camarata, M. (1994). A comparison of conversation based to imitation based procedures for training grammatical structures in specifically language impaired children. *Journal of Speech and Hearing Research, 37*, 1414–1423.

Campos, J.J., Mumme, D.L., Kermoian, R., & Campos, R.G. (1994). A functionalist perspective on the nature of emotion. In N.A. Fox (Ed.), *The development of emotion regulation: Biological and behavioral considerations* (pp. 284–303). Monographs of the Society for Research in Child Development, 59, Serial No. 240.

Caparulo, B.K., & Cohen, D.J. (1983). Developmental language studies in the neuropsychiatric disorders of childhood. In K.E. Nelson (Ed.), *Children's language* (Vol. 4, pp. 423–463). Hillsdale, NJ: Lawrence Erlbaum Associates.

Chen, S.H.A., & Bernard-Optiz, V. (1993). Comparison of personal and computer-assisted instruction for children with autism. *Mental Retardation, 31*(6), 368–376.

Clark, M.D. (1993). A contextual/interactionist model and its relationship to deafness research. In M. Marschark & M.D. Clark (Eds.), *Psychological perspectives on deafness* (pp. 353–362). Hillsdale, NJ: Lawrence Erlbaum Associates.

Colby, K.M. (1973). The rationale for computer-based treatment of language difficulties in nonspeaking autistic children. *Journal of Autism and Childhood Schizophrenia, 3*(3), 254–260.

Cole, P.M., Michel, M.K., & Teti, L.O. (1994). The development of emotion regulation and dysregulation: A clinical perspective. In N.A. Fox (Ed.), *The development of emotion regulation: Biological and behavioral considerations* (pp. 73–100). Monographs of the Society for Research in Child Development, 59, Serial No. 240.

Coldwell, R.A. (1991a). Computers in use with autistic children: Some case studies. In *Proceedings of the Ninth Australian Computers in Education Conference at Bond University* (pp. 94–100). Brisbane, Australia.

Coldwell, R.A. (1991b, September). Intellectually handicapped children: Development of hieroglyphic symbols. *Australian Educational Computing*, 10–12.

Csikszentmihalyi, M. (1990). *Flow.* New York: Harper & Row.

Csikszentmihalyi, M. (1993). *The evolving self.* New York: HarperCollins.

de Villiers, J., de Villiers, P., & Hoban, E. (1994). The central problem of functional categories in the English syntax of oral deaf children. In H. Tager-Flusberg (Ed.), *Constraints on language acquisition: Studies of atypical children* (pp. 9–48). Hillsdale, NJ: Lawrence Erlbaum Associates.

Durand, V.M. (1992). New directions in educational programming for students with autism. In D.E. Berkell (Ed.), *Autism: Identification, education, and treatment* (pp. 273–293). Hillsdale, NJ: Lawrence Erlbaum Associates.

Fogel, A. (1993). *Developing through relationships.* Chicago: University of Chicago Press.

Fox, N.A. (1994). Dynamic cerebral processes underlying emotion regulation. In N.A. Fox (Ed.), *The development of emotion regulation: Biological and behavioral considerations.* Monographs of the Society for Research in Child Development, 59, Serial No. 240.

Frith, U. (1989). *Autism: Explaining the enigma.* Oxford, England: Basil Blackwell.

Grandin, T. (1995). *Thinking in pictures.* New York: Doubleday.

Green, S., & Clark, A. (1991). The microcomputer support for language through learning. *Communication, 25*(3), 12–14.

Haley, K., Camarata, S., & Nelson, K.E. (1994). Positive and negative social valence in children with specific language impairment during imitation based and conversation based language intervention. *Journal of Speech and Hearing Research, 37,* 378–388.

Heimann, M. (1992). Inlärning—en sällsynt företeelse [Learning—a rare event]. *Nordisk Psykologi, 44*(3), 203–211.

Heimann, M. (1995, July). *On the effect of multimedia computer programs: Gains made by children with autism in reading, motivation and communication skills.* Paper presented at the symposium on cognitive and social aspects of communication disabilities. Convenors: E. Hjelmquist & I. Lundberg. IV European Congress of Psychology, Athens, Greece.

Heimann, M., Nelson, K.E., Gillberg, C., & Kärnevik, M. (1993). Facilitating language skills through interactive micro-computer instruction: Observations on seven children with autism. *Scandinavian Journal of Logopedics and Phoniatrics, 18,* 3–8.

Heimann, M., Nelson, K.E., Tjus, T., & Gillberg, C. (1993). The impact of an interactive micro-computer instructional system on language learning for children with autism and multiple handicaps [Summary]. In *Proceedings of the 2nd European Conference on the Advancement of Rehabilitation Technology.* Stockholm, Sweden: The Swedish Handicap Institute.

Heimann, M., Nelson, K.E., Tjus, T., & Gillberg C. (1995). Increasing reading and communication skills in children with autism through an interactive multimedia computer program. *Journal of Autism and Developmental Disorders, 25,* 459–480.

Heimann, M., Tjus, T., & Nelson, K.E. (1995, March). *Multimedia facilitation of processing and learning in varied children's skill domains.* Poster presented at the Biennial Meeting of the Society for Research in Child Development, Indianapolis, IN.

Jordan, R., & Powell, S. (1990a). Improving thinking in autistic children using computer presented activities. *Communication, 24,* 23–25.

Jordan, R., & Powell, S. (1990b). Teaching autistic children to think more effectively. *Communication, 24,* 20–23.

Kinsbourne, M. (1987). Cerebral-brainstem relations in infantile autism. In E. Schopler & G.B. Mesibov (Eds.), *Neurobiological issues in autism* (pp. 88–111). New York: Plenum.

Koegel, L.K., & Koegel, R.L. (1995). Motivating communication in children with autism. In E. Schopler & G.B. Mesibov (Eds.), *Learning and cognition in autism* (pp. 73–87). New York: Plenum.

Lepper, M.R., Woolverton, M., Mumme, D.L., & Gurtner, J-L. (1993). Motivational techniques of expert human tutors: Lessons for the design of computer-based tutors. In S.P. Lajoie & S.J. Derry (Eds.), *Computers as cognitive tools* (pp. 75–105). Hillsdale, NJ: Lawrence Erlbaum Associates.

Light, J. (1988). Interaction involving individuals using augmentative and alternative communication systems: State of the art and future directions. *Augmentative and Alternative Communication, 4*, 66–82.

Lotter, V. (1978). Follow-up studies. In M. Rutter & E. Schopler (Eds.), *Autism, a reappraisal of concepts and treatment* (pp. 475–495). New York: Plenum.

Malone, T.W., & Lepper, M.R. (1987). Making learning fun: A taxonomy of intrinsic motivations for learning. In R.E. Snow & M.J. Farr (Eds.), *Aptitude, learning, and instruction: III. Conative and affective process analyses* (pp. 223–253). Hillsdale, NJ: Lawrence Erlbaum Associates.

Maratsos, M., & Chalkley, M.A. (1980). The internal language of children's syntax: The ontogenesis and representation of syntactic categories. In K.E. Nelson (Ed.), *Children's language* (Vol. 2). Hillsdale, NJ: Lawrence Erlbaum Associates.

Marschark, M. (1993). Origins and interactions in the social, cognitive, and language development of deaf children. In M. Marschark & M.D. Clark (Eds.), *Psychological perspectives on deafness* (pp. 7–26). Hillsdale, NJ: Lawrence Erlbaum Associates.

Nelson, K.E. (1977). Facilitating children's syntax acquisition. *Developmental Psychology, 13*, 101–107.

Nelson, K.E. (1980). Theories of the child's acquisition of syntax: A look at rare events and at necessary, analytic, and irrelevant components of mother–child conversation. *Annals of the New York Academy of Sciences, 345*, 45–67.

Nelson, K.E. (1982). Experimental gambits in the service of language acquisition theory. In S.A. Kuczaj (Ed.), *Language development, syntax and semantics* (pp. 159–199). Hillsdale, NJ: Lawrence Erlbaum Associates.

Nelson, K.E. (1987). Some observations from the perspective of the rare event cognitive comparison theory of language acquisition. In K.E. Nelson (Ed.), *Children's language* (Vol. 6, pp. 289–331). Hillsdale, NJ: Lawrence Erlbaum Associates.

Nelson, K.E. (1989). Strategies for first language teaching. In M.L. Rice & R.L. Schiefelbusch (Eds.), *The teachability of language* (pp. 263–310). Baltimore: Paul H. Brookes Publishing Co.

Nelson, K.E. (1991). On differentiated language learning models and differentiated interventions. In N. Krasnegor, D. Rumbaugh, R. Schiefelbusch, & M. Studdert-Kennedy (Eds.) *Biological and behavioral determinants of language acquisition development* (pp. 399–428). Hillsdale, NJ: Lawrence Erlbaum Associates.

Nelson, K.E., Camarata, S.M., Welsh, J., Butkovsky, L., & Camarata, M. (1996). Effects of imitative and conversational recasting treatment on the acquisition of grammar in children with specific language impairment and younger language-normal children. *Journal of Speech and Hearing Research, 39*, 850–859.

Nelson, K.E., Carter, W., & Prinz, P.M. (in review). *Deaf children's writing gains through microcomputer exploration of intermixes of sign language, graphics, and text.*

Nelson, K.E., & Heimann, M. (1995). *DeltaMessages—a multimedia program for language learning* (Computer software program). Warriors Mark, PA: Super Impact Images, and Göteborg, Sweden: Topic Dos Hb.

Nelson, K.E., Heimann, M., Abuelhaija, L., & Wroblewski, R. (1989). Implications for language acquisition models of children's and parents' variations in imitation. In G.E. Speidel & K.E. Nelson (Eds.), *The many faces of imitation in language learning.* New York: Springer-Verlag.

Nelson, K.E., Loncke, F., & Camarata, S. (1993). Implications of research on deaf and hearing children's language learning. In M. Marschark & M.D. Clark (Eds.), *Psychological perspectives on deafness* (pp. 123–151). Hillsdale, NJ: Lawrence Erlbaum Associates.

Nelson, K.E., & Nelson, K. (1978). Cognitive pendulums and their linguistic realization. In K.E. Nelson (Ed.), *Children's language* (Vol. 1). Hillsdale, NJ: Lawrence Erlbaum Associates.

Nelson, K.E., Perkins, D., & Lepper, M. (1996). *Learning as a rare event.* Unpublished manuscript, Pennsylvania State University, State College.

Nelson, K.E., & Prinz, P.M. (1991). *ALPHA Interactive Language Series/Gator Super Sentences* (Computer software program). Warriors Mark, PA: Super Impact Images.

Nelson, K.E., Prinz, P.M., Prinz, E.A., & Dalke, D. (1991). Processes for text and language acquisition in the context of microcomputer-videodisc instruction for deaf and multihandicapped deaf children. In D.S. Martin (Ed.), *Advances in cognition, education, and deafness* (pp. 162–169). Washington, DC: Gallaudet University Press.

Newby, K. (1994). *The relationship between social valence and target acquisition in two types of language intervention.* Unpublished thesis, Pennsylvania State University, State College.

Olswang, L.B., Bain, B.A., & Johnson, G.A. (1992). Using dynamic assessment with children with language disorders. In S.F. Warren & J. Reichle (Eds.), *Communication and language intervention series: Vol. 1. Causes and effects in communication and language intervention* (pp. 187–216). Baltimore: Paul H. Brookes Publishing Co.

Panyan, M.V. (1984). Computer technology for autistic children. *Journal of Autism and Developmental Disorders, 14*(4), 375–382.

Prinz, P.M., Nelson, K.E., Loncke, F., Geysels, G., & Willems, C. (1993). A multimodality and multimedia approach to language, discourse, and literacy development. In B.A.G. Elsendoorn & F. Coninx (Eds.), *Interactive learning technology for the deaf* (pp. 121–132). Berlin: Springer-Verlag.

Prizant, B.M., & Wetherby, A.M. (1989). Enhancing language and communication in autism. In G. Dawson (Ed.), *Autism: Nature, diagnosis & treatment* (pp. 282–309). New York: Guilford Press.

Reynell, J. (1985). *Reynell Developmental Language Scales.* Los Angeles: Webster Psychological Corporation.

Romanczyk, R.G., Ekdahl, M., & Lockshin, S.B. (1992). Perspectives on research in autism: Current trends and future directions. In D.E. Berkell (Ed.), *Autism: Identification, education, and treatment* (pp. 21–51). Hillsdale, NJ: Lawrence Erlbaum Associates.

Romski, M.A., & Sevcik, R.A. (1989). An analysis of visual-graphic symbol meanings for two nonspeaking adults with severe mental retardation. *Augmentative and Alternative Communication, 5*, 109–114.

Romski, M.A., & Sevcik, R. (1991). Patterns of language learning by instruction: Evidence from nonspeaking persons with mental retardation. In N. Krasnegor, P. Rumbaugh, R. Schiefelbusch, & M. Studdert-Kennedy (Eds.), *Biological and behavioral language development* (pp. 429–445). Hillsdale, NJ: Lawrence Erlbaum Associates.

Salomon, G. (1993). On the nature of pedagogic computer tools: The case of the writing partner. In S.P. Lajoie & S.J. Derry (Eds.), *Computers as cognitive tools* (pp. 179–196). Hillsdale, NJ: Lawrence Erlbaum Associates.

Salomon, G., Globerson, T., & Guterman, E. (1989). The computer as a proximal zone of development: Internalized reading-related metacognitions from a writing partner. *Journal of Educational Psychology, 81*, 620–627.

Schofield, J.W., Evans-Rhodes, D., & Huber, B.R. (1990). Artificial intelligence in the classroom: The impact of a computer-based tutor on teachers and students. *Social Science Computer Review, 8*, 24–41.

Siegler, R.S. (1991). *Children's thinking.* Englewood Cliffs, NJ: Prentice Hall.

Slobin, D.I. (1985). Cross-linguistic evidence for the language-making capacity. In D.E. Slobin (Ed.), *The cross-linguistic study of language acquisition* (Vol. 2, pp. 1157–1256). Hillsdale, NJ: Lawrence Erlbaum Associates.
Tager-Flusberg, H. (1989). A psycholinguistic perspective on language development in the autistic child. In G. Dawson (Ed.), *Autism: Nature, diagnosis & treatment* (pp. 92–115) New York: Guilford Press.
Tager-Flusberg, H. (1994). Dissociations in form and function in the acquisition of language by autistic children. In H. Tager-Flusberg (Ed.), *Constraints on language acquisition: Studies of atypical children* (pp. 175–194). Hillsdale, NJ: Lawrence Erlbaum Associates.
Taube, K., Tornéus, M., & Lundberg, I. (1984). *Läsning och skrivning. Handläggning för kartläggning och utveckling*. Stockholm: Psykologiförlaget. [in Swedish]
Thelen, E. (1988). Dynamic approaches to the development of behavior. In J.A. Kelso, A.J. Mandell, & M.F. Schlesinger (Eds.), *Dynamic patterns in complex systems* (pp. 348–369). Singapore: World Scientific.
Thelen, E., & Smith, L.B. (1994). *A dynamic systems approach to the development of cognition and action*. Cambridge, MA: MIT Press.
Underwood, J.D.M., & Underwood, G. (1990). *Computers and learning*. Oxford, England: Basil Blackwell.

# Index

Page numbers followed by "*f*" denote figures; those followed by "*t*" denote tables.